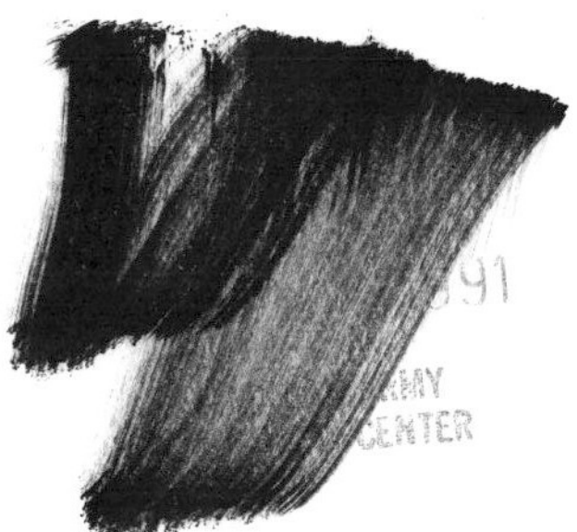

LASERS IN OTOLARYNGOLOGY-HEAD AND NECK SURGERY

Edited by

R. KIM DAVIS, M.D.

Associate Professor of Surgery
Division of Otolaryngology—Head and Neck Surgery
The University of Utah School of Medicine
Salt Lake City, Utah

1990
W.B. SAUNDERS COMPANY
Harcourt Brace Jovanovich, Inc.

Philadelphia • London • Toronto • Montreal • Sydney • Tokyo

W. B. SAUNDERS COMPANY
HARTCOURT, BRACE JOVANOVICH, INC.

The Curtis Center
Independence Square West
Philadelphia, PA   19106–3399

Editor: W. B. Saunders Staff
Designer: Paul Fry
Production Manager: Carolyn Naylor
Manuscript Editor: Terry Russell
Illustration Coordinator: Brett MacNaughton
Indexer: Dorothy Stade

LASERS IN OTOLARYNGOLOGY   ISBN 0-7216-3124-X

Printed in the United States of America

Last digit is the print number: 9 8 7 6 5 4 3 2 1

CONTRIBUTORS

Bruce N. Patrick Benjamin, D.L.O., FRACS, FAAP
Lecturer in Diseases of the Ear, Nose, and Throat
The William Blano Centre
Sydney, Australia
LASER SURGERY IN MULTIPLE RESPIRATORY PAPILLOMATOSIS

Kenneth N. Buchi, M.D.
Assistant Professor of Medicine
Department of Internal Medicine
Division of Gastroenterology
University of Utah School of Medicine
Salt Lake City, Utah
ENDOSCOPIC ESOPHAGEAL LASER THERAPY

Jean Marc Brunetaud, M.D.
Associate Professor of Gastroenterology
  and Biomedical Engineering
Centre Multidisciplinaire de Traitement
  par Laser
Centre Hospitalier et Universitaire de Lille
  Lille, France
ENDOSCOPIC ESOPHAGEAL LASER THERAPY

R. Kim Davis, M.D., FACS
Associate Professor of Surgery
Division of Otolaryngology–
  Head and Neck Surgery
Department of Surgery
University of Utah School of Medicine
Salt Lake City, Utah
LARYNGEAL CANCER: THE ROLE OF LASER SURGERY; LASER SURGERY FOR BENIGN
CONDITIONS IN THE ORAL CAVITY AND OROPHARYNX; LASER SURGERY FOR ORAL
CAVITY AND OROPHARYNGEAL CANCER; LASER THERAPY: FUTURE DIRECTIONS

Scott Dinehart, M.D.
Assistant Professor
Department of Otolaryngology and Department of Dermatology
University of Arkansas for Medical Sciences
Little Rock, Arkansas
LASERS IN FACIAL PLASTIC AND RECONSTRUCTIVE SURGERY

John A. Dixon, M.D.

Professor of Surgery
Senior Consultant
Utah Laser Institute
University of Utah School of Medicine
Salt Lake City, Utah

LASERS IN OTOLARYNGOLOGY: A PERSPECTIVE

James A. Duncavage, M.D., FACS

Associate Professor
Vanderbilt University Medical Center
Nashville, Tennessee

LASER SURGERY FOR BENIGN LARYNGEAL LESIONS;
ENDOSCOPIC LASER ARYTENOIDECTOMY

John G. Hunter, M.D.

Assistant Professor of Surgery
Director, Utah Laser Institute
University of Utah School of Medicine
Salt Lake City, Utah

LASERS IN OTOLARYNGOLOGY: A PERSPECTIVE

Leland P. Johnson, M.D.

Associate Clinical Professor of Surgery
Department of Surgery
Division of Otolaryngology–Head and Neck Surgery
University of Utah School of Medicine
Salt Lake City, Utah

NASAL AND PARANASAL SINUS APPLICATIONS OF LASERS

Glenn W. Knox, M.D.

Resident
Department of Otolaryngology–Head and Neck Surgery
Vanderbilt University Medical Center
Nashville, Tennessee

ENDOSCOPIC LASER ARYTENOIDECTOMY

David R. Nielsen, M.D. FACS Otologist

Southwest Otologic Institute
Phoenix, Arizona

OTOLOGIC APPLICATIONS OF LASER SURGERY

Robert H. Ossoff, D.M.D., M.D., FACS

Guy M. Maness Professor and Chairman
Department of Otolaryngology–Head and Neck Surgery
Vanderbilt University Medical Center
Nashville, Tennessee

LASER SURGERY FOR BENIGN LARYNGEAL LESIONS; ENDOSCOPIC LASER
ARYTENOIDECTOMY

James L. Parkin, M.D., M.S., FACS

Hetzel Professor and Chairman
Division of Otolaryngology–Head and Neck Surgery
Department of Surgery
University of Utah School of Medicine
Salt Lake City, Utah
OTOLOGIC APPLICATIONS OF LASER SURGERY

David S. Parsons, M.D., FAAP

Colonel, United States Air Force Medical Corps
Chief of Pediatric Otolaryngology
Associate Clinical Professor of Pediatrics and Otolaryngology
University of Texas Health Sciences Center
San Antonio, Texas
ANESTHETIC CONSIDERATIONS IN LASER SURGERY

Stanley M. Shapshay, M. D.

Chairman,
Department of Otolaryngology–Head and Neck Surgery
Lahey Clinic, Burlington
Clinical Associate Professor of Otolaryngology
Boston University School of Medicine
Boston, Massachusetts
LASER BRONCHOSCOPY

Michael H. Stevens, M.D.

Professor of Surgery
Department of Surgery
Division of Otolaryngology–Head and Neck Surgery
University of Utah School of Medicine
Salt Lake City, Utah
LASER SURGERY FOR BENIGN CONDITIONS IN THE ORAL CAVITY AND OROPHARYNX

Milton Waner, M.B., B.Ch.(Rand), FCS(SA)

Associate Professor
Department of Otolaryngology
University of Arkansas for Medical Sciences
Little Rock, Arkansas
LASERS IN FACIAL PLASTIC AND RECONSTRUCTIVE SURGERY

PREFACE

Laser therapy in otolaryngology–head and neck surgery is an exciting and rapidly expanding field. I have had the special opportunity of being tutored by Drs. Strong and Jako in the initial applications of the CO_2 laser, stimulated and encouraged in laser applications over many years by Dr. Stanley M. Shapshay, and exposed to a vast array of new lasers and techniques at the Laser Institute of the University of Utah under the direction of Dr. John A. Dixon. With this background, I am honored and excited to edit this book of current laset practice.

With the recent advances in laser technology and applications, it has become difficult for most surgeons to keep abreast of all the new developments. Additionally, it is difficult to find essential background information from any single source to allow an adequate basis for assessment of current laser techniques. Being involved in medical education, I am particularly aware of the critical need for surgeons to learn safe surgical techniques carefully and, more important, to understand in depth the indications and contraindications for any procedure. This book is an attempt to address both of these areas.

The book is extensively illustrated in the manner of a surgical atlas. Its scope, however, is beyond surgical description alone and focuses on procedures in which current laser therapy confers a distinct advantage. The contributing authors are nationally and internationally known authorities with extensive experience in the laser therapies included in the book. They have graciously agreed to describe their operative techniques and have been willing to share their wisdom and experience concerning indications and contraindications for potential laser surgeries. I greatly appreciate their clear descriptions and their candor.

The book begins with the perspectives of one of the true pioneers in laser therapy, Dr. John A. Dixon. Attention is then focused on the critical interplay between anesthetic techniques and laser surgery. The underlying principle in the book is that of developing foundations for safe laser applications. Subsequent chapters deal with the different specialty areas of otolaryngology, with attention being given to the areas of greatest laser use. Realizing that laser technology is rapidly evolving, I hope this book provides a solid foundation of knowledge in laser therapy and allows the reader to understand and appreciate new developments as they come.

I want to thank the contributing authors for their time and expertise. Special thanks are given to Julian Maack for his patient and excellent work with illustrations, and to Illene Harris for her excellent and cheerful work in preparing the manuscripts.

Most especially, I want to express my love and appreciation to my wife JoNell and to my children Kimberly, Neal, Tamralyn, Cyndi, Mindy, and Eric for their patience, understanding, and constant support.

R. KIM DAVIS, M.D.

Contents

CHAPTER 1

LASERS IN OTOLARYNGOLOGY: A PERSPECTIVE

John A. Dixon

John G. Hunter

Laser applications in otolaryngology were described in the late 1960s and early 1970s by such pioneers as Strong, Jako, Vaughan, and Andrews.[1,2] Although new surgical techniques are developed slowly, 20 years of laser use in otolaryngology hardly qualifies this treatment modality as new. Broad observations are largely subjective; however, such perspectives may be useful in establishing a current orientation and in projecting future directions.

A review of the early publications discussing lasers in the field of otolaryngology indicates a number of expectations or goals advanced for laser therapy, most of which have been realized. These are listed in Table 1–1.

Certainly many patients have benefited by the application of lasers to lesions previously considered inoperable. The surgeon has benefited greatly by endoscopic and freehand applications that supplement standard surgical instrumentation. Multiple procedures can be performed with lasers that are markedly less invasive than nonlaser surgeries undertaken heretofore. In selected instances there is good evidence of shortened hospital stay and reduced health care cost.

Still, it is difficult to validate the impressions of superior results with laser therapy in the absence of controlled trials with statistically significant, interpretable data. A few numbers, however, are available to give broad indications of clinical trends. As with the evaluation of all new procedures or medications, an initial wave of optimism is followed by pessimism engendered by increased knowledge of limitations and complications. In the more than 20 years of laser application, opinions of laser use have gone through at least three such fluctuations and now appear to be stabilizing somewhat. What can be measured?

The major society that surgeons who employ lasers belong to is the American Society for Laser Medicine and Surgery. It was organized in 1977 with 31 members. This organization now

Table 1–1. INITIAL GOALS FOR LASER THERAPY

Improved patient therapy	Less invasive procedures
Wider choice of surgical tools	Shortened hospital stay
Treatment of previously inoperable lesions	Reduced health care cost

has 1358 members and is growing at a rate of approximately 50 per cent per year. Of those members, otolaryngologists compose approximately 10 per cent and are the sixth most numerous practitioners represented, following those practicing dermatology, research, general surgery, gastroenterology, and gynecology.

The number of publications in the laser surgery field has increased also. The March 1978 issue of Index Medicus lists 11 publications under the heading of Laser, Therapeutic Applications. The March 1988 issue lists 128 publications under the same title.

Lasers have been employed in otolaryngology at the University of Utah since 1978, when argon laser therapy for nasal telangiectasia was instituted.[3] In subsequent years carbon dioxide (CO_2), neodymium:yttrium-aluminum-garnet (Nd:YAG), copper vapor, gold vapor, and argon pumped dye lasers, as well as other types, have been added and provide a broad range of instruments for surgeons at the University of Utah Laser Institute. The frequency of laser applications in otolaryngology at the Institute appears in Figure 1–1. As can be seen, the frequency of use is characterized by a rather rapid increase followed by a plateau. In 1987, a decrease in laser use occurred. Since 1988, however, laser applications have increased considerably.

Because of the great variability in the descriptions of otolaryngologic procedures it is difficult to determine the exact percentage in which the laser is used as the primary instrument. This appears to have reached a high point of approximately 15 per cent in 1984 and 1985. In 1990 it would be approximately 9 per cent.

These figures and trends are subject to various interpretations. It is possible to speculate that initial expectations for laser use were not fulfilled so that usage has declined and the future role of lasers is problematic. Discussion with surgeons involved, however, indicates a more probable interpretation: the use of lasers as a surgical technique has matured. This is primarily true for the Nd:YAG, CO_2, and argon lasers employed for thermal tissue effects. In some of the initial investigative periods, protocols were designed to compare lasers with standard techniques. Many of these studies showed no substantial benefit of laser therapy. These studies clarified the role of lasers and reduced the total number of applications.

It is evident that there are many complications associated with laser use. A partial list of these appears in Table 1–2. A better understanding of the frequency and magnitude of such complica-

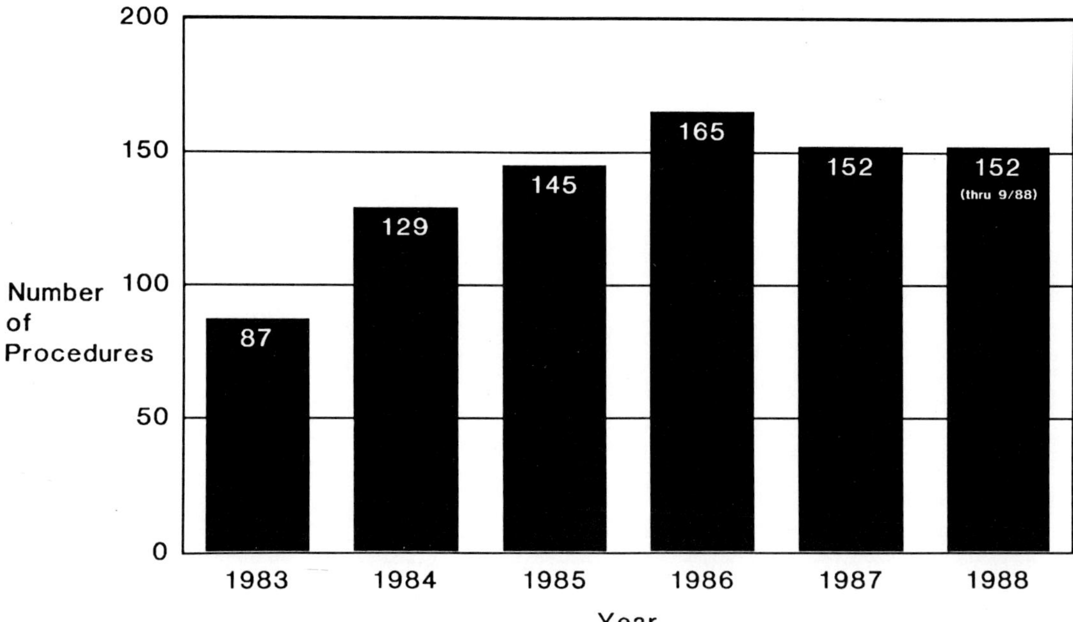

FIGURE 1–1. Number of otolaryngology laser procedures, University of Utah Laser Institute, 1983 to 1988.

Table 1–2. COMPLICATIONS OF LASER SURGERY

Burns	Endotracheal fires and explosions
Scarring	Eye injury
Hemorrhage	Electrical shock—electrocution
Perforations	Swelling and obstruction

tions has undoubtedly influenced the number of laser applications and made it possible for the surgeon to evaluate more specifically the risk-benefit ratio of a specific laser application.

Comparative studies are under way in a number of anatomic areas where conventional surgical techniques are available. These should be useful in future evaluation of the role of lasers. In a number of unique instances, however, such as the treatment of hereditary hemorrhagic telangiectasia (HHT), choanal atresia, and hemangiomas, lasers have provided an approach to hitherto untreatable lesions.

Laser surgery in otolaryngology began with a few courageous advocates. Applications were attempted for a variety of lesions, and many more surgeons became involved. After the initial surge of enthusiasm for and use of lasers, indications and contraindications became more clear, resulting in a decline in the frequency of laser applications. An analysis of the proportion of indications for laser use in which lasers are the only modality or the treatment of choice suggests that for continuous application thermal lasers the frequency is between 9 and 15 per cent. In these cases, even surgeons who may be critical of the broad applications of lasers are strong in their support for laser treatment of this selected group of lesions. Continued prospective, controlled, randomized trials will undoubtedly clarify further the indications for laser use. All of the previous comments relate to the commonly available CO_2, argon, and Nd:YAG lasers, which depend primarily on thermal effects of laser-tissue interaction to produce desired results. Other light-tissue interaction mechanisms may prove to be clinically useful.

Various proposed mechanisms of laser interactions are represented in Figure 1–2. Photothermal interactions have been thoroughly explored, utilizing lasers at relatively low power density (100 to 1000 watts/cm^2) for relatively long periods of time (milliseconds to seconds).

A considerable amount of work applicable to otolaryngology has been carried out regarding photochemical reactions (see Chapter 13). In this application, an exogenous chromophore, such as Photofrin II, is utilized to sensitize the cells, tumor, or vessels targeted. Following this, laser energy is applied (frequently in the milliwatt range) for long periods of time (frequently in the 6 to 8 minute range). Although there is some thermal component of this interaction, the primary mechanism of action is photochemical. Numerous compounds are available with photosensitizing capabilities. Many of these await U.S. Food and Drug Administration (FDA) approval and the development of lasers with appropriate wavelengths. Although delayed by uncertainties about photosensitizer availability, a number of photochemical feasibility studies in head and neck tumors have indicated good cancer palliation. Further refinement of specificity of the various drugs and methods for introduction of light to the tumor site are in process.

Recent investigations in photoablative and electromechanical mechanisms of laser-tissue interaction have been extremely interesting. High energy pulsed lasers (megawatts and gigawatts per square centimeter) have been applied to tissue for extremely short durations (nanosecond to femtosecond) with interesting results.[4] It appears that in some cases chemical bonds may be directly broken, producing a relatively nonthermal ablative effect.[5] In other instances, energy densities are achieved that strip the electrons from atoms, resulting in the formation of a plasma.[6] By a third mechanism, shock waves are created, producing nonthermal fragmentation of tissue.

In one study performed on the Mark III free electron laser at the University of Utah Laser Institute, investigators utilized in vivo rat bone as the target. The free electron laser is a tunable device, allowing ready change from one wavelength to another. Wavelengths from 2.8 to 3.2 microns were utilized, with pulse energies of 25 to 50 mJ/pulse and pulse duration of 500 fem-

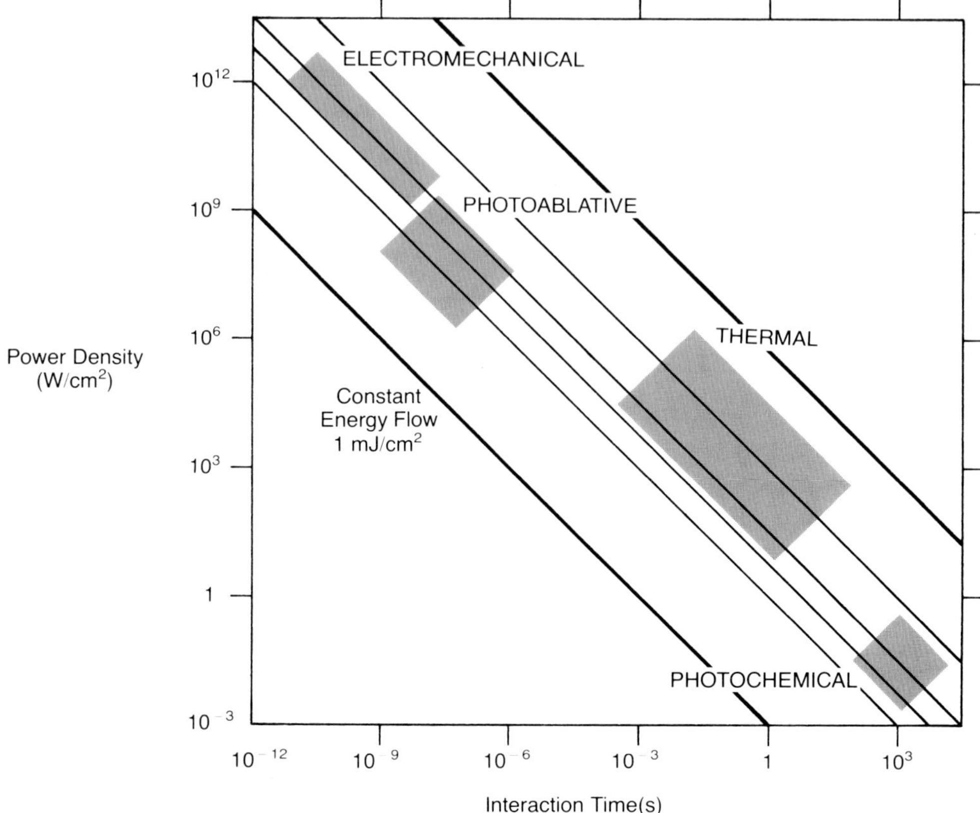

FIGURE 1–2. Mechanisms of laser-tissue interactions.

toseconds. Bone was selected for the test object because of the high pulse energy of the free electron laser and the possibility of producing electromechanical effects without thermal injury. Additional in vitro studies using chicken bone compared standard bone saw, CO_2 laser, and the free electron laser; results appear in Figure 1–3. The clean, precise incision with the free electron laser is evident.

Studies were carried out in vivo utilizing rat femurs, and healing of bone incisions was observed. The zone of thermal injury and necrosis is evident in Figure 1–4 where the CO_2 laser was used. The precise cut, 50 microns wide, with only a 5 to 10 μm zone of thermal injury at the incision site is evident with the free electron laser (Fig. 1–5).

Utilizing variations in available wavelengths, average power, peak power, pulse energy, and repetition rate, it appears that a myriad of laser-tissue interactions may become available with the use of photochemical, photothermal, photoablative, or electromechanical mechanisms. Clarification of the interaction of these variables is just beginning and will undoubtedly require a considerable amount of time. It is evident that experience with standard lasers and delivery systems, such as fibers and endoscopes, will be invaluable in adapting these new techniques for much greater specificity in tissue ablation with reduction in complications.

The increase in the clinical use of lasers and the complexities of laser research necessitated the formation of various organizational structures within institutions utilizing lasers for achieving the most efficient management, utilization, and operation. These organizations range from the simplest form, as exemplified by a one or two person supervision of laser schedules, safety, and credentials, to a multidiscipline, multisurgeon, multi–basic science institute to manage multiple optical laboratories, lasers, and installations, as well as clinical programs.

At the clinical level, the most common organizational form is a laser division headed by a surgeon with laser experience, who may also be the laser safety officer, and a nurse or staff person.

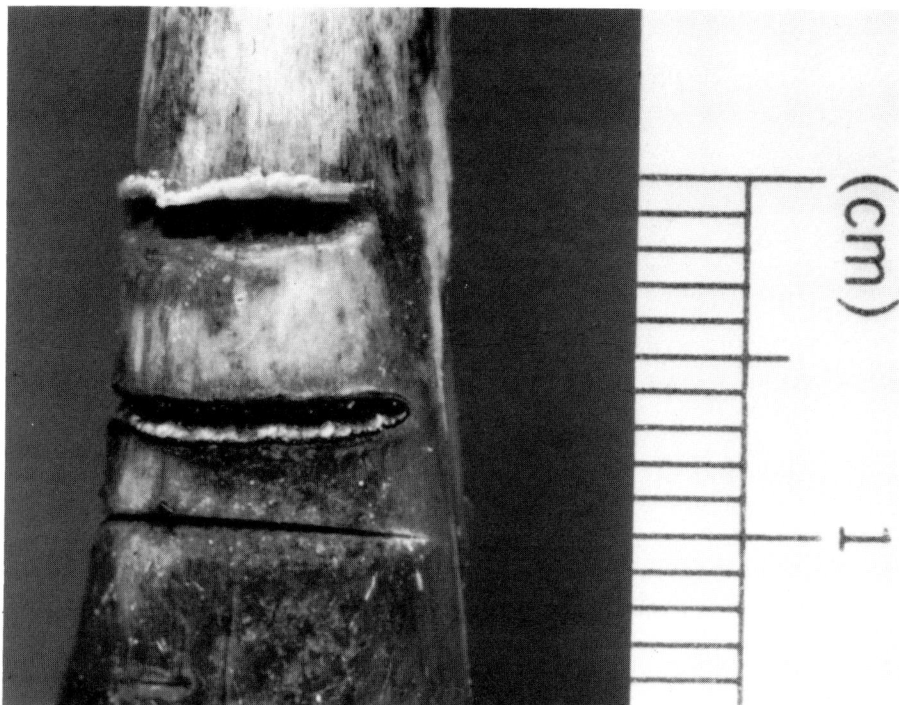

Figure 1–3. In vitro study of chicken femur. *Top,* Standard bone saw. *Center,* CO_2 laser. *Bottom,* Free electron laser (3.1 μ, 50 mJ/pulse).

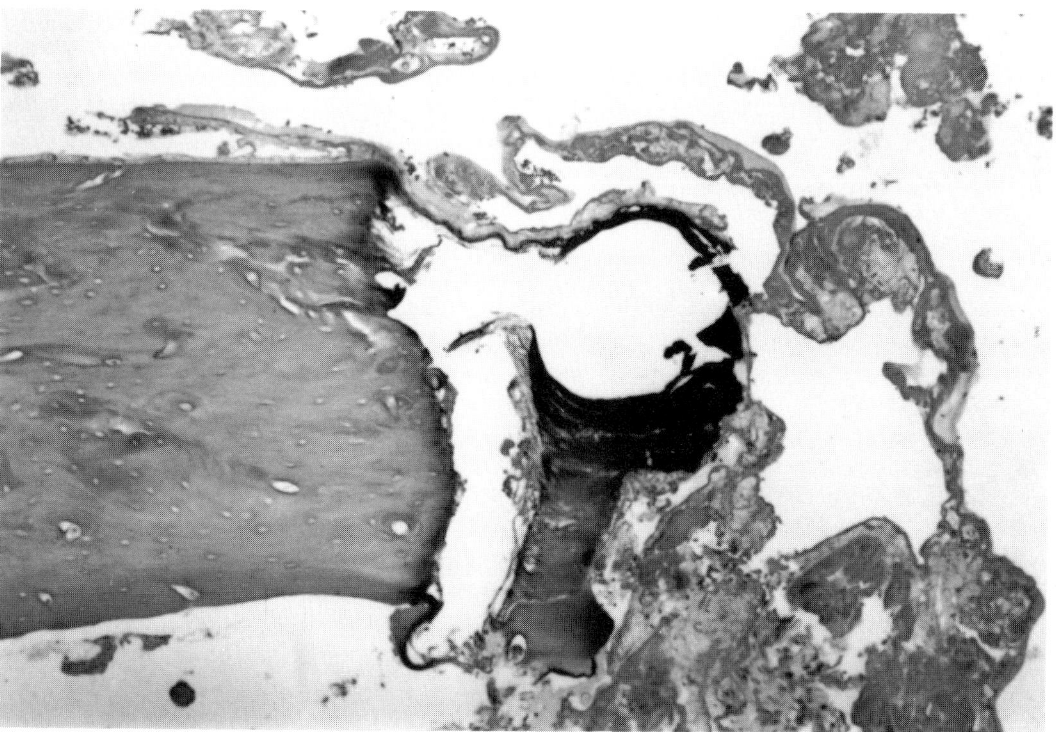

Figure 1–4. Rat femur 10 days after incision with continuous CO_2 laser. Note separation of necrotic carbonized bone.

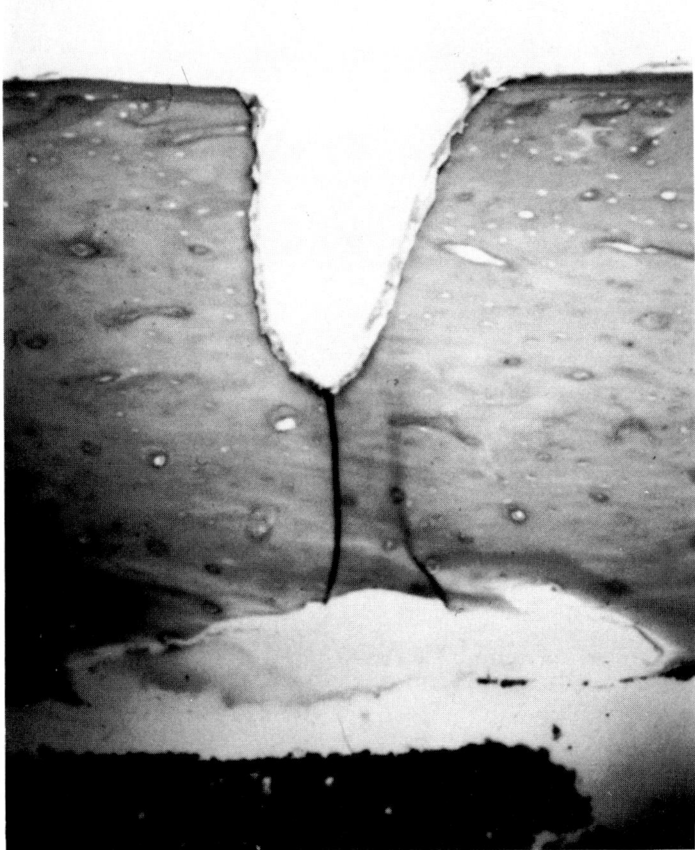

FIGURE 1–5. In vivo rat femur 10 days after incision with free electron laser (3.1 μ, 50 mJ/pulse). Note absence of thermal injury and necrotic bone. (Lines at bottom are staining artefacts.)

These fundamental positions may be expanded dramatically in larger clinical operations. On these individuals fall the multiple tasks of laser acquisition, installation, and maintenance. In addition, the vital functions of accreditation for use of lasers are evidently within their purview. Nearly all clinical programs require a minimal amount of laser training and supervision during initial applications. All applications must be carefully reviewed, documented, and recorded.

A considerable division concerning accreditation has arisen between the surgeons who use lasers occasionally in their practice and so-called laser surgeons. The former group have taken the position that the prime source of all accreditation in each field is the existing specialty board of that discipline: surgeons using lasers should be examined and certified by the existing board of their specialty, with inclusion of questions concerning lasers or laser applications and some indication of laser proficiency indicated on their certification. This group appears to include the majority that is most influential in the laser accreditation field. A minority group has incorporated an American Board of Laser Surgery giving examinations for certification in the laser field. This board has not yet been approved by the American Board of Medical Specialists or the various sections of the American Medical Association. It appears likely that, especially in otolaryngology, the utilization of existing boards will prevail and the development of a laser surgery board will be counterproductive and confusing to hospital administrators and those responsible for accreditation.

It appears inevitable that laser education will simply become part of established residency programs. In the interim, laser training must be attained by participation in a number of short-term laser courses provided by various academic institutions coupled with preceptorship-type experience during initial applications. It is probable that within the next 4 to 5 years all such training will be superseded by standard residency-type training. It is thus necessary for laser program directors or safety officers to be flexible and utilize a great deal of individual observation during this transition period.

The multidisciplinary organizational form is exceedingly important for involvement of basic scientists. There is little in the training of surgeons to equip them for study in the application of highly complicated concepts involving theoretic and quantum physics. The major advances in the field of laser applications appear to be accomplished by teams of investigators, involving surgeons, photobiologists, physicists, chemists, microscopists, bioengineers, medical engineers, mathematical modelers, spectroscopists, fiberopticists, and specialists in laser instrumentation. Such specialists usually have major projects of their own that they are pursuing. The persuasive skill of the surgical investigator is tested in ''borrowing'' some time from these individuals and convincing them that great good can come from their participation in and the successful conclusion of a surgical project.

A major problem in such investigative groups is that of communication. Just as surgery has developed highly specialized fields with their own jargon, so have the basic scientists in the physical sciences developed an exclusive vocabulary. It is a real challenge for the surgeon to be able to communicate clearly to such individuals the nature of a surgical objective and the specific problems to be solved. On the other side, the physicist has a great deal of difficulty understanding the physicians' physiologic or anatomic explanation and deriving from that, in technical terms, the objectives to be achieved by the research project.

With research lasers costing hundreds of thousands to millions of dollars each, it becomes absolutely essential that investigators learn to work in a joint laboratory with sharing of time on costly laser devices. The dedicated use of a research instrument by a single individual or discipline is no longer possible. Such accommodations are quite foreign to the usual investigative practices of the clinician and the basic scientist but are essential to rapid advances in research and development. Future advances in surgical laser techniques may well depend on developments in biochemistry, physics, or electrical engineering. Much of the information sought by physicians is already available in these areas and simply needs to be extracted and applied.

It is difficult to predict where the next clinical advances will be made in the application of lasers in otolaryngology. Optimization of existing instrumentation is evidently possible with smaller, portable, less expensive reliable power sources. Although fiber delivery systems have been made less expensive and more efficient, the long-sought-after, small flexible fiber for delivery of CO_2 or infrared energy still eludes researchers. Investigations into infrared wavelengths, such as those utilized in the erbium:YAG laser, which is heavily absorbed by water, may be fruitful. Here again, fiber transmission of laser energy has proved to be a problem. Investigations of sapphire fibers suggest that these may be made in small flexible units that can withstand the high pulsed energy of modern surgical lasers.

Minor modifications in the wavelengths of lasers that operate by thermal means, such as the 1.34 μm Nd:YAG continuous wave (CW) laser, appear to have, at best, marginal advantages over existing techniques. More likely to be beneficial are instruments such as the flashlamp pumped dye laser or high energy pulsed lasers (e.g., the free electron laser).

In all of the attempts to evaluate the role of lasers in otolaryngology it becomes important to maintain realistic expectations. Some initial reports on lasers made extravagant claims that lasers would be utilized for the majority of surgical procedures, that blood loss would be dramatically decreased, and that all procedures could be done without incisions. Many of these claims have proved unfounded. Surgeons not acquainted with the superficial coagulation capabilities of the CO_2 laser have attempted to transect large vessels with disastrous consequences. Judgment is essential. It is becoming evident that lasers are extremely useful surgical instruments for highly selected and well-defined indications. Training of the surgeon is necessary to facilitate understanding and application of lasers in an effective fashion. The exact percentage of cases in which the laser is applicable is unclear at this time.

Just as a surgeon has many differently shaped hemostatic clamps on the surgical tray during an incision procedure, existing and newly developed lasers will provide additional instruments for highly selected applications that will continue to expand the surgical equipment options. The challenge to the otolaryngologist in applying lasers is to continually investigate, utilize, and evaluate developments in the dynamic area of laser technology.

References

1. Strong MS, Jako GJ: Laser surgery in the larynx. Ann Otol Rhinol Laryngol 81:781, 1972.
2. Vaughan CW, Strong MS, Jako GJ: Laryngeal carcinoma: Transoral treatment utilizing the CO_2 laser. Am J Surg 136:490, 1978.
3. Parkin JL, Dixon JA: Laser photocoagulation in hereditary hemorrhagic telangiectasia. Otolaryngol Head Neck Surg 89:204, 1981.
4. Dixon JA, Straight RC, Dayton MT: Free electron laser fragmentation of biliary calculi. Lasers Surg Med 7:88, 1987.
5. Trokel SL, Srinivasan R, Braren B: Excimer laser surgery of the cornea. Am J Ophthalmol 96:710, 1983.
6. Steinert RF, Puliafito CA, Kittrell C: Plasma shielding by Q-switched and mode-locked neodymium:YAG lasers. Ophthalmology 90:1003, 1983.

CHAPTER 2

ANESTHETIC CONSIDERATIONS IN LASER SURGERY

David S. Parsons

Anesthetic techniques for rigid endoscopy have advanced rapidly in keeping with changes in surgical techniques and improved equipment. Not many years ago, rigid endoscopies were performed with little or no anesthesia. Today, methods vary because of the wide range of patient ages, from premature neonates to geriatric patients. Alterations in technique for induction and maintenance of anesthesia must also be based on the patient's general health and pulmonary status, the preoperative diagnosis, and the intended surgical procedure. Identification of the possible choices for delivery of anesthesia is a critical decision for the otolaryngology and anesthesia teams. A wide variety of anesthetic approaches are available, and the method most advantageous must be selected to achieve the best and safest result.

Endoscopy requires excellent communication between the anesthesiologist and the otolaryngologist, as both desire access to the same critical space—the patient's airway. Although their ultimate goal (the well-being of the patient) is the same, the means to achieve this goal are sometimes in conflict, and mutual understanding, communication, and compromise are essential to realize the optimal outcome.

Advances in endoscopic surgery, specifically laser microlaryngoscopy and telescopic endoscopy, have changed the approaches to general anesthesia; new methods currently are being utilized. The choice of technique depends not only on the anesthetic agents available, the methods of ventilation to be used, and the age and general state of the patient, but also mostly on the procedure to be performed and the requirements of the surgeon. The ideal requirements for anesthesia include safety, simplicity, rapid induction, prompt comfortable recovery, an immobile unobstructed view of the larynx, satisfactory control of the airway and ventilation, no time restriction for the surgical procedures or for photographic documentation, conditions that allow for observation of the dynamics of the larynx, and prevention of aspiration[1] (Fig. 2–1).

Although local anesthesia alone is still used in selected cases of rigid endoscopy, the sophistication of anesthesia has improved so that most procedures are performed with general anesthesia. General anesthesia facilitates the endoscopic procedure, reduces trauma to the invaded anatomic structures, eliminates psychologic trauma, and ensures the complete cooperation of the patient. It also allows an unhurried and accurate evaluation of the problem. The otolaryngologist and anesthesiologist should have a variety of anesthetic techniques available for different situations. These

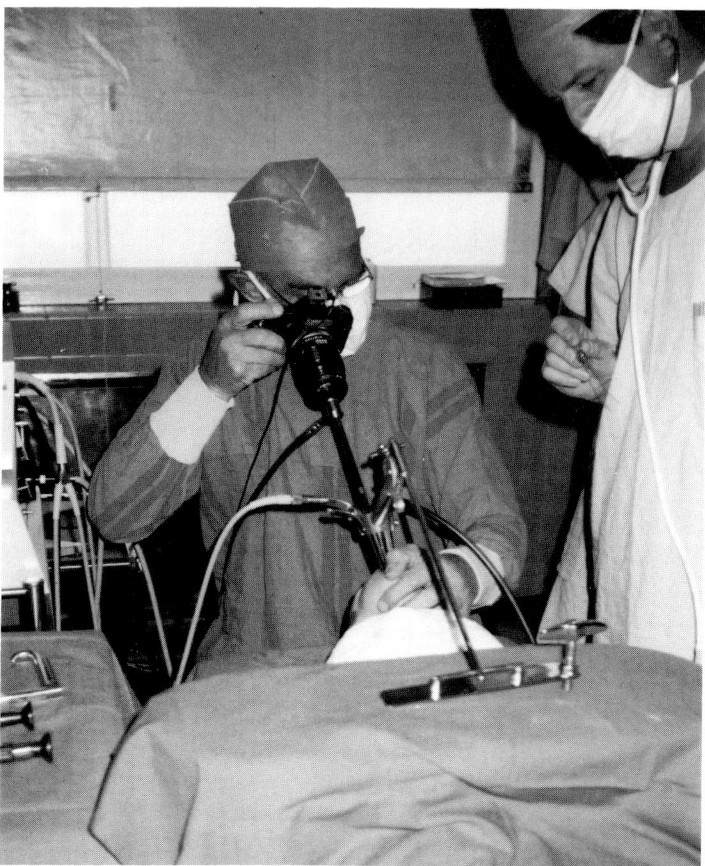

FIGURE 2–1. The larynx of a small infant is suspended for direct laryngoscopy. Anesthesia is given by insufflation, and the child is breathing spontaneously. The procedure is carried out in an unhurried fashion with photographic documentation. The laryngoscope is suspended utilizing the Benjamin modified suspension support (Karl Storz) and is resting on an overtable, which is attached to the operating table. The light source is supplied by the Benjamin-Havas light clip.

should include the apneic technique; jet ventilation, which may include both laryngoscopic jetting and midtracheal jetting; intubation techniques; and spontaneous respiration for children.

The role of the endoscopist has changed dramatically over the past 25 years. At present, he or she is regarded as a true consultant, and his or her opinion is sought in the investigation and management of congenital or acquired airway and intrathoracic problems. Removal of a foreign body 25 years ago was a traumatic situation for the anesthesiologist, the endoscopist, and the patient. In contrast, today this procedure carries little morbidity or mortality and is usually controlled as a rather uneventful happening.

Advances in endoscopy are aided by the use of computed tomography (CT) and magnetic resonance imaging (MRI). Improved methods have been developed for diagnostic laryngoscopy, bronchoscopy, and esophagoscopy because of such new equipment as the flexible fiberoptic illumination with intense xenon light sources, more sophisticated ventilating bronchoscopes (which include rigid pediatric instruments from 2.5 to 6.0 mm in diameter), a wide selection of high quality pediatric laryngoscopes, carbon dioxide (CO_2) and 532 nm potassium-titanyl-phosphate (KTP-532) lasers and their various delivery systems, telescopes with various viewing angles (from 0 to 120 degrees), and dependable techniques for photography and documentation.[28] The advances in endoscopic equipment have also aided the anesthesiologist immensely.

This chapter discusses multiple techniques of general anesthesia for patients of different ages, the medications, and how these techniques can be matched to the various surgical approaches being used for today's laser endoscopies.

LOCAL ANESTHESIA

Local anesthesia endoscopy is most often performed in the office setting. Utilization of this technique in the operating room environment is not uncommon, particularly for laser surgery. Patients who are selected for local anesthesia should have intravenous sedation. The benefits of this sedation include greater controllability and a more calm, cooperative patient. Narcotic agents are an important part of local anesthesia management. Fentanyl (Sublimaze) is the shortest acting of the commonly used narcotics and is among the most potent. However, in the office setting it should be restricted to low doses or not used at all because of the potential for significant side effects. Although the side effects of fentanyl are manageable by reversal with naloxone (Narcan), naloxone itself can produce severe side effects, including pulmonary edema, respiratory depression, and electrocardiographic (ECG) changes. Morphine is the classic analgesic with sedative effects, but it produces significant nausea. It can potentially sensitize the cardiac sinus, producing reflex bradycardia. The effects of morphine can also be reversed with naloxone.

The use of tranquilizers is advantageous. Although diazepam (Valium) is an excellent medication for calming with minimal effects on the cardiac system when used alone, it has the distinct disadvantage of having no commercially available antagonist and has a long half-life with a pattern of erratic peaks and valleys. It causes pain when given intravenously to the awake patient. Midazolam (Versed) is now the benzodiazepine most frequently used in the perioperative period. It is 2 to 2.5 times as potent as diazepam, has a rapid onset when administered intravenously, is a profound amnestic, and is easily titratable. It can, however, cause respiratory depression. Other frequently used, intravenously administered supplementary agents include fentanyl, meperidine (Demerol), morphine, hydroxyzine (Vistaril), diazepam, and ketamine (Ketalar).

Norton and Strong believe that general anesthesia is clearly the management of choice for procedures of significant magnitude.[2]

PREMEDICATION

Preoperative planning is absolutely critical to avoid conflict and confusion when the anesthesiologist and the endoscopist both need access to the airway. This is particularly important if specialized equipment, such as an operating microscope or a laser, is being used.

Premedication objectives are related to ensuring a relaxed patient with minimal fear of the proposed surgery. Giving premedication with respiratory depressant effects, such as narcotics or barbiturates, should be avoided. Diazepam, 0.1 mg/kg orally, may help a patient to remain calm prior to surgery. However, a variety of studies over the years confirm that careful preoperative counseling is the most important factor in reducing fear and anxiety in patients. The usual anticholinergic agents are atropine, scopolamine, and glycopyrrolate (Robinul), but these have depressant effects on lysosomes and ciliary activity. They also increase the viscosity of secretions that can contribute to patchy atelectasis. Edelist uses glycopyrrolate in preference to atropine, as it does not produce as much tachycardia.[3] It is given intramuscularly 45 minutes prior to the operative procedure. If the patient has ischemic heart disease, propranolol, 0.5 to 1.0 mg intravenously, is given to prevent both hypertension and the tachycardiac response to laryngoscopy.[3] The newer short-acting beta blocking agents are often used instead of propranolol.

A common mistake by endoscopists who are not accustomed to working with children is having the child with nothing by mouth for a prolonged period of time prior to the procedure. Most pediatric anesthesiologists require periods of gastric emptying of no more than 4 hours prior to the procedure; they encourage the child to take clear liquids up to that time. Some anesthesiologists even recommend nothing by mouth for only 2 to 3 hours for small infants. Excessive premedication should be avoided in a child. The concept that medication can replace physician-patient rapport is particularly fallacious in the case of the pediatric patient. Induction of anesthesia can be done rectally, by inhalation, or intravenously, depending on the age of the child, the existence of an intravenous line, and the rapport between the patient and the anesthesiologist.[2]

GENERAL ANESTHESIA

Induction and Maintenance

Monitoring is of major significance because portions of the airway are often compromised during surgery. Airway stimulation produces significant cardiac responses and is discussed below. An ECG oscilloscope is mandatory in view of the known propensity for cardiac arrhythmias and other abnormalities to occur during suspension laryngoscopy.[4] In addition to the usual monitoring of vital signs such as body temperature and blood pressure, arterial oxygen saturation is continuously monitored by means of a pulse oximeter or a transcutaneous oxygen (Tc_{O_2}) monitor. Analysis of Tc_{CO_2} and ST segment are available and offer improved safety in monitoring the patient with a compromised airway. Verification of neuromuscular blockade is confirmed with a nerve stimulator.

Induction of general anesthesia in the adult or older child must be tailored to the patient; most often this is accomplished with a short-acting barbiturate and is maintained with an inhalation agent. However, if the patient has a significant upper airway obstruction, such as papilloma, an inhalation induction agent is often preferable, with maintenance of spontaneous ventilation. The otolaryngologist may wish to view the larynx during this period of spontaneous ventilation before paralysis is initiated.

Induction of anesthesia, in most cases, is accomplished via the intravenous route. Thiopental sodium 2.5 per cent is most frequently used. Ketamine should rarely be used because of the excitement it frequently induces, leading to an increased metabolic oxygen requirement, hypercapnia, venous engorgement, and laryngospasm.[2]

Neuromuscular blockade is accomplished using intermediate-acting nondepolarizing agents, such as atracurium or vecuronium, which result in a period of relaxation of approximately 20 to 30 minutes. Repeated doses of a short-acting agent, such as succinylcholine, with a duration of action of 3 to 4 minutes, can result in an increased incidence and severity of cardiac rhythm irregularities, and continuous infusions may produce a phase II or prolonged block.[5]

The patient is intubated with the smallest caliber endotracheal tube that can adequately support ventilation. The tube is protected from laser impact by wrapping it with aluminum tape or by using tubes that have been coated with a protective material (Xomed Laser-Shield, Jacksonville, FL) to prevent intraoperative laser-induced fires. Use of red rubber Rusch tubes instead of polyvinyl chloride (PVC) tubes has gained popularity for laser surgery because the red rubber tubes are less flammable and require greater laser energy to ignite than do PVC tubes. The products of combustion are also less toxic. The PVC tubes, when ignited in a high ambient oxygen environment, burn like a blowtorch, whereas the red rubber tubes tend only to smolder, char, and possibly melt.[31] The cuff is filled with saline, which acts as a heat sink, and is covered with moist surgical cottonoids. Adding methylene blue to the saline often aids the surgeon in detecting a cuff perforation. Whenever an artificial airway is used for laser endoscopy, the fractional concentration of oxygen in inspired gas (FiO_2) is maintained at 40 per cent or less, if possible, to decrease the risk of fire in the upper airway as a result of inadvertent laser impact on the endotracheal tube.[6]

When utilizing general anesthesia, one of the decisions that must be made is whether to use spontaneous or controlled ventilation. If using controlled ventilation, succinylcholine has been the preferred agent in the past for paralysis, although recent reports[7,8] recommend use of the intermediate-acting nondepolarizing relaxants atracurium besylate or vecuronium bromide. Pediatric anesthesiologists at the author's institution do not recommend succinylcholine for children and prefer the latter two drugs. The second decision is whether an inhalation agent can be used. If jet ventilation is chosen and there is no satisfactory scavenging system, total intravenous anesthesia must be provided. This is usually accomplished with an ultra-short-acting barbiturate for hypnosis used with fentanyl for analgesia and midazolam for amnesia. Communication between the endoscopist and the anesthesiologist is crucial to avoid possible pneumothoraces when jetting is used.[9,29]

Warner and colleagues[11] report that 5 of 20 patients given total intravenous anesthetics required prolonged mechanical ventilation for respiratory depression and, therefore, added enflurane to the inhaled mixture delivered by a conventional anesthetic circuit. They believe the addition of the inhaled anesthetic lowers the requirement for fixed drugs and decreases the incidence of unacceptable respiratory depression at the end of the procedure.

Induction of anesthesia can result in transitory hypertension within the systemic and pulmonary circulation. Cardiovascular reactions are provoked by stimulation of the epiglottis or larynx during either laryngoscopy or endotracheal intubation and by carbon dioxide accumulation owing to impaired ventilation. These are the main provocative factors for hemodynamic changes, which, although transitory, have been associated with serious complications in susceptible patients. Sørensen and associates state that stimulation due to instrumentation of the larynx is the main determinant for the hemodynamic changes registered during laryngoscopy.[10] Their study evaluated two sets of patients. One set of patients was intubated, and a direct laryngoscopy was performed. The second group was not intubated, but received the apneic technique with a laryngoscope placed for 30 to 45 seconds followed by 15 seconds of ventilation; the cycle was repeated. In the patients with the irregular respiratory pattern, significant rises in the arterial partial pressure of carbon dioxide (Pa_{CO_2}) occurred, which should make the otolaryngologist aware that both instrumentation and the apneic technique can predispose the patients to respiratory or cardiac problems.[10]

After induction, multiple methods of ventilation can be selected, including spontaneous respirations in children weighing less than 35 kg, proximal or distal laryngoscopic jet ventilation, midtracheal jet ventilation, or controlled ventilation through an endotracheal tube. Johnson and coworkers[9,29] utilize jet ventilation for operative laryngoscopy with a 3.5 mm diameter pediatric chest tube (Argyle, Brunswick Co). Benjamin uses a 2.8 mm outside diameter soft tube (Benjet, Tuta Laboratories, Sydney, Australia) with four pedals to prevent tracheal mucosal injury caused by a whipping motion of the distal tube with jetting[1] (Fig. 2–2). This technique is particularly beneficial for vocal cord injections under general anesthesia. It is also effective for laser surgery.[1]

Johnson induces and maintains anesthesia with incremental doses of fentanyl, a short-acting narcotic; thiopental, an ultra-short-acting barbiturate; and succinylcholine, an ultra-short-acting depolarizing skeletal muscle relaxant. He also uses topical 4 per cent lidocaine (3 to 5 ml) at the glottis. The patient is ventilated employing a high concentration oxygen jetting system at the rate of approximately 10 to 16 inhalations per minute with a pressure of 15 to 20 pounds/in^2 (psi). Johnson's experience shows that alveolar ventilation is maintained and, when the ventilation is at adequate levels, Pa_{CO_2} is kept in a range below the preanesthetic levels. Pa_{O_2} values are generally approximately 200 mm Hg.[9,29] Benjamin's technique is quite similar.[1] The primary advantage of these techniques versus those utilizing the standard cuffed endotracheal tube is the excellent visualization of the larynx. The open-ended bronchoscope can be passed, and these tubes remain in place while ventilation is continued uninterrupted. Johnson uses the apneic technique only when removing tissue from the vocal cords or obtaining bronchial washings. Contraindications to the use of jetting include the presence of poor pulmonary compliance, obesity, and obstructive airway disease.[9,29]

The midtracheal jet technique must always allow the free egress of air. Jetting should never be commenced until the laryngoscope is placed to view the glottic opening and ensure that a clear expiratory phase is possible. Caution should be used during laser excision of vocal cord lesions if lower airway packing is placed over the jet tube, as this can prevent the free egress of air. Benjamin discourages the use of any packing with midtracheal jetting. Again, communication between the endoscopist and the anesthesiologist is crucial to avoid possible pneumothoraces.

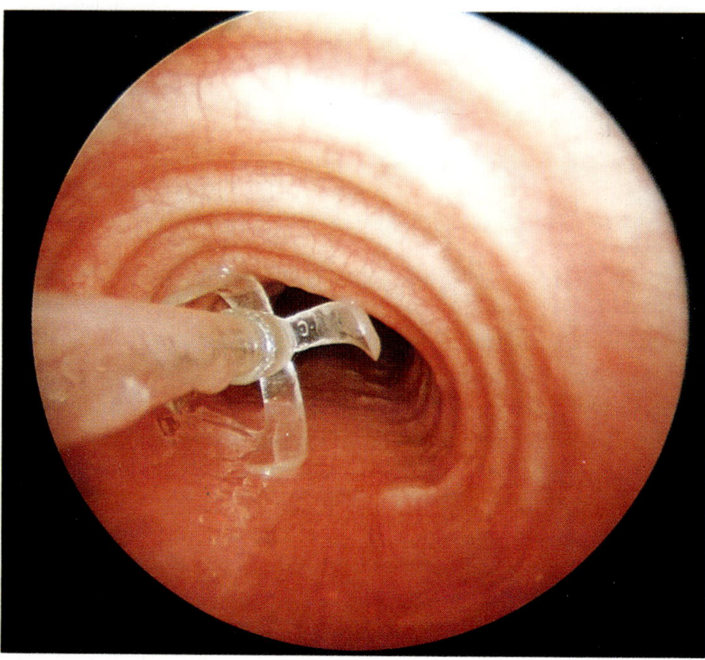

Figure 2–2. The Benjamin jet ventilation tube (Benjet). The tip is placed in the midtrachea, and the four petals prevent mucosal irritation by the whipping motion induced with each jet blast.

A catheter placed through the cricothyroid membrane for jetting results in increased complications because of the rather frequent occurrence of subcutaneous and mediastinal emphysema. Proximal or distal jetting mounted on the laryngoscope itself can produce problems by blowing gas into the stomach, moving the vocal cords during each jet burst and blowing tumor particles or papilloma down into the lower respiratory tract.[9,29]

The need for denitrogenation of anesthetized patients has been well understood for 25 years. All patients should receive ventilation with oxygen before induction of anesthesia. This can either be 100 per cent oxygen breathing or multiple deep breaths of 100 per cent oxygen immediately before induction.[12] The author uses laryngoscopes for intubation that have a large side bore catheter and insufflates 100 per cent oxygen during intubation, whether it be with an endotracheal tube or a midtracheal jet catheter.

Studies conducted in children show that the continuous oxygen flow during intubation is important.[13] There is a decrease in oxygen tension of 7.1 per cent when oxygen insufflation is used; without oxygen insufflation, the oxygen tension drops 33 per cent. The investigators concluded that the oxygen insufflation during laryngoscopy and intubation for spontaneously breathing, anesthetized infants effectively minimizes the decrease in Tc_{O_2} from prelaryngoscopic levels. This makes instrumentation of the airway safer. A decrease in Pa_{O_2} during the period of laryngoscopy by anesthesia is a common and expected occurrence. This happens especially in children because of their increased oxygen utilization, smaller functional residual capacity, and greater cardiac output. It is often a challenge to intubate children, particularly small infants. Hypoxemia in combination with vagal stimulation produced by the laryngoscopy can lead to bradycardia, premature ventricular contractions, and ultimately cardiovascular collapse.[13]

The effects of fentanyl are well studied.[14,15] Kautto examined the impact of fentanyl on arterial pressure and heart rate increases during laryngoscopy.[14] His study shows that using fentanyl during anesthesia induction decreases the amount of fentanyl required during the operation. Fentanyl supplementation in low doses (2 μg/kg) significantly attenuates the arterial pressure and heart rate increases, but larger doses (6 μg/kg) completely abolish these responses. Kautto further stated that sympathoadrenal responses to laryngoscopy and intubation may predispose to cardiac arrhythmias and increased myocardial oxygen consumption.[14] These can be dangerous to the patient with hypertension and/or ischemic heart disease. Thiopental induction is often supplemented with small doses of fentanyl to achieve a good tolerance of the endotracheal tube; less thiopental is therefore required.

In humans, fentanyl causes hypotension in about 25 per cent of patients anesthetized with nitrous oxide and oxygen. In patients with limited cardiac reserve, fentanyl in massive doses is widely used as a sole anesthetic because of its benign effect on the myocardium and cardiovascular dynamics. In Kautto's study systolic pressure gradually decreased after intubation to 18 per cent below the preoperative value.[14] The heart rate did not increase significantly in the group given fentanyl. This may reflect the analgesic effect of fentanyl and the parasympathetic action in the presence of sympathoadrenal stimulation caused by the laryngoscopy and the intubation.

Fentanyl is known to cause bradycardia in humans, and its effects can be reversed with naloxone. It can also cause a significant dose-dependent ventilatory depression.[14]

Podolakin and Wells stress that the dosage of fentanyl usually given can be inadequate in some patients.[15] They cited patients with severe ischemic heart disease who developed profound bradycardia at the time of laryngoscopy but who also had their vocal cords sprayed with topical lidocaine. They recommended that the dose of fentanyl should be at least 50 μg/kg, and they no longer advise the use of lidocaine on the cords. They cited other studies on the incidence of arrhythmias during tracheal intubation, which can be as high as 90 per cent.[15] The large doses of fentanyl that they recommended require postoperative ventilation, and the author uses such amounts for only patients with severe ischemic heart disease.

It has been shown that laryngoscopy and intubation stimulate reflex circulatory responses. The initiation of these reflex changes in heart rate and rhythm can cause cardiac arrest. The use of potent narcotics for cardiac anesthesia, in particular fentanyl, has been widely accepted as a safe, reliable, and reproducible method for maintaining stable cardiac function. Doses of 20 to 30 μg/kg, although adequate for producing a level of anesthesia to prevent tachycardia and hypotension, proved inadequate in prevention of reflex tachycardia at the time of laryngoscopy. Podolakin and Wells subsequently increased their induction dose of fentanyl to at least 50 μg/kg in selected patients.[15]

Virtually all rigid endoscopic laser procedures are performed under general anesthesia. Modern techniques are versatile, controlled, and safe. They should allow an unhurried, precise, and complete examination without stress to the patient, the anesthesiologist, or the endoscopic surgeon.

Benjamin used a technique in children weighing less than 35 kg that has become almost universally accepted.[16] He recommended induction with thiopental sodium and inhalation of nitrous oxide and oxygen by the face mask with subsequent addition of halothane. A Guedel airway is placed whenever the patient is ventilated via mask. Anesthesia is deepened and lidocaine, up to 5 mg/kg, is used topically on the cords. The patient breathes spontaneously throughout the procedure. The face mask is briefly removed and the administration of the anesthetic gases is temporarily suspended while a momentary direct laryngoscopy is performed. If the airway is potentially compromised, a quick telescopic view can be obtained to determine the extent of the obstruction.[16] A constant flow of oxygen is, however, important during this brief direct laryngoscopy; at the author's institution, the laryngoscopes have a wide bore cannula on the left side to allow continuous insufflation of either 100 per cent oxygen or oxygen and anesthetic gases.

Benjamin then suspends the patient for microlaryngoscopy (see Fig. 2–1). The exposure of the larynx is now ideal, as there is *no* anesthetic tube in place to obstruct the view of the surgeon (Fig. 2–3). Anesthesia is continued by insufflation of gases through a wide bore metal cannula, which fits into a channel on the left side of the laryngoscope (Fig. 2–4). The gases are released close to the glottic opening and are maintained at a high concentration while the child continues to breathe spontaneously throughout the procedure. For patients weighing more than 35 kg, Benjamin uses the Benjet midtracheal jet ventilation (Fig. 2–5; see Fig. 2–2). The microlaryngoscope is suspended but never on the patient's chest. An overtable that can be connected directly to the operating table is utilized, allowing maximum patient and table mobility[1,16] (see Fig. 2–1).

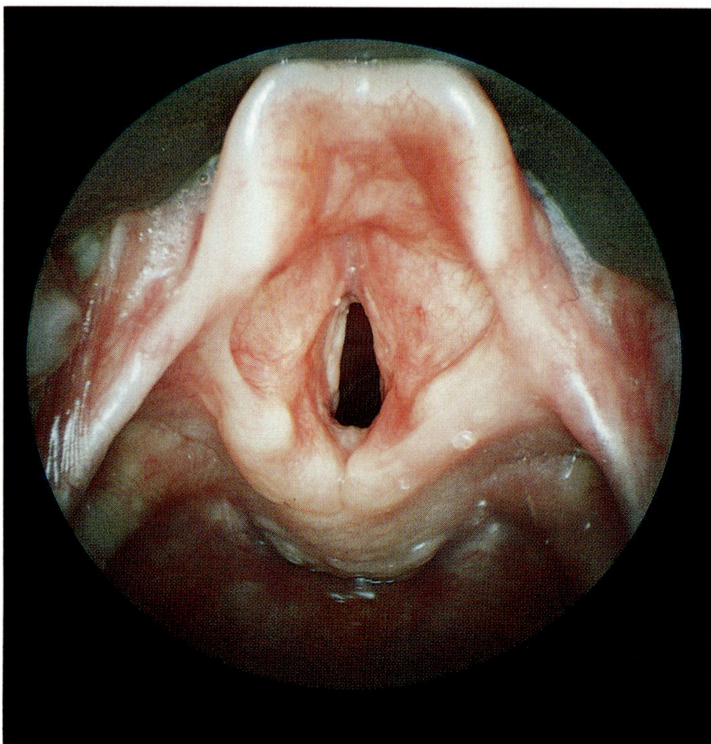

FIGURE 2–3. A normal pediatric larynx without an artificial airway in place. The child is suspended, and a Benjamin pediatric laryngoscope (Karl Storz) is used. This is a standard pediatric view utilizing a 0 degree telescope for optimal visualization.

The use of *no* anesthesia has little application today and is only occasionally necessary in sick neonates. It may sometimes be preferable to intubate a baby with a difficult airway problem, such as severe Pierre Robin syndrome, without general anesthesia.[1]

Cohen and Geller stated that, in evaluating the infant airway, no anesthesia is safer than too little.[17] In the newborn, they use oxygen insufflation for direct laryngoscopic examination; they then make the determination as to whether or not an infant is given general anesthesia for bronchoscopy. In the evaluation of the stridulous infant, they stated that observation of the dynamic function of the larynx is an essential part of the examination and paralysis obliterates the ability to see normal vocal cord motion.[17] Benjamin prefers to evaluate vocal cord mobility at the completion of endoscopy but agrees that continuous insufflation of oxygen as the patient is awakening is essen-

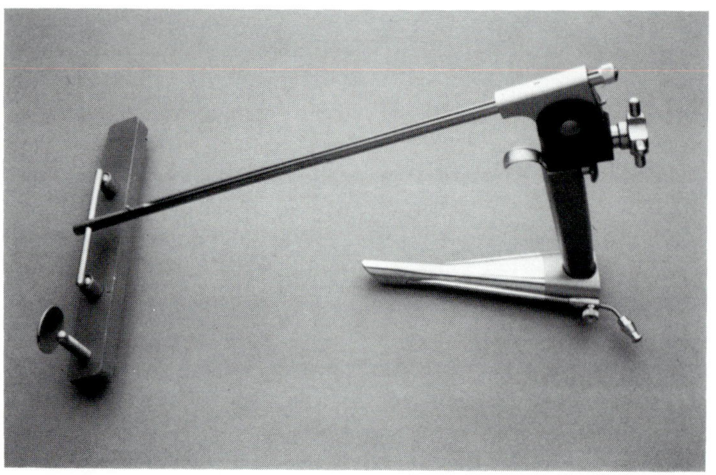

FIGURE 2–4. The Benjamin pediatric laryngoscope with a wide bore metal cannula on the left side for administration of anesthetic gases. The suspension device is the Benjamin modification.

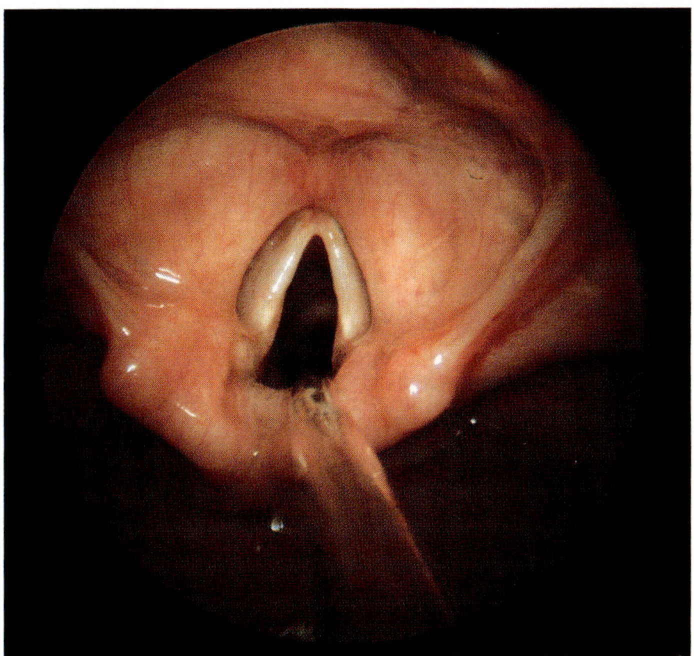

FIGURE 2–5. The normal larynx of an adolescent with a Benjet in place. Notice the excellent visualization with almost no impairment from the tube. Laser surgery is possible with standard precautions to prevent fires. The tube can be elevated by the laryngoscope into the anterior commissure for posterior glottic vaporizations.

tial.[16] Cohen and Geller stress that paralysis with succinylcholine, before the determination of vocal cord mobility is made, can lead to the inability to ventilate the obstructed patient with loss of control of the airway, hypercapnia, hypoxia, and cardiac arrest.[17] After the determination that the patient can be safely paralyzed, succinylcholine is given and the larynx and subglottic area are examined. The child remains apneic during this part of the examination. Hyperventilation with 100 per cent oxygen is necessary at the time of administration of the muscle relaxant to create a reservoir of pulmonary oxygenation.[17] The author does not use succinylcholine in children, but, for those weighing less than 35 kg, spontaneous ventilation is allowed throughout the procedure.

The apneic technique is successfully utilized by a large number of surgeons. Like any method, it has potential problems that must be understood by both the otolaryngologist and the anesthesiologist. During apnea, the patient's Pa_{CO_2} level rises rapidly (3 mm/minute).[18] This rise in carbon dioxide concentration can lead to hypertension and cardiac irritability, and therefore the apneic technique is contraindicated in many patients. The technique is most appropriate when the surgeon knows that the patient has a borderline airway and believes that any trauma caused by endotracheal intubation may precipitate the need for a tracheotomy. Occasionally a better understanding of the laryngeal disorder is required when contemplating which size of endotracheal tube to use or when assessing the possible need for a tracheotomy. The obvious disadvantage is the time constraint under which one must work. For practical purposes, this technique severely limits the surgeon's ability to capture optimal operative photography, perform extensive or complicated microsurgery, and present effective intraoperative teaching.

Induction of general anesthesia for the apneic technique is the same as that described above. Appropriate monitoring is utilized. If there are no extensive papillomas or tumors involving the larynx, the surgeon may elect to proceed directly to the apneic technique. If there is an extensive mass, the bulk of the disease is removed with an endotracheal tube in place; this reduces the number of apneic cycles required. When the bulk of the mass is small enough for removal with two or three apneic cycles, the procedure is converted to the apneic anesthetic technique.[19] Laryngoscopes such as the Lindholm, Benjamin Slimline, or Benjamin pediatric (Karl Storz Endoscopy-America, Inc.) provide optimal binocular vision and can be suspended from an overtable utilizing the Benjamin modification suspension apparatus (Fig. 2–6; see Fig. 2–4). The operating laser

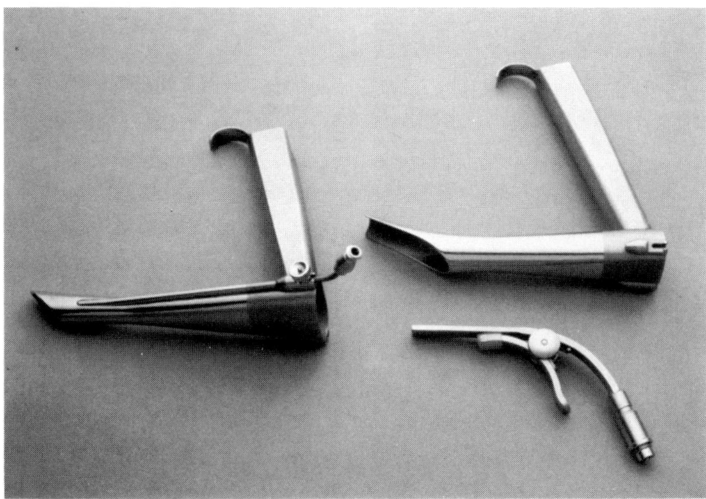

FIGURE 2-6. The Benjamin pediatric laryngoscope *(left)* and the Lindholm laryngoscope *(top right)* have side ports available for anesthetic or oxygen insufflation, jetting, or suction. The Benjamin-Havas clip *(bottom right)* attaches to the light cable and can be changed easily when switching laryngoscopes.

microscope is then brought into position, and the larynx is viewed using a 400 mm focal length lens. An endotracheal tube is then placed through the laryngoscope, between the vocal folds and into the trachea. The anesthesiologist is asked to hyperventilate the patient with 100 per cent oxygen and halothane (Fluothane) or isoflurane (Forane) inhalation agents. Neuromuscular blockade is confirmed with a nerve stimulator. After the patient has been hyperventilated for approximately 30 seconds to 2 minutes and the oxygen saturation, in routine cases, is approximately 99 to 100 per cent by the pulse oximeter or greater than 300 mm Hg on the transcutaneous oxygen monitor, the endotracheal tube is removed. The laryngoscope and the operating microscope are not moved. The remaining disease is then vaporized from those areas of the larynx where laser surgery was not previously possible. All flammable material is clear of the airway during this portion of the procedure.[20]

Venturi jet ventilation can be safe and efficient with minimal complications when properly performed. Premedication recommendations for Venturi jet ventilation include oral diazepam, morphine, and atropine.[19,30] Children with papillomatosis are not premedicated as a rule, and uncooperative children are given methohexital (Brevital) rectally. Infants and neonates with congenital anomalies are usually just given atropine. Anesthesia induction is standard. If ventilation is adequate and the oximeter reveals adequate oxygen saturation, intravenous fentanyl and a muscle relaxant, such as succinylcholine or atracurium, are administered. After adequate muscle relaxation is achieved, as shown by stimulation of the ulnar nerve, the laryngoscope is placed and jetting is begun through an injector needle mounted in the light channel of the laryngoscope. Infants and children are ventilated at jet pressures starting at 5 to 10 psi, which are increased until adequate chest rise and fall are noted. Adults are begun at 20 psi, and pressures are increased until the adequate chest rise and fall are observed. All patients are monitored by oximetry, and the anesthesia is maintained with a jet mixture of inhalation agents and oxygen. Exhaled gases are salvaged by an exhaust system, and intravenous fentanyl is given intermittently. The anesthetic gases are removed for awakening; 100 per cent oxygen is administered; and the effects of atracurium, if used, are reversed with atropine and neostigmine.[19]

Miyasaka and colleagues also discussed a jet injector (Sanders) technique for bronchoscopy in children and believe that it is an acceptable technique.[21] However, they discussed many important points that must be well understood if this technique is to be utilized. There are so many variables for the otolaryngologist to recognize that this procedure probably should be discouraged if it is not performed on a routine basis, particularly in children with stiff or sick lungs.

Crockett and associates believe that appropriate patient selection must exclude patients with poor pulmonary compliance or obese patients.[19] In these situations, jet ventilation should be terminated and the patient intubated. Any patient with near total glottic obstruction, such as might be seen with papilloma, is not a candidate for this procedure. Failure to recognize such obstructive problems can result in subcutaneous emphysema, pneumothorax, or pneumomediastinum. In cases of severe papilloma, the author believes that the patient should be intubated first and the mass debulked before jetting is initiated (Fig. 2–7). Crockett and associates also expressed concern about the blasting of tissue and blood into the distal trachea and the abnormal forced movements of the cords.[19]

During CO_2 laser bronchoscopy greater protection against ignition of endotracheal tubes is possible by utilizing oxygen with helium.[26] This combination agent is less flammable than the combination of nitrogen and oxygen. The use of nitrous oxide during laser endoscopic surgery is contraindicated because it supports combustion and exposes patients to an unnecessary risk of fire or explosion. Mixtures of nitrous oxide and oxygen support combustion of endotracheal tube fires ignited by a CO_2 laser just as readily as does 100 per cent oxygen. Endotracheal explosion is the most common serious complication of CO_2 laser surgery. The elimination of nitrous oxide from anesthetic gases should lessen the occurrence of this disaster.[22]

High frequency jet ventilation delivered through a wide bore needle inserted into the trachea through the cricothyroid membrane can be employed. This has the advantage of general anesthesia without a tube in the glottis. Adequate respiratory function can be maintained in most patients without difficulty. Experience has demonstrated, however, that high frequency jet ventilation may be associated with a number of rather compelling problems. The needle must be introduced percutaneously, and the development of a hematoma, pneumomediastinum, pneumothorax, or subcutaneous emphysema is well documented. Further, the whipping action of the needle with each rush of air can be traumatic to the tracheal mucosa.[23]

When using rigid endoscopic techniques, Shapshay and Beamis prefer general anesthesia for better control of the airway and for patient comfort.[24] Light general anesthesia using intravenous medications (thiopental sodium and neuroleptanesthetic agents) is preferred for patients with major airway obstruction.[24] Spontaneous respiration is preferred in children; when this is not possible because of excessive coughing or hypoventilation, the jet ventilation or intubation technique is

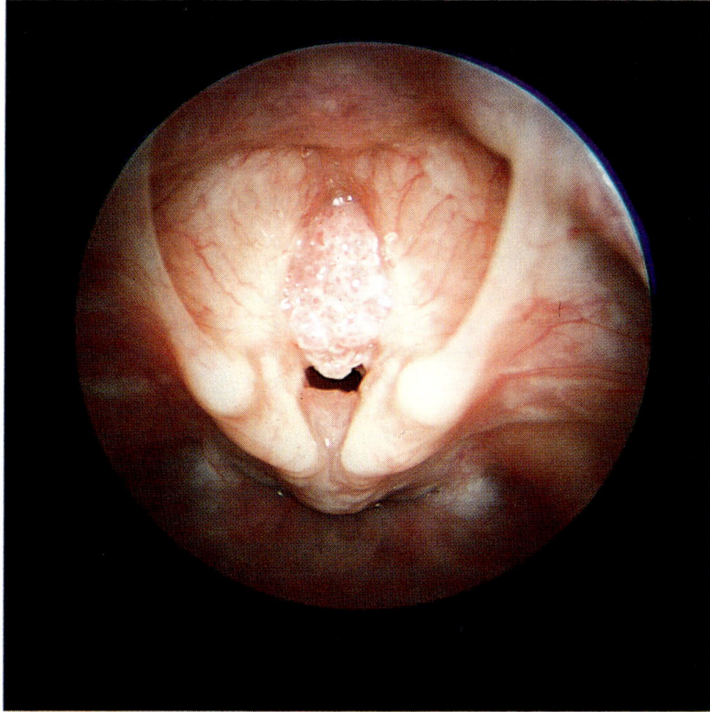

FIGURE 2–7. Obstructive papillomatosis can be treated by laser directly if the child is breathing spontaneously. When Venturi jet ventilation is used the mass of the papilloma must be resected manually prior to utilization of the laser. This requires placement of an endotracheal tube through the papilloma.

employed. When spontaneous ventilation is utilized, an early sign of lightening of the anesthesia is observed by noting movement of the true vocal cords.[3]

Of the choices of anesthetic agents, the most commonly used for inhalation anesthesia are the nonexplosive drugs enflurane (Ethrane), halothane, and isoflurane. Use of noncombustible agents is mandatory when either cautery or laser techniques are planned.

Complications

The otolaryngologist must not forget that ventricular arrhythmias can develop with topical epinephrine or halogenated hydrocarbons, particularly in the presence of hypercapnia and endogenous catecholamine release.[2]

Nitrous oxide presents another problem that is all too frequently overlooked. Although this drug is among the weakest of the anesthetics, it does decrease cardiac output in the damaged heart. Equally important is the tendency of the nitrous oxide to diffuse into the air-filled endotracheal cuff during prolonged procedures, with resultant increases in cuff pressures; this causes ischemic compression of the tracheal mucosa.[2]

Operating room contamination with nitrous oxide and volatile anesthetic agents is a controversial and unresolved subject. Concerns exist regarding the incidence of spontaneous abortions in pregnant women, possible congenital abnormalities in children born to operating room personnel, and an increased incidence of liver disease or reticuloendotheliosis in the operating room staff. Edelist recommends removal of the gases, such as with a scavenging system, or not using inhalational agents.[3]

Occasionally, the intense pressure of the laryngoscope blade on the supraglottis during suspension laryngoscopy stimulates deep laryngeal receptors and induces severe cardiac arrhythmias, such as premature ventricular contractions or bigeminy. Myocardial ischemia and infarction have also been reported.[25] The occurrence of ventricular arrhythmias must not be ignored, as the patient is at increased risk for intra- or postoperative myocardial infarction. Both the superior laryngeal nerve and the cardioinhibitory fibers of the vagus nerve contribute to the reflex circuit that produces arrhythmias. The laryngoscope must be withdrawn and the patient hyperoxygenated. Usually the arrhythmia clears promptly. If reinsertion and suspension of the laryngoscope causes a repetition of the arrhythmia, it is wise to terminate the procedure and reschedule it. On the next occasion, the superior laryngeal nerve should be blocked prior to induction of general anesthesia, or the reflex may be abolished by the administration of lidocaine, 50 to 100 mg intravenously, immediately after induction.[2]

The incidences of laryngeal spasms are relatively high, as are those of postoperative edema of the larynx. Edelist recommended the use of lidocaine on the cords at the termination of the procedure to prevent immediate postoperative laryngospasm.[3] Pre- or intraoperative intravenous steroids appear to be beneficial in reducing postoperative airway edema. The author uses steroids only when excessive mucosa trauma is anticipated or is observed to have occurred.

Care must be taken to remove desiccated carbonaceous debris that accumulates on the lasered papilloma or tumor. Hydrodesiccated debris can become superheated and, if allowed to accumulate, can create a fire hazard in a high oxygen concentration environment. Other potential complications include flammable endotracheal or tracheotomy tubes, misdirection of the laser with tissue damage, and rupture of the endotracheal tube cuffs.

Awakening and Postoperative Management

In the techniques described above, it is necessary to reverse the nondepolarized neuromuscular blockade. The patient should be awakened with continuous oxygen insufflation. Monitoring is critical during this period. Removal of endoscopic equipment or reversal of the muscle relaxant effects can cause laryngospasm. The anesthesiologist will usually be in control of the patient at this time and must be ready for this possibility. A gastric tube should be routinely inserted before the patient's anesthetic state is lightened to empty the stomach of both air and secretions if jetting or mask ventilation was provided.[2] Humidified air by face shield will be required in the recovery room, and treatments with nebulized racemic epinephrine may be necessary. Patients who had intraoperative arrhythmias must be monitored postoperatively for resolution of the arrhythmia and for evidence of myocardial ischemia.

Hypoxemia related to persistent hemorrhage, accumulation of secretions or debris, and anesthesia-induced respiratory depression are common denominators for most intra- and postoperative complications.[24] Respiratory depression attributable to muscle relaxants or central nervous system depressants must be diagnosed and treated and adequate oxygenation assured.[26]

The majority of complications are evident within 1 to 2 hours after the procedure. It is critical that recovery room personnel understand both the anticipated and the unexpected reactions that can occur.

If topical lidocaine was utilized to prevent laryngospasm, the surgical team should be aware of the potential for toxic serum lidocaine concentrations. Although the incidence of this has been low, it can represent a significant postoperative complication.[27]

Airway edema in any patient can be life threatening but is especially dangerous in a small child. The tiny airways become severely obstructed with minimal edema, particularly in the child with preexisting compromise, such as subglottic stenosis or glottic webs. Although the majority of the author's laser airway procedures are performed on an outpatient basis, those patients who remain hospitalized often require intensive care unit (ICU) monitoring. Endoscopic procedures, even in small babies, can be performed safely with minimal morbidity.

Additional Pediatric Considerations

Pediatric laryngoscopy developed from the general principles of adult laryngoscopy, which were then applied to infants and children.[28] The requirements and anatomy of these smaller patients, however, are quite different. The infant larynx is higher, softer, more easily displaced, and more easily irritated with a great tendency to spasm. Improved understanding in pediatric endoscopy has led to the development of new endoscopic instruments and significant modifications of anesthetic techniques.[16]

Most endoscopy in infants and children is performed under general anesthesia. The techniques of anesthesia must encompass the full range of laryngeal, bronchoesophagologic, and microsurgical procedures and must be suitable for children of all ages, from premature neonates through adolescents. There is a vast difference in the requirements for diagnostic endoscopy, laser therapy, and anesthesia in a tiny premature infant as compared with those for an older child or adult.

In 1983, Benjamin recommended that anesthesia for endoscopy in children under 10 years of age (usually less than 35 kg) begin with thiopental, be followed by spontaneous respiration induction using inhalations of nitrous oxide and oxygen, and eventually replace the nitrous oxide with halothane. Topical agents such as lidocaine, up to a maximum of 5 mg/kg, halt unwanted reflex activity when sprayed on the larynx and cervical trachea. This technique avoids the use of an endotracheal tube during laryngoscopy[16] (see Fig. 2–3). A thorough bronchoscopy can often be performed utilizing only a telescope placed through the laryngoscope down to the level of the mainstem bronchi, and occasionally into the segmental bronchi, without the use of a bronchoscope (Fig. 2–8). An endotracheal tube is introduced for esophagoscopy and for an examination of the nasopharynx and nasal cavity.

Anesthetic gases are discontinued toward the end of Benjamin's laryngoscopy technique, and oxygen alone is insufflated so that an unhurried assessment of the return of vocal cord movements can be made. The general dynamics of the glottis and supraglottis are observed. This method is of great value in determining the presence of pathologic changes such as vocal cord paralysis or

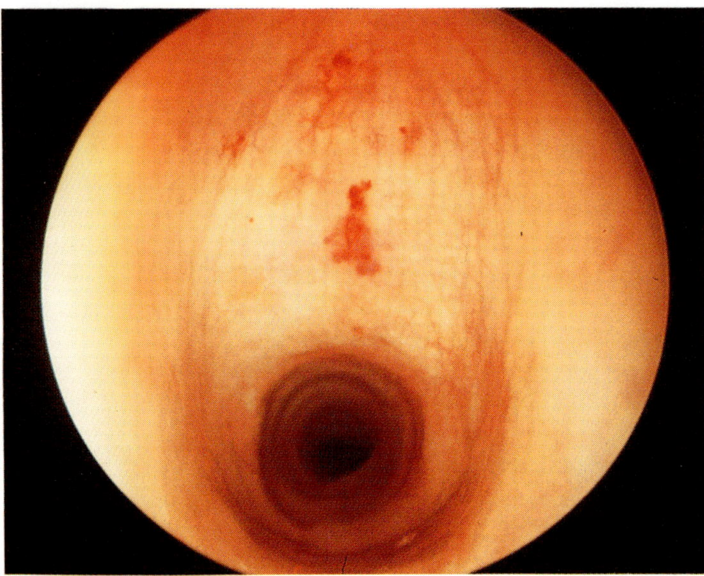

FIGURE 2–8. Tracheal stenosis with complete tracheal rings is photographed from the level of the true vocal cords. The stenosis is severe, and a bronchoscope cannot be passed into the trachea. A 2.7 mm diameter telescope is passed; the complete examination is performed as the child breathes spontaneously, with insufflation of anesthetic gases given through the side ports of the laryngoscope.

laryngomalacia, if static anatomic evaluation is insufficient. These techniques give clear, unobstructed access to all parts of the larynx without the need for an anesthetic tube, making this technique ideal for laser surgery (see Fig. 2–3).

Unless an adequate scavenging system is available, the surgeon may be concerned about the potential for personal inhalation injury if a large number of endoscopies are performed utilizing this technique; this risk is controversial and unproved. This author utilizes a face mask on the surgeon with high flow oxygen when using spontaneous insufflation to prevent inhalation complications.

This technique has been used satisfactorily in neonates who do not require ventilatory support. The author has been able to keep the children adequately anesthetized for prolonged periods of evaluation with telescopes, laser procedures, and photographic documentation.

Utilizing an endotracheal tube in a child obstructs visualization of the posterior commissure, the arytenoids, the posterior vocal cords, and the subglottis. It severely impairs the surgeon's ability to visualize glottic movement. However, for the child who requires ventilatory support, laryngoscopy must be performed with the endotracheal tube in place. Short periods of apnea can be utilized but only with optimal monitoring and experienced otolaryngologic and anesthetic teams.

With neonates or premature infants, meticulous care is needed to minimize possible trauma from transport to or from the operating room and from handling. It is important to conserve body heat and to maintain hydration during endoscopic examination. Particular attention must be given to the gentle handling of the delicate mucosa of the pharynx, larynx, and tracheobronchial tree. Endoscopic examination of the upper airway and esophagus can be comprehensively and safely performed, even in premature infants weighing less than 1000 grams.[28] Teamwork among the nursing staff, the anesthesia team, and the endoscopist is absolutely vital. It is essential that specialized pediatric endoscopic and anesthesia services be localized in selected hospitals that can provide adequate intra- and postoperative care for these patients.

Additional Adult Considerations

In adults, general anesthesia is commonly administered using one of four techniques: endotracheal intubation; midtracheal jet ventilation, with the Benjet or Johnson 3.5 mm diameter chest tube; proximal or distal laryngoscopic jetting; or the apneic technique. Laser application to the anterior vocal cords can be accomplished with an endotracheal tube in place, but the tube must be wrapped with reflective tape or be coated with a laser retardant to prevent flash fires. The smallest diameter tube possible is recommended. The Benjet tube offers excellent visualization but is not available in a laser-retardant tube. Small tubes can be manipulated well away from the target area. Caution must still be utilized, as these tubes can create a flash fire after several direct laser impacts. Although insufflation via a catheter with spontaneous respirations is possible in adults and adolescents, the author's experience has been that larger patients are poorly anesthetized, and midtracheal jet ventilation is preferred for patients weighing more than 35 kg. Jetting should not be used in patients with pulmonary compromise, including chronic obstructive pulmonary disease (COPD) or severe obesity. Jetting is not recommended in the geriatric population.

The apneic anesthesia technique affords improved visualization of the larynx and subglottis because the view is unencumbered by any form of artificial airway. This unobstructed view allows a more thorough removal of diseased tissue, especially in the posterior commissure and subglottis. The risk of fire is almost eliminated. The jetting risk of physically disseminating papilloma particles or tumor into the lower tracheobronchial tree or toward the surgeon does not exist. Use of a pulse oximeter or a transcutaneous oxygen monitor is important for optimal safety.

Weisberger and Miner believed that mechanical ventilation should be resumed if oxygen saturation is equal to or less than 97 per cent or if the transcutaneous monitor reading is less than 150 mm Hg.[20] They do not extend the apnea longer than 3.5 to 4 minutes at a maximum. For children less than 5 years of age, they limit the apnea to 30 seconds to 2 minutes. The laser is then placed on standby; the operating microscope arm is pivoted to the side; and an unwrapped endotracheal tube or small ventilating bronchoscope is inserted into the trachea through the laryngoscope, which is still in its original suspended position. At this point, the end tidal CO_2 is determined, and the patient is again hyperventilated with 100 per cent oxygen and the inhalation agent to bring arterial saturation back to 99 to 100 per cent. The above is repeated if additional diseased tissue must be removed. At the end of the procedure, the cords are sprayed with topical lidocaine (no more than 5 mg/kg) to minimize the incidence of laryngospasm as the patient awakens from anesthesia. Weisberger and Miner stated that the benefits of this procedure are that it can be performed on an outpatient basis and that no vocal cord motion occurs as with jet ventilation or spontaneous respiration.[20] They term the technique intermittent apneic anesthesia.

This author does not utilize laryngoscopic mounted jet ventilation, either proximally or distally, for any type of endoscopy. This jet ventilation technique does dramatically dry the glottis and supraglottis, causes significant motion of the laser target area, allows jetted gas expansion of the esophagus and stomach, and blows tumor or possible live virus debris into the tracheobronchial tree.

EQUIPMENT

The benefit of utilizing multiple laryngoscopes during a procedure should be understood. A right-sided slotted laryngoscope with an excellent light source is beneficial for use in patients of any age, from premature infants to adults, for instrumentation or intubation. A laryngoscope with side channels capable of handling insufflation of oxygen or anesthetic gases is important. On laryngoscopes with bilateral side channels, one side can be used for insufflation or jetting of gases while the other side is used for suctioning of laser-induced smoke. The anterior commissure scope feature is essential for some examinations. A laryngoscope should be available that can examine the entire larynx, including the epiglottis, without distorting normal relationships; the Lindholm laryngoscope can be placed in the vallecula, and both surfaces of the epiglottis can be examined as well as the supraglottis (Fig. 2–9). Rapid changing of the laryngoscopes can create anesthetic problems; therefore, the light cables and anesthesia cannulas must be easy to switch without significant interruption of respirations. The Benjamin-Havas light clip (see Fig. 2–6) enables changing of

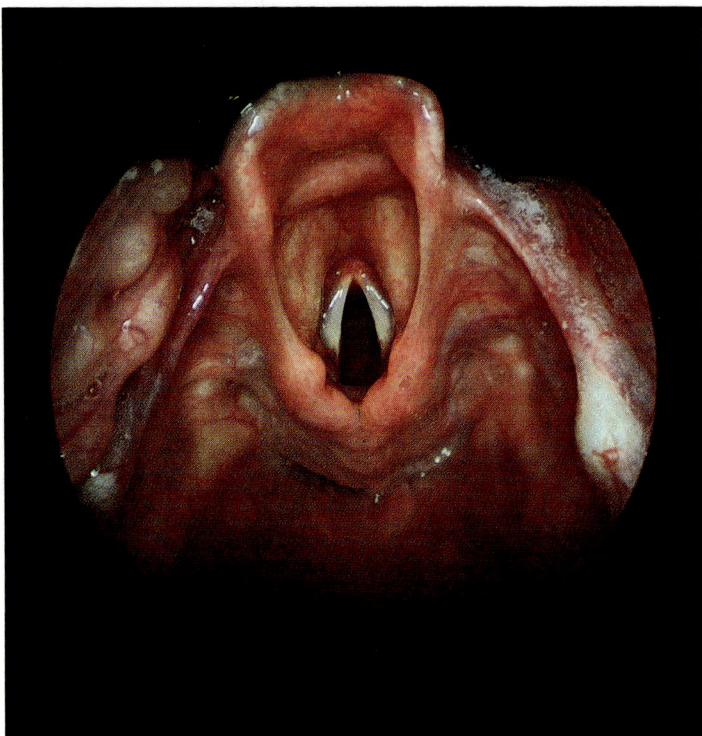

FIGURE 2–9. This is a typical view obtained utilizing a Lindholm laryngoscope (Karl Storz) with a 0 degree telescope. Note the excellent panoramic view of the entire hypopharynx and laryngeal structures. The telescope can be advanced below the cords without interruption of anesthesia, and various angled scopes can be used to evaluate the undersurface of the cords.

laryngoscopes easily and rapidly. The suspension device should be simple to operate and a type that can be attached and secured by the primary endoscopist without assistance (see Figs. 2–1, 2–4). Anesthetic techniques, such as spontaneous insufflation, apnea, or jetting, allow evaluation of the larynx, subglottis, and tracheobronchial tree with telescopes of various angles from 0 to 120 degrees.[28]

The anesthesia technique should also allow optimal documentation whenever possible. Television monitoring, from either the telescope or microscope, is a tremendous teaching aid; equipment is now available that will allow videorecording and the production of slides or computer image prints.

References

1. Benjamin B: Anesthesia for laryngoscopy. Ann Otol Rhinol Laryngol 93:338, 1984.
2. Norton ML, Strong MS: Anesthesia for endoscopic diagnoses and surgery. Otolaryngol Clin North Am 14:687, 1981.
3. Edelist G: Anaesthesia for endoscopy and laser surgery. Can Anaesth Soc J 31:S1, 1984.
4. Strong MS, Vaughan CW, Mahler DL, et al.: Cardiac complications of microsurgery of the larynx. Laryngoscope 84:908, 1974.
5. Goudsouzian NG: Muscle relaxants in children. *In:* A Practice of Anesthesia for Infants and Children. Edit. Ryan FE. New York, Appleton-Century-Crofts, 1986, p 105.
6. Davis RK, Simpson GP: Safety with the carbon dioxide laser. Otolaryngol Clin North Am 16:801, 1983.
7. Brutinel WM, McDougall JC, Cortese DA: Bronchoscopic therapy with the neodymium-yttrium-aluminum-garnet laser during intravenous anesthesia. Chest 84:512, 1983.
8. Vourc'h G, Tannieres ML, Toty L, Personne C: Anaesthetic management of tracheal surgery using the neodymium-yttrium-aluminum-garnet laser. Br J Anaesth 52:993, 1980.
9. Johnson JT, Chang JL, Myers EN: Jet ventilation for operative laryngoscopy. Laryngoscope 92:1194, 1982.
10. Sørensen MB, Jacobsen E: Pulmonary hemodynamics during direct diagnostic laryngoscopy. Acta Anaesthesiol Scand 25:51, 1981.
11. Warner ME, Warner MA, Leonard PF: Anesthesia for the Nd-YAG laser resection of major airway obstructing tumors. Anesthesiology 60:230, 1984.
12. Gold MI, Muravchick S: Arterial oxygenation during laryngoscopy and intubation. Anesth Analg 60:316, 1981.

13. Ledbetter JL, Rasch DK, Pollard TG, Helsel P, Smith RB: Reducing the risks of laryngoscopy in anesthetized infants. Anaesthesia 43:151, 1988.
14. Kautto UM: Attenuation of the circulatory response to laryngoscopy and intubation by fentanyl. Acta Anaesthesiol Scand 26:217, 1982.
15. Podolkin W, Wells DG: Precipitous bradycardia induced by laryngoscopy in cardiac surgical patients. Can J Anaesth 34:618, 1987.
16. Benjamin B: Technique of laryngoscopy. Int J Pediatr Otorhinolaryngol 13:299, 1987.
17. Cohen SR, Geller KA: Anesthesia in pediatric endoscopy: The surgeon's view. Otolaryngol Clin North Am 14:705, 1981.
18. Smith RB: Anesthesia for endoscopy. Trans PA Acad Ophthalmol Otolaryngol 28:167, 1975.
19. Crockett DM, McCabe BF, Scamman FL, Lusk, RP, Gray SD: Venturi jet ventilation for microlaryngoscopy: Technique, complications, pitfalls. Laryngoscope 97:1326, 1987.
20. Weisberger EC, Miner JD: Apneic anesthesia for improved endoscopic removal of laryngeal papillomata. Laryngoscope 98:693, 1988.
21. Miyasaka K, Sloan IA, Froese AB: An evaluation of the jet injector (Sanders) technique for bronchoscopy in paediatric patients. Can Anaesth Soc J 27:117, 1980.
22. Sosis M: Nitrous oxide is contraindicated in endoscopic surgery. Can J Anaesth 34:539, 1987.
23. Vivori E: Anaesthesia for laryngoscopy. Br J Anaesth 52:638, 1980.
24. Shapshay SM, Beamis JF: Safety precautions for bronchoscopic Nd-YAG laser surgery. Otolaryngol Head Neck Surg 94:175, 1986.
25. Wenig DL, Raphael N, Stern JR, Shikowitz MJ, Abramson AL: Cardiac complications of suspension laryngoscopy. Arch Otolaryngol Head Neck Surg 112:860, 1986.
26. Eisenman TS, Ossoff RH: Anesthesia for bronchoscopic laser surgery. Otolaryngol Head Neck Surg 94:45, 1986.
27. Labedzki L, Ochs HR, Abernethy DR, Greenblatt DJ: Potentially toxic serum lidocaine concentrations following spray anesthesia for bronchoscopy. Klin Wochenschr 61:379, 1983.
28. Benjamin B: The role of the paediatric endoscopist. J Laryngol Otol 100:1397, 1986.
29. Johnson JT, Myers EN: Recent advances in operative laryngoscopy. Otolaryngol Clin North Am 17:35, 1984.
30. Godden DJ, Wilky RF, Fergusson RJ, Wright DJ, Crompton GK, Grant IWB: Rigid bronchoscopy under intravenous general anesthesia with oxygen Venturi ventilation. Thorax 37:532, 1982.
31. McLeskey CH: International Anesthetic Research Society 1988 Review Course Lectures. IARS 62nd Congress, San Diego, CA March 5–9, 1988, p 135.

CHAPTER 3

LASER SURGERY FOR BENIGN LARYNGEAL LESIONS

James A. Duncavage

Robert H. Ossoff

HISTORICAL PERSPECTIVE

The use of lasers for laryngeal surgery began in Boston in the late 1960s. It was thought then that a laser might offer an advantage over other conventional therapeutic modalities in treating cancer of the larynx. This driving force for the development of an instrument to treat cancer of the larynx started with the use of the argon laser to excise laryngeal tissue. It was soon found that the argon laser lacked the necessary precision for laryngeal surgery. It is now known why the argon laser was imprecise. The argon laser is a visible laser whose tissue coefficients are affected by tissue pigments. A precise cut through tissue cannot be obtained if the laser energy is absorbed by many different chromophores. As early excitement with the argon laser was fading, a new laser, the neodymium in glass laser, became available experimentally. Again, the researchers were unable to produce a precise cut, through experimentation on the canine vocal cord. They did find that applying a dark material, in this case copper sulfate, to the vocal cord surface allowed the neodymium in glass laser energy to be absorbed on the vocal cord surface. The imprecise nature of the resultant laser injury forced the investigators to abandon this laser.

An experimental laser wavelength produced by American Optical became the next focus of interest. This was a gas laser using carbon dioxide. The original experimental model was approximately the size of a telephone booth. It had an articulating arm, but lacked a system to deliver the laser energy through a microlaryngoscope. The development of the micromanipulator by Bredemeier[1] overcame the obstacle of delivery of laser energy from the laser to the larynx.[2] The carbon dioxide (CO_2) laser was found to allow precise injury to the canine vocal cord. This opened the door to clinical use of the CO_2 laser.[3] The CO_2 laser has now become an accepted surgical instrument for treatment of diseases of the larynx. It has allowed for the improvement of certain surgical procedures and also enabled the development of new surgical procedures.

LASER APPLICATIONS IN THE LARYNX

The treatment of mucosal diseases of the larynx is undergoing a transition. The introduction of the operating microscope to laryngology has allowed for a precise way to diagnose and treat laryngeal pathologic conditions. With the introduction of microlaryngeal instrumentation, precision was improved by binocular control of the surgical field. Today, videostroboscopy offers the laryngologist an opportunity to study the larynx in a slow motion view. This, coupled with an understanding of the histologic features of the larynx, can allow formation of a treatment plan for mucosal disease of the larynx that will address the underlying pathologic condition.

The principles applied to evaluation of patients with benign mucosal diseases are directed at identifying a predisposing cause of the problem. This information can usually be gained from the history. A more specific voice history, when necessary, can be obtained by a speech pathologist. When the history indicates that the benign laryngeal pathologic change is due to vocal misuse or vocal irritation, treatment is nonsurgical. Every attempt is made to eliminate the irritants, and voice therapy is prescribed to correct the vocal misuse.

If surgical treatment of the benign mucosal lesion is chosen, a decision is usually made to use either conventional or CO_2 laser surgery techniques.

A decision to use the CO_2 laser is based on the advantages of this surgical tool versus the disadvantages. The advantages are precision, with less tissue manipulation; better visibility resulting from hemostasis of the microcirculation of the laryngeal epithelium; and a hands off surgical technique. The disadvantages are all related to a common source (i.e., thermal damage). Thermal properties of the laser could cause combustion of the endotracheal tube.[4,5] Lateral thermal heat spread could injure the vocal ligament or spread to the vocalis muscle.[6]

If the CO_2 laser is chosen as the surgical instrument for the laryngeal surgery, certain precautions are necessary. Special microlaryngoscopes with a dedicated suction channel must be used along with instruments that are finished in a special way to prevent accidental laser beam reflection.[7] Communication among members of the anesthesia and the operating teams is mandatory. The anesthesiologist must select an endotracheal tube that permits safe use of the laser in the airway. The nurses must have the room arranged properly for laser use and have done a preoperative check of the laser prior to bringing the patient into the operating room.

The surgeon alone has the ability to obtain the desired surgical goal when using the laser. To be successful, the surgeon must remember certain principles of CO_2 laser surgery. The surgeon must understand the relationship between watts of laser energy delivered to tissue and the area over which the energy is delivered. This is described as power density (watts per area). In addition, the intimate association of the power density and time of laser energy delivery is expressed as radiant exposure. The concept of radiant exposure must be fully understood. The movement of laser energy as heat, away from the area of laser impact is called lateral thermal energy spread.[8] To limit heat damage within the larynx, the single most important concept for the laryngeal surgeon to remember is to avoid the delivery of laser energy to the larynx in a continuous application. Therefore, the shortest time pulse that will produce the desired surgical effect should be selected. Typically, when the CO_2 laser is used in the larynx at a 400 mm focal distance and a spot size of 0.8 mm, 4 to 6 watts and 0.1 second are selected as the laser settings on the module.

Two other concepts, both related to lateral thermal spread of laser energy, deserve mentioning. If the CO_2 laser is to be used to create an incision through the squamous epithelium of the vocal cord, it is better to deliver the energy in a skipping technique to produce a serrated cut (Fig. 3–1). This skipping of laser energy delivery lessens the chance of uneven depth of laser cutting. The other technique is shaving (Fig. 3–2). If one imagines a vocal cord nodule to be approximately 0.4 mm in diameter, and the 400 mm focal distance, CO_2 laser beam diameter to be 0.8 mm, it would be safer to the surrounding vocal cord epithelium to allow only the lateral one half of the laser beam to impact on the nodule and let the medial one half pass through the glottis and be absorbed by an underlying operating platform.

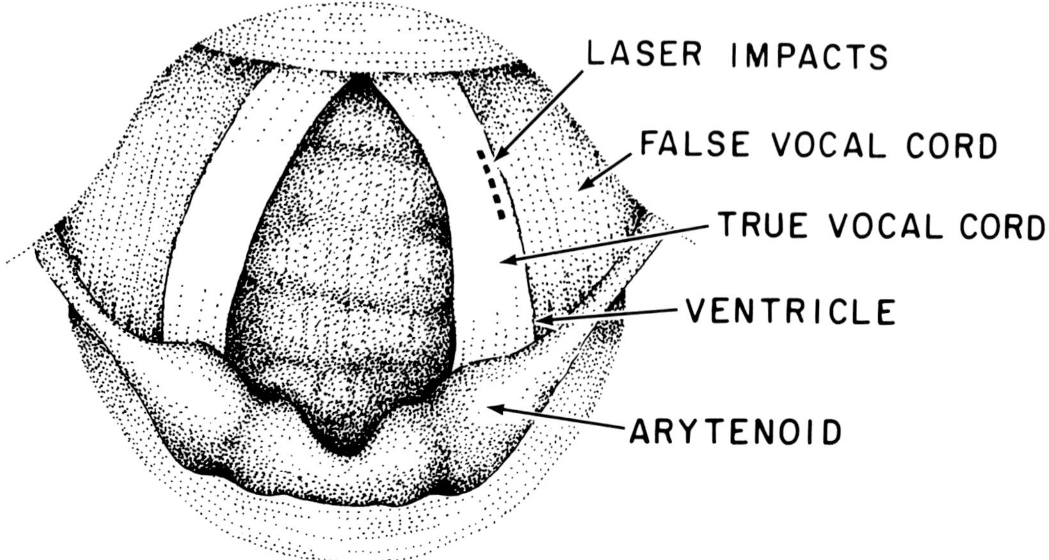

Figure 3–1. Skipping technique.

Vocal Cord Nodules

The treatment of all vocal cord nodules involves identification of the underlying vocal abnormality and correction through voice therapy. If voice therapy corrects the underlying vocal abnormality, but the nodule does not regress, surgery to remove the nodule is an option for the patient. The CO_2 laser excision of nodules offers the advantage of precise removal of the nodule, sparing most of the squamous epithelium of the vocal fold. The one disadvantage is that no surgical specimen is obtained.

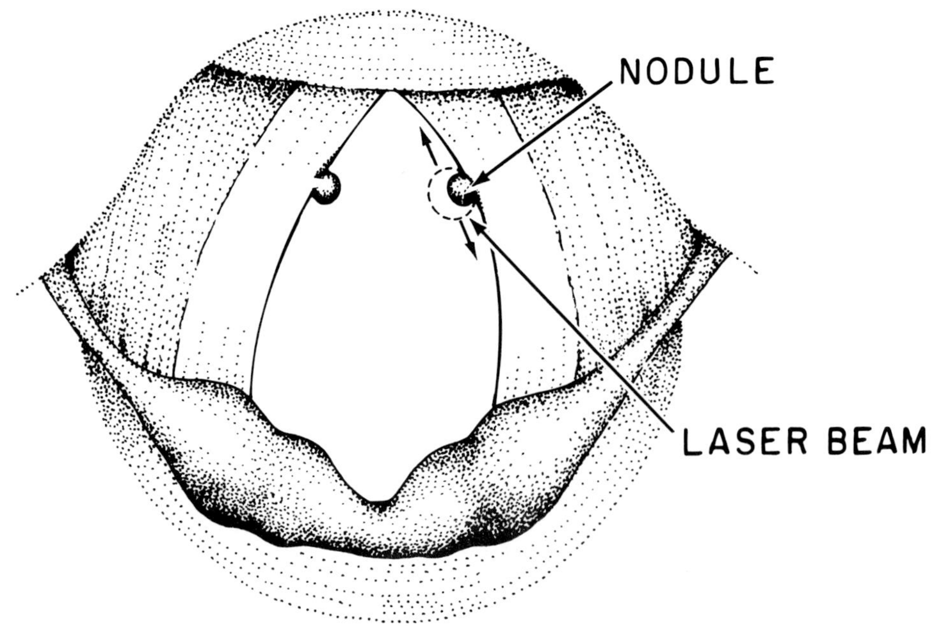

Figure 3–2. Shaving technique.

The surgical technique requires endotracheal intubation with an appropriate laser-safe tube or ventilation via a Venturi technique. The use of the Venturi technique produces some passive movement of the vocal folds, which can be circumvented by lasering when the patient is apneic. A special laser microlaryngoscope is used with suspension. The patient is completely paralyzed. The operating microscope is set at 10 × magnification. Moist cottonoid pledgets are placed in the subglottis to protect the endotracheal tube cuff. A mixture of helium and oxygen is delivered to the patient by the anesthesiologist. An operating platform is placed inferior to the vocal fold nodule. A test firing of the laser on the operating platform discloses the orientation of the aiming laser beam with the CO_2 laser beam. The laser is set at 4 watts and 0.1 second pulse length, and the laser energy is delivered in either a single pulse with each foot pedal depression or repeat pulses with each foot pedal depression.

The laser energy is delivered to the nodule to produce vaporization. The technique of shaving is used to precisely vaporize the nodule without causing any injury immediately lateral to the nodule. The delivery of laser energy lateral to the nodule could result in injury to the vocal ligament, resulting in an adynamic segment of vocal fold during phonation. The end point for the laser vaporization is reached when the epithelia anterior and posterior to the nodule are even with the nodule. Next, the charred, black debris should be removed. This is best accomplished by gently removing the moist cottonoid pledgets from the subglottis and wiping over the lasered area.

Immediately postoperatively the patient is allowed to breathe by face mask with humidified room air or 40 per cent oxygen. An electrocardiogram (ECG) is obtained if any arrhythmias were observed intraoperatively or if the patient has cardiac symptoms.[9] The patient is advised to maintain voice rest for approximately 7 days. The patient may talk but only for brief periods in a relaxed, quiet voice. The patient is to avoid all inhalation irritants. The patient is seen for a follow-up examination at 2 weeks postoperatively. At this time, epithelial regeneration over the surgical defect should be complete. Some edema will remain at 2 weeks, and a second visit at 1 month will find the vocal folds appearing normal.

Vocal Fold Polyps

Two types of polyps are observed involving the vocal folds. One is the isolated vocal fold polyp. The other form is polypoid degeneration of the vocal folds.

An isolated vocal fold polyp, although caused by vocal injury, must be removed surgically. Any underlying vocal misuse and vocal fold irritants are identified from the patient's history. Appropriate steps are taken to eliminate the misuse and irritants preoperatively.

The operative set-up for removal of a polyp is exactly the same as that described for treatment of nodules. This includes a laser-safe tube and protection of the tube cuff. In addition, 1 : 1000 solution of topical epinephrine (Adrenalin) should be available.

The removal of the polyp with the CO_2 laser is technically different from the removal of nodules. After the cottonoid pledgets are placed to protect the tube cuff, a suitably sized operating platform is placed beneath the polyp. The laser setting variables for excising a polyp are 6 watts, 0.1 second, and single or repeat laser pulses. The polyp is grasped with a suitable laser microlaryngeal forceps. Initially, no traction is placed on the polyp. The CO_2 laser is used in a skipping technique to serrate from the anterior to posterior vocal fold in a straight line. Only epithelium is vaporized. If tension is placed on the polyp before the incision is begun, the resultant laser incision leaves a defect in the underlying vocal ligament and vocalis muscle. To avoid cutting into the vocal fold, traction should be exerted medially only after the vocal epithelium has been vaporized. After the vocal epithelium has been vaporized, a blunt probe or microsuction is used to identify the vocal ligament. If the vocal ligament is identified, laser impacts can be directed medially away from this important structure. Sometimes, a technique called the third hand technique is used to excise large bulky polyps of the larynx. Briefly, this technique allows the hand used for the laser micromanipulator to be free for use in the larynx. This may be necessary when lateral retraction of the vocal ligament is necessary and the other hand is pulling the polyp medially. If the laser beam is imagined to function as a stationary band saw blade, moving the area to be incised across this beam will produce the cutting effect necessary to excise the polyp. In many instances, after excision of the polyp, bleeding is troublesome. Topical epinephrine on a cottonoid pledget will stop the bleeding and allow safe extubation at the end of the procedure.

The postoperative management of the patient with a polyp is identical to that described for nodules.

The treatment of polypoid degeneration of the vocal folds is much more involved. Most patients are women and heavy smokers. Attempts at eliminating smoking are many times unsuccessful. A voice assessment and voice therapy evaluation preoperatively are mandatory for this group of patients.

A brief review of the surgical treatment of polypoid degeneration of the vocal folds helps in understanding the present treatment options. In the past, patients underwent staged removal of vocal fold epithelium for polypoid degeneration. The introduction of the CO_2 laser resulted in a one stage removal of the vocal fold epithelium. The CO_2 laser was used to vaporize the squamous epithelium of both vocal folds. A 2 mm anterior strut of epithelium was saved on one true vocal fold to prevent anterior webbing.

The next advancement was to save the vocal fold epithelium and remove only the Reinke's space fluid and the resultant excessive squamous epithelium. The only controversy about this technique regards how to make the initial incision, with a knife or via the CO_2 laser. Either a microlaryngeal knife or the CO_2 laser can be used to cut through the squamous epithelium of the vocal fold. The incision is made laterally toward the thyroid cartilage and only through the epithelium. The advantage of the CO_2 laser is that hemostasis allows better visualization. The disadvantage is the lateral heat dissipation to the epithelium. The risk of deep injury is minimal owing to the fluid in Reinke's space, which absorbs the CO_2 laser energy. After the incision is made, a microflap of epithelium is elevated using a blunt straight and blunt right angled probe. Then the mucinous fluid is suctioned from the subepithelial space. After the fluid is removed, the squamous epithelium is in close approximation with the vocal ligament. The redundant epithelium is retracted laterally and excised with a microlaryngeal scissors. The authors have not found it necessary to use the CO_2 laser to tissue-weld the epithelial flap in place, although others have reported doing so.

The immediate postoperative care of the patient is the same as that described for patients with nodules. Plans for patient care during the 3 week postoperative period must be coordinated with the voice therapist preoperatively. This is necessary because during the initial postoperative time the voice may not be suitable for communication unless a voice therapist works with the patient over the initial 3 week postoperative period.

Stenosis

The CO_2 laser has been used to successfully treat patients with a stenosis of the larynx. The CO_2 laser is well adapted for treatment of stenosis because of the laser's ability to be coupled to an operating microscope. The use of the laser to treat stenoses many times must be augmented by stents, dilations, intralesional steroid injections, and microflaps of trap door configuration. The micro–trap-door flap has been developed because of the CO_2 laser's advantages of precision and hands off technique.[10]

Certain types and locations of laryngeal stenoses respond well to laser excision. The soft tissue supraglottic stenoses can be treated effectively with vaporization or excision. In the authors' series, three of three patients with a supraglottic stenosis responded well to laser excision.[11]

The glottic level stenoses can be divided into anterior and posterior types. The anterior glottic webs respond well to CO_2 laser vaporization. The authors found that four of five patients had improvement in airway patency. When using the CO_2 laser for anterior commissure stenoses, avoidance of lateral thermal damage is important. An attempt should be made to work at short laser pulses and the lowest power setting that will vaporize the scar band. The authors believe that early utilization of the voice may help in preventing reformation of the scar.

The posterior commissure and subglottic stenosis do not respond favorably to CO_2 laser excision. In the authors' series, only 3 of 10 such lesions had a favorable response and airway improvement. If these are more closely examined, some useful information becomes apparent. If the stenosis involves only the posterior commissure, and at least one arytenoid is mobile, the use of the micro–trap-door flap can be successful in improving the airway. The micro–trap-door flap, as described by Dedo and Sooy in 1984, is basically a biologic tissue dressing that promotes reepithelization and provides separation of opposing denuded surfaces. The technique uses a CO_2 laser and a 400 mm focal distance. A tracheotomy is usually present. If not, it is recommended that a tracheotomy be done before the laser procedure. Palpation of both arytenoids should be done at the time of surgery. At least one arytenoid must be mobile, and the associated posterior cricoarytenoid muscle must be innervated. To judge innervation, it is helpful to videotape the vocal cords preoperatively. The micro–trap-door flap requires binocular visualization to judge depth. The scar band between the two arytenoids is palpated. The mucosal lining of the stenosis is preserved. The CO_2 laser is set at 4 to 6 watts, at 0.1 second pulses, and is used to vaporize the subepithelial scar. Judgment is required to know when to stop inferiorly. This is determined by palpation and visualization. When the inferiormost extent of the scar has been vaporized, micro-scissors are used to cut the attachments of the epithelial flap on the right and left sides. The flap is then gently laid into position. The authors believe that the tracheotomy is beneficial, in that it diverts airflow away from the micro–trap-door flap. This may allow the flap a better chance of remaining in proper position.

The soft granulation tissue scars of the subglottic airway are left to the early formation of a mature scar. Experience with tracheal stenosis has shown that the early granulation proliferative form of a stenosis responds well to laser vaporization.[12]

The postoperative management of the patient with laryngeal stenosis includes a planned return to the operating room in approximately 4 to 6 weeks for a reevaluation and possible decannulation. Patients are maintained on a broad spectrum, systemic antibiotic for a minimum of 2 weeks. Humidification is recommended for home care.

Microspot Technique

Improvements in delivery system technology have led to the development of a 400 mm focal distance micromanipulator with a target tissue spot size of approximately 0.4 mm. This smaller surface area over which the laser energy is delivered to tissue should decrease the lateral thermal damage compared with that resulting from an 0.8 mm spot size.

To understand the potential use of the microspot, it is necessary to review the concepts of phonosurgery. The principles of phonosurgery entail the concept of the larynx as a precise organ of phonation. The vibrating surface of the vocal fold is the squamous epithelium. This epithelium flows smoothly over the underlying vocalis muscle. The mucosal epithelial waves flow from the infraglottic surface of the vocal fold to the superior surface of the vocal fold. A scarred segment produces an adynamic segment. The microspot, being much smaller by a factor of one half than the original 0.8 mm CO_2 laser microlaryngeal spot, allows for more precise laser vaporization, thereby decreasing the possibility of development of an adynamic vocal fold segment. This microspot could allow for more precise removal of stenoses. In addition, a hemostatic incision on the vocal fold to create a microflap may be desirable. However, at present, no videostroboscopy studies are available comparing the microspot technique with conventional laryngeal surgery or conventional CO_2 laser laryngeal surgery. Until these studies are available, the advantages of the microspot remain theoretic.

Granulomas

The treatment of granulomas requires a careful history to pinpoint any vocal misuse or dietary problems contributing to esophageal reflux. A complete physical examination of the larynx is also done, with attention to the vocal processes.

When there is a doubt that the lesion is a benign granuloma, a biopsy is taken. In patients who are smokers and consumers of alcoholic beverages, a biopsy should be done to establish a diagnosis of benign chronic inflammation. In this situation, when the patient will be under a general anesthetic and will have a biopsy, a frozen section is obtained. If the frozen section reveals no evidence of cancer, the chronically inflamed tissue is vaporized with the CO_2 laser. This requires reintubation with a laser-safe tube and adherence to all CO_2 laser safety precautions. Prior consent from the patient should have been obtained. This treatment philosophy is directed at establishing a diagnosis, but also allows for the treatment during the same anesthesia.

When vaporizing the chronically inflamed tissue, care should be taken to avoid exposure of the underlying arytenoid cartilage. From CO_2 laser wound studies it is evident that the CO_2 laser energy sterilizes the wound. This may help in allowing reepithelization to occur. Postoperatively, the patient is placed on a nonirritating diet and advised to stop smoking and drinking alcoholic beverages. A voice therapist advises the patient on voice care. Medical management with a histamine$_2$ (H_2) antagonist is also used in most cases of granuloma.

If the office examination of the patient with a granuloma appears to disclose no findings that are suggestive of malignancy, a strict medical plan is indicated. The plan consists of patient information for diet management and a consultation with the voice therapist to identify and correct any vocal misuse. Esophagography should be scheduled, with information given to the radiologist that reflux of gastric acid is suspected. An antacid regimen is started. If the esophagogram indicates reflux, the patient is advised to have a consultation with a gastroenterologist. If the patient shows no signs of improvement, a decision to perform a biopsy and to use CO_2 laser treatment of the chronically inflamed tissue is contemplated after 3 to 6 months of medical therapy. The treatment of granulomas of the larynx is difficult. Definitive diagnosis is essential for effective therapy. Therefore, the biopsy is an important part of the treatment. If the biopsy specimen is benign, the surgical treatment of the granuloma can be done when the biopsy is performed. No studies have been done to determine the ideal management of this disease.[13]

References

1. Bredemeier HC: Laser accessory for surgical applications. U.S. Patent 3,659,613, issued 1972.
2. Jako GJ: Laser surgery of the vocal cords: An excellent study with carbon dioxide laser on dogs. Laryngoscope 82:2204, 1972.
3. Strong MS, Jako GJ: Laser surgery in the larynx; early clinical experience with continuous CO_2 laser. Ann Otol Rhinol Laryngol 81:791, 1972.
4. McGill TJI, Friedman EM, Healy GB: Laser surgery in the pediatric airway. Otolaryngol Clin North Am 16:865, 1983.
5. Duncavage JA, Ossoff RH, Rouman WC, et al.: Injuries to the bronchi and lungs caused by laser-ignited endotracheal tube fires. Otolaryngol Head Neck Surg 92:639, 1984.
6. Durkin GE, Duncavage JA, Toohill RJ, et al.: Wound healing of true vocal cord squamous epithelium following CO_2 laser ablation and cup forcep stripping. Otolaryngol Head Neck Surg 95:273, 1986.
7. Strong MS, Vaughan CW, Healy GB, et al.: Recurrent respiratory papillomatosis: Management with the CO_2 laser. Ann Otol Rhinol Laryngol 85:508, 1976.
8. Ossoff RH, Karlan MS: Instrumentation for CO_2 laser surgery of the larynx and tracheobronchial tree. Surg Clin North Am 64:973, 1984.
9. Strong MS, Vaughan CW, Mahler DL, et al.: Cardiac complications of microsurgery of the larynx: Etiology, incidence and prevention. Laryngoscope 84:908, 1974.
10. Duncavage JA, Piazza LS, Ossoff RH, Toohill RJ: The microtrapdoor technique for the management of laryngeal stenosis. Laryngoscope 97:825, 1987.
11. Duncavage JA, Ossoff RH, Toohill RJ: CO_2 laser management of laryngeal stenosis. Ann Otol Rhinol Laryngol 94:565, 1985.
12. Healy GB, McGill TJI, Friedman EM: Carbon dioxide laser in subglottic hemangioma. Ann Otol Rhinol Laryngol 93:370, 1984.
13. Benjamin B, Croxson G: Vocal cord granulomas. Ann Otol Rhinol Laryngol 94:538, 1985.

CHAPTER 4

Laser Surgery in Multiple Respiratory Papillomatosis

Bruce Benjamin

"Warts in the throat" were described in the seventeenth century.[1] In 1880 papillomas were specified by Mackenzie as the most common benign tumors of the larynx in children.[2] The term juvenile laryngeal papillomatosis prevailed into the 1960s. It was considered that papillomas were confined to the laryngeal mucosa, were found in patients under 15 years of age, and had a strong tendency to regress at puberty.

It is now clear that papillomas occur at any age,[3–7] about two thirds of patients being younger than 15 and one third older than 15 years of age. The highest incidence is before the age of 5 years.[4,7] Papillomas occur most commonly in the larynx, but may be found elsewhere in the upper respiratory tract[8] from the nasal mucosa to the lung parenchyma and even in the esophagus. There is no relationship between puberty and the age of onset, the rate of control, or the rate of recurrence;[5,6] the patient should be treated without regard to his or her age, as there is no tendency for regression at puberty. Although unexpected remissions occur, the disease is notorious for frequent recurrences. The more accurate term recurrent respiratory papillomatosis is preferred.[5]

The human papilloma virus (HPV) causes respiratory papillomas.[3,9,10] Batsakis and colleagues postulate that "an activation of a persistent viral infection, coupled with an unknown promoter, is the etiologic basis for laryngeal papillomas."[3] There is convincing evidence of an etiologic relationship between condylomata acuminata and some laryngeal papillomas.[10]

Papillomas are not neoplastic,[11] but are benign squamous lesions that tend to occur in clusters and are composed of a vascular connective tissue core covered by stratified squamous epithelium with little or no tendency to invade submucosal tissue. They are usually multiple, sessile, and spread over a wide area, but may be pedunculated and localized.

There are often multiple sites of involvement in the upper aerodigestive tract.[3] The potential for spread in the respiratory tract explains the progression that occasionally occurs into the lung parenchyma, where the deposits of squamous papilloma appear as multiple cystic spaces on a chest x-ray film. Pulmonary parenchymatous spread is multicentric, relentlessly progressive, and eventually fatal.

Malignant degeneration is exceedingly rare,[12] unless radiotherapy had been used in an ill-judged attempt to control the disease. Radiotherapy is contraindicated.

The natural history of untreated papillomas over a long period of time has not been studied, but it is clear that the growth rate may be irregular and unpredictable, with remissions and exacerbations occurring for no apparent reason.[4,6,7] Although spontaneous resolution may occur, there is usually a tendency for recurrence and progression, in some cases despite all forms of treatment. The potential to compromise function of the larynx and cause airway obstruction sometimes makes them a serious threat to life.

The variety of treatments employed in the management of recurrent respiratory papillomatosis demonstrates that there is no known cure. Nevertheless many forms of treatment have been advocated,[6,7,13] including the use of a vaccine made from the patient's papillomas, radiotherapy, ultrasound, injection of hormones, homeopathy, steroids, vidarabine (Vira-A), local treatment with podophyllum, systemically administered magnesium and calcium, tetracyclines, and cytotoxic treatment with topical 5-fluorouracil or with systemic bleomycin.[14] No lasting success has been reported with these adjunctive forms of treatment. Recently photodynamic therapy utilizing hematoporphyrin derivative and a gold vapor laser, originally developed for the treatment of cancer, has been reported as promising therapy that may be effective against papilloma virus in the respiratory tract.[15]

There is no treatment that has been shown to eradicate the disease. The basis of management is to maintain an adequate airway by removal of papillomas. Many techniques have been used, including naked eye endoscopic removal with forceps, electrocautery, cryosurgery, laryngofissure for direct removal, endoscopic microlaryngeal removal, and more recently laser surgery. Tracheotomy was commonly performed some years ago, but should be avoided when possible, as papillomas are likely to grow at the tracheostoma either because of surgical incision into the tissues or as a result of activation of papilloma virus when squamous metaplasia occurs. Good anesthetic and surgical technique minimizes the necessity for tracheotomy, which need be considered only if the airway is in danger of being obstructed because of rapid growth of the papillomas or because of noncompliance of the patient with treatment.

The CO_2 laser is preferred as the surgical modality of choice by most laryngologists,[4,5,7,13] as it allows precise removal of papillomas in virtually all areas with minimal trauma and scarring in the larynx.

CLINICAL FEATURES

Papillomas in pediatric and adult patients occur in much the same manner.[4,7] Alteration of voice is present in more than 90 per cent of patients, and about 25 per cent have some degree of increasing respiratory obstruction when first seen. There is huskiness or hoarseness in adults and older children and a weak or feeble cry in infants. The presenting features sometimes lead to misdiagnosis, especially in children with noisy breathing, the patients being mistakenly treated for asthma, bronchitis, or "croup." On average, children have voice or obstructive symptoms for about 12 months before the correct diagnosis is made, whereas adults have symptoms for about 5 months. Some infants have symptoms from their papillomas in the first few months of life.[5,6,7,13] Some actually have papillomas present from birth, but it seems illogical to postulate that the papillomas are acquired by the baby during passage through a birth canal with HPV lesions. It is more likely that in those mothers with condylomata acuminata the virus is carried to the respiratory mucosa of the baby by blood-borne transfer.

There is a strong tendency for papillomas to occur in the larynx itself,[3–7] and approximately half the patients have lesions that are confined to the larynx;[7] further, there is good evidence that patients with laryngeal disease only have more localized and milder disease,[7] so that control can be achieved with fewer operations. The other half of the patients not only have papillomas in the larynx, but also have disease involving other areas of the aerodigestive tract, including the trachea or bronchi, the oropharynx, and the esophagus. In the larynx, the anterior glottis, especially the region of the anterior commissure, is a site of predilection; during the course of treatment it is the site where papillomas are most difficult to eradicate and yet avoid scarring, which can cause an anterior web. It is uncommon for the mucosa of the posterior glottis to be involved.

DIAGNOSIS

In adults and older children the diagnosis is strongly suspected clinically by indirect examination of the larynx using mirror laryngoscopy. Flexible fiberoptic laryngoscopy is used in patients if mirror laryngoscopy is inadequate after local anesthesia, if the mouth cannot be satisfactorily opened, and if cooperation can be obtained from some younger children.

Improved radiologic imaging techniques of the larynx and upper airways[1] using conventional plain radiography, high kilovoltage and beam filtration radiography, or, in selected cases, xeroradiography are available[16] and may outline the size and sites of papillomas to assist in the preoperative assessment of airway compromise.

Final histopathologic proof of diagnosis must be made from biopsy material obtained at direct laryngoscopy.

ANESTHETIC TECHNIQUES

In modern practice general anesthesia is used almost universally for laryngoscopy, microlaryngoscopy, microlaryngeal operations, and laser surgery;[16,17] the chosen anesthetic technique must ensure safety and yet allow maximum visual and surgical access. Some techniques require the use of an endotracheal tube, and some do not; others use a modified tube for high pressure jetting.

For adults a relaxant technique with controlled ventilation is preferred, and for pediatric endoscopy spontaneous respiration with inhalation anesthesia is preferred. In all patients general anesthesia is supplemented by spraying a measured amount of topical lidocaine on the larynx and upper trachea.

The choice of technique depends on the anesthetic agents available, the method of ventilation to be used, the state of the patient's general health, the procedure to be performed, and the requirements of the surgeon. Demanding problems may confront the endoscopist and the anesthesiologist, sometimes quite unexpectedly, so that understanding and teamwork are essential to safely share access to a limited airway.

The problem of laser ignition and combustion of a tube[5,7,16] during microlaryngeal laser surgery under general anesthesia in adults has not been satisfactorily solved. The anesthesia tube can be wrapped in aluminum foil or coated with a so-called laser-safe coating to provide some protection, but the cuff and the unprotected parts of the tube may be at risk if the foil does not adhere to the tube or if the coating does not give dependable protection. Most metal tubes are thick walled, are cumbersome, inflict trauma on the larynx and trachea, and do not provide optimal exposure. The Laser-Flex cuffed tracheal tube is satisfactory; it is made of spiraled stainless steel with a soft plastic distal segment and two cuffs that are inflated with isotonic saline. Indiscriminate or careless laser surgery with a metal tube or an aluminum-wrapped tube has caused overheating of the metal, with consequent thermal burn of the soft tissues. A safe method is that in which no anesthetic tube is used. This technique is readily available for infants and children, but cannot be satisfactorily applied to adults.

For adults there are many jetting techniques that depend on regular bursts of high pressure oxygen or an oxygen and nitrous oxide mixture. During jet ventilation, according to the surgeon's preference, the tip of the jetting device can be in the proximal opening of the laryngoscope, in the subglottic region, or in the midtrachea. General anesthesia with a muscle relaxant achieves nearly ideal conditions when a peroral translaryngeal endotracheal catheter of small diameter is used for gas exchange. The Benjamin jet anesthesia tube (Benjet tube) is a small (2.8 mm external diameter) jet tube for use in adults. It is easy to introduce and remove, cannot be kinked or obstructed, and is unobtrusive in the larynx. The surgeon has an excellent view of the field, as the tube usually lies inconspicuously in the posterior commissure but can be displaced by the laryngoscope to the anterior commissure for work in the posterior larynx. During laser surgery the tube is protected by a moist cottonoid pledget, and its position in the subglottic region and trachea is constantly noted so that it will not be struck by the laser beam. Although potentially flammable after laser ignition in a low flow oxygen environment, a tube of such small diameter can be easily displaced into the anterior or posterior part of the larynx so that, with vigilance by the operator, the laser beam may be used at a safe distance. This jet technique has been used for laryngoscopy, microlaryngoscopy, and microlaryngeal surgery for over 10 years without complication.[17] No tube has been ignited, and there have been no barotrauma complications. However, anesthetic techniques that use high pressure jet ventilation should be employed only by an experienced anesthesiologist and surgeon who are able to recognize the potential complications. Jet ventilation should not increase the potential risk of seeding new growth of papillomas.[4]

In infants and children a general anesthetic inhalation technique relying entirely on spontaneous respiration using oxygen, nitrous oxide, halothane, and topical anesthesia does *not* require an endotracheal tube. The gases are insufflated into the larynx through a narrow cannula in the laryngoscope. A similar method relies on insufflation into the oropharynx via a tube passed through one nasal cavity, but it may be difficult to maintain a steady level of anesthesia. This spontaneous respiration technique gives unrestricted access to all parts of the airway and has the ultimate advantage that no anesthetic tube is used and the danger of laser ignition of the tube is completely avoided.

Particular care should be taken, especially in infants and children, to maintain the airway during induction of anesthesia for the initial examination in patients who have suspected or known papillomas, even though airway obstruction may not be apparent or may appear to be minimal at preoperative assessment. Progressive obstruction may occur as the depth of anesthesia is increased. It is therefore safer to commence anesthesia in the operating room when an endotracheal tube, a laryngoscope, and a bronchoscope are readily available.

ENDOSCOPIC TECHNIQUE

The initial assessment of new patients includes examination under anesthesia of the nasal cavities, nasopharynx, oropharynx, trachea, bronchi, and esophagus to ascertain the location and spread of the tumors using the appropriate rigid instrument and telescope for each anatomic site. There are three stages in endoscopy of the upper respiratory tract:[16]

Direct Laryngoscopy. Examination with the naked eye viewing through an open tube laryngoscope is the initial diagnostic procedure for lesions of the larynx and the pharynx. The Lindholm laryngoscope is recommended for a panoramic view of the larynx and the pharynx in adults and children as young as 6 months of age. There are many different examining and operating laryngoscopes available according to the personal preference of the surgeon, each having its own advantages and disadvantages.

The adult Holinger anterior commissure laryngoscope gives access if the anatomy of the teeth, pharynx, and neck makes laryngoscopy difficult; but it is not applicable to microlaryngoscopy, as its narrow barrel allows only monocular vision.

The pharynx and larynx are systemically evaluated. External pressure on the neck and gentle repositioning of the laryngoscope allow various areas to be more prominently displayed. One or other vocal fold can be "rolled" to see its undersurface, and the false cord can be partly pushed aside to see more of the upper surface of the vocal fold.

Laryngoscopy with Telescopes. This stage requires image magnification using rigid telescopes to provide a more precise and comprehensive evaluation. All areas are evaluated using Hopkins rigid rod lens telescopes passed either through a hand-held laryngoscope or a laryngoscope suspended in position by a laryngoscope holder. The distribution of papillomas in the laryngopharynx, subglottis, and tracheobronchial tree is noted.

A 0 degree straight-ahead telescope gives a close-up, wide-angled magnified image. Using a 30 or a 50 degree angled telescope the laryngeal ventricles, the anterior and posterior commissures,

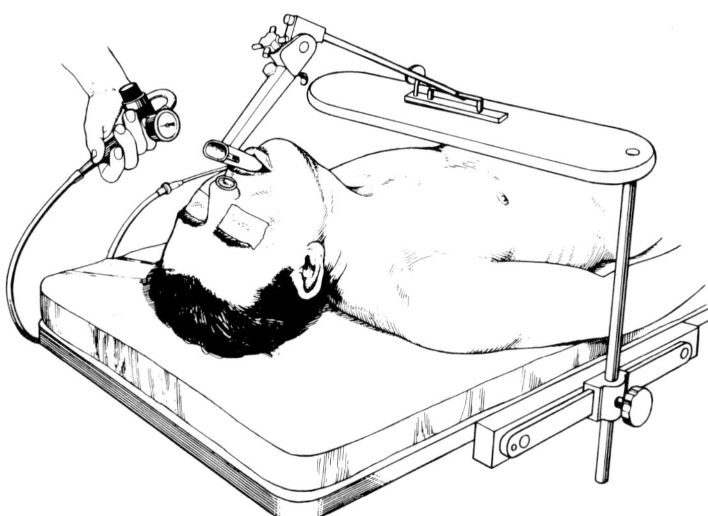

Figure 4–1. Microlaryngoscopy.

and the anterior subglottic region can be inspected in detail. Telescopes allow more extensive and complete examination of the pharynx, larynx, and trachea than is possible with microlaryngoscopy; after a microlaryngoscope is fixed in position, using the microscope only, examination of the upper airways other than the larynx is limited, and the ventricles and subglottic region cannot be fully inspected.

The most difficult areas in which to detect papillomas are the ventricles, the extreme anterior commissure, under a laryngeal web, and in a scarred and distorted larynx. This survey of the oropharynx, larynx, and subglottic region with rigid telescopes should be a routine part of diagnostic laryngoscopy in a patient being assessed for papilloma before proceeding to suspension microlaryngoscopy and laryngeal laser surgery.

Microlaryngoscopy. Microlaryngoscopy offers variable magnification, brilliant illumination, binocular vision, precise surgical manipulation, and the use of both hands. When positioned, the microlaryngoscope is supported by a self-retaining laryngoscope holder, the foot of which rests on a table above the patient's chest; the overtable is firmly attached to the operating table (Fig. 4–1).

TREATMENT

Multiple papillomas in the pharynx, larynx, and upper airways require treatment, with the exception of solitary papillomas, which are often seen on the mucosa of the soft palate, uvula, or pillars of the tonsils and which seldom require removal.

The object of treatment in obstructive cases (Fig. 4–2) is to maintain a clear airway, at least sufficient to avoid tracheotomy; in some infants and children operations may be required as often as every 1 or 2 weeks. The object of treatment in nonobstructive cases (Fig. 4–3) is repeated removal, often every 3 to 6 months, in an attempt to achieve ''control'' by eradication of all papillomas.

The rate of papilloma growth and the frequency of operations for removal are highly variable from patient to patient, and the same patient may require frequent operations at one time and removal at longer intervals at a later time. Some patients are free of disease for months or even many years and then have a recurrence. Cure can never be assumed. The best outlook is for a prolonged remission, which can occur at any time in any patient. There is no treatment that has been shown to consistently and permanently eradicate the disease. Adjunctive treatment, including administration of interferon,[13,18,19] does not appear to have a significant effect on papilloma

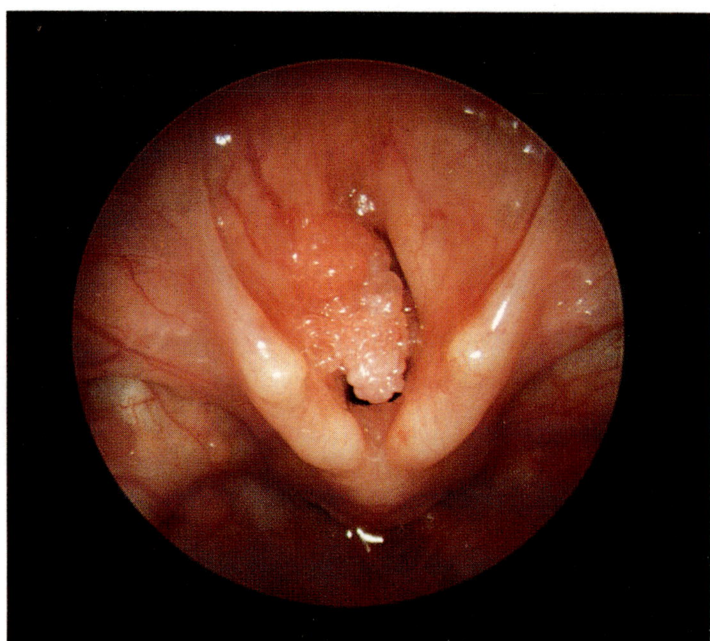

FIGURE 4–2. Obstructive papillomas in a child.

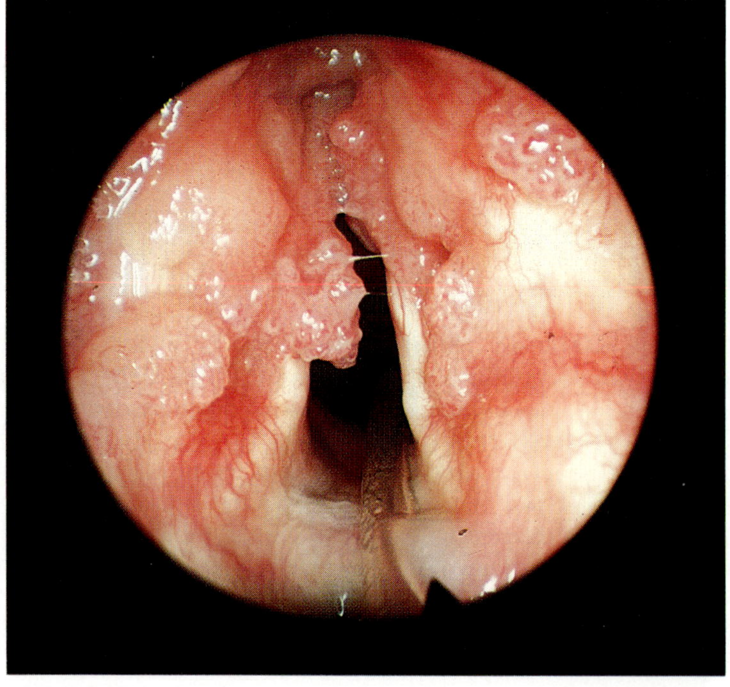

FIGURE 4–3. Widespread papillomas in an adult.

Optimal treatment depends on good exposure and good surgical equipment. The quality of the anesthetic induction and surgical technique is critical. Use of the CO_2 laser allows removal of visible disease with minimal damage to surrounding tissues. At the first examination precise and comprehensive panendoscopic assessment of the upper aerodigestive tract is necessary to ascertain the location and spread of the papillomas. In those cases in which airway obstruction is severe a substantial amount of papilloma should be removed with large cup forceps on one side only, both for diagnosis and to improve the airway.

Tracheotomy should be avoided if possible. Skilled anesthetic technique and frequent operations permit surgical maintenance of a good airway during periods of active exacerbation. Tracheotomy is necessary only if the airway cannot be safely maintained for repeated surgical removal or if there is noncompliance with the treatment regimen.

Microlaryngoscopy and Laser Surgery

The operating microscope with a 400 mm objective lens and the laser attached is positioned so that the laser beam has clear access through the mouth of the laryngoscope (Fig. 4–4). A laser with a small diameter beam is advantageous in pediatric work.

Accessory instruments for laser surgery include metal laser mirrors, anterior commissure protectors, moist cottonoids, tooth protectors, and smoke and steam evacuators.

For an anatomic site with difficult access, such as the laryngeal ventricle or the subglottic region, the laser beam can be reflected onto the lesion using a small metal mirror. Small metal commissure protector ''paddles'' are used to protect one vocal cord for work near the anterior commissure. Treatment with the CO_2 laser, although not curative itself, is particularly suitable for

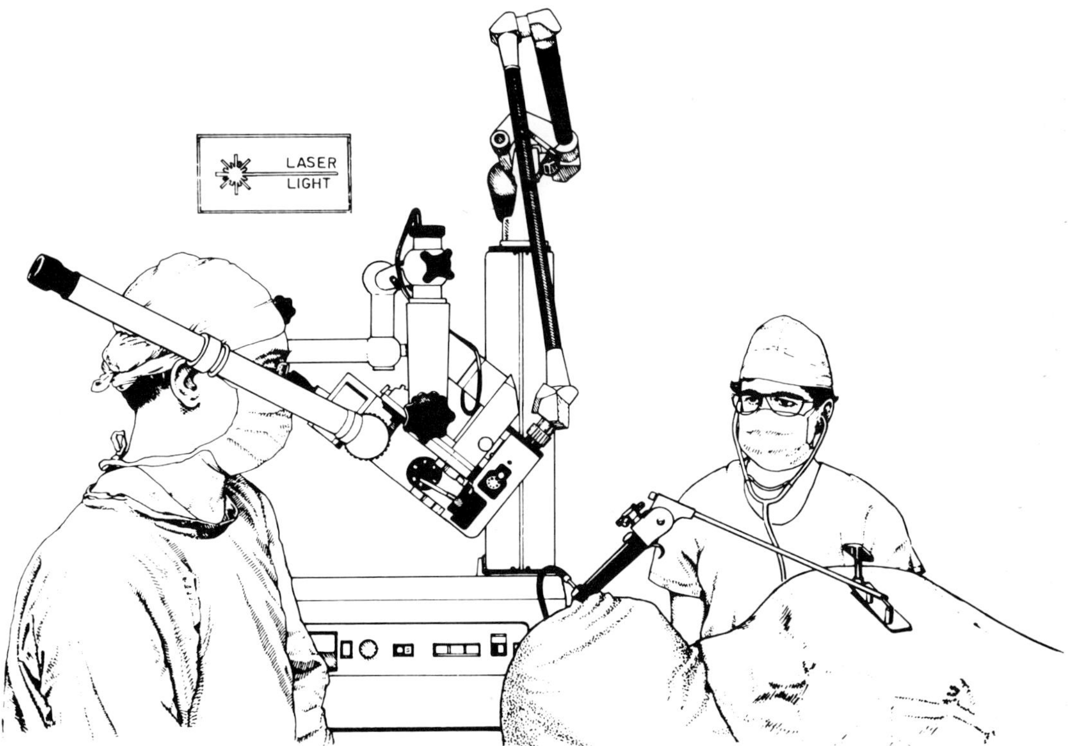

Figure 4–4. Microlaryngoscopy.

laryngeal papillomas and is used in almost every case. Multiple sites can be treated at one operation with due care to prevent scarring and web formation. Papillomas are vaporized using the micromanipulator for constant visual control of the beam. In this way there is a virtual absence of bleeding, minimal reactive edema, and little postoperative pain. Cup forceps, angled left, right, or upward, are sometimes required to remove residual papillomas from areas where visualization and access is limited after laser surgery and in conjunction with it.

The use of cup forceps alone provokes troublesome, nuisance bleeding in the operative field. The CO_2 laser with variable spot size is unquestionably advantageous in papilloma removal. Clear access for laser beam therapy can be obtained in the oral cavity, the pharynx, the nasal cavities, and the tracheobronchial tree, in addition to the larynx. The bronchoscopic coupler is essential for laser treatment of tracheal and bronchial papillomas. Subglottic or upper tracheal lesions are treated by laser directly if possible through a subglottiscope with the laser coupled to the operating microscope.

In adults the Benjamin Slimline binocular operating microlaryngoscope or in children the Healy subglottiscope is used to separate the vocal cords and expose the operative site. If the lesions are in the middle or lower trachea (Fig. 4–5), or the bronchi, the laser is coupled to a bronchoscopic adaptor for microsurgical application in the tracheobronchial tree.

Papillomas in the pharynx are seen most often on the mucosa of the soft palate, the tonsillar pillars, and the posterior nasopharyngeal wall; they are sometimes found on the upper surface of the soft palate on the floor of the nasopharynx. In the latter site they are best exposed using a Dott-Dingman cleft palate gag and best seen and assessed with a 120-degree retrograde telescope.[16] Papillomas in a tracheotomy stoma can be removed from the outside with the laser on the microscope or the regular handpiece.

During removal of papillomas the mucosa adjacent to the base of papillomas is removed to give a free margin, except near vital structures. The lesions are removed to a shallow depth only, to the level of the submucosa; sometimes the fibers of the vocalis muscle can be seen, but they should

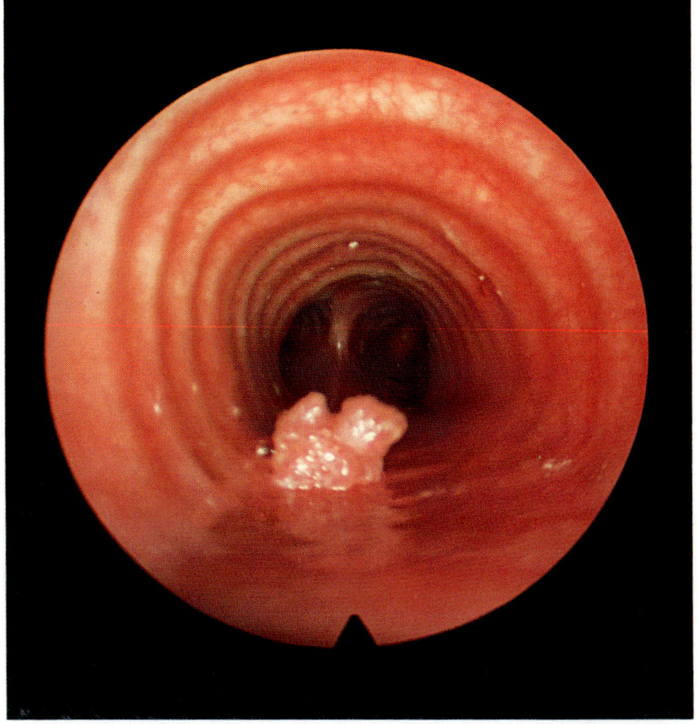

FIGURE 4–5. Papillomas in the trachea.

not be exposed. Care must be taken to avoid injury to normal laryngeal structures, as the potential for adhesions and web formation (especially at the anterior commissure) is great, and more so if the surgeon is inexperienced. The tip of a suction tube should be held close to the site of laser surgery to remove smoke or steam, so that the steam (at 100°C) will not cause a secondary burn of nearby mucosa. Laser energy is used in short rather than prolonged bursts to allow cooling and prevent unwanted heat coagulation. Small, wet neurosurgical cottonoid pledgets are used to protect adjacent tissues, the subglottic region, and the surface of the anesthetic tube. Gentle technique, avoidance of excessive endoscopic or laser trauma, and in selected cases use of a postoperative moist air atmosphere minimize postoperative stridor and respiratory distress.

COMPLICATIONS

Possible complications of treatment include the following:

- Scar formation has been noted at the anterior commissure or occasionally the posterior commissure or in the ventricle (Fig. 4–6).

- Laryngocele resulting from obstruction of the neck of the saccule by disease or by reaction to surgery has been reported.

- "Seeding" of the stoma or of the trachea at traumatized areas of mucosa after tracheotomy is a well-known complication and an obvious reason to avoid tracheotomy if at all possible.

- Pulmonary papillomatosis appears to be a complication of the disease, not of treatment. Multiple, small cystic lesions occur where papilloma masses obstruct small airways and are seen on plain chest x-ray films or computed tomography (CT) scan. There is no known reason for pulmonary seeding; it is seen only in patients whose laryngeal disease has required tracheotomy. There is no known treatment.

Anterior glottic webbing and ignition of a combustible anesthetic tube require further discussion.

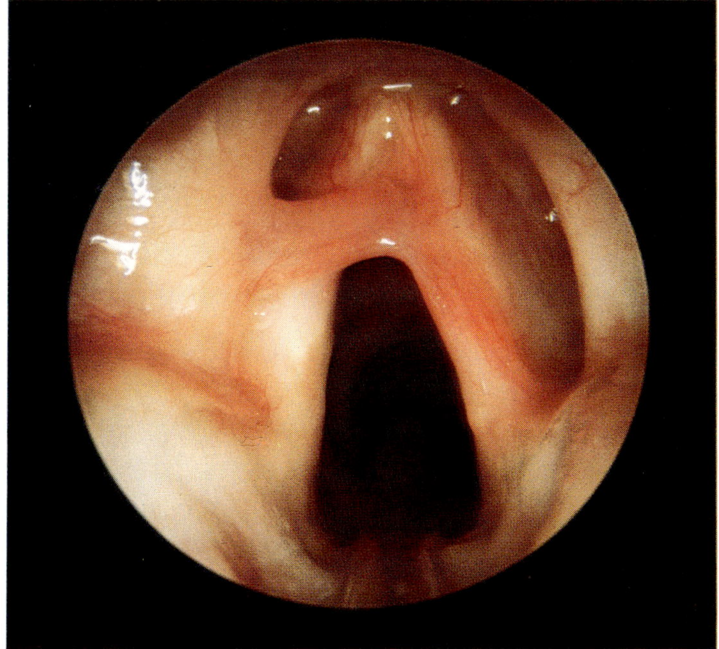

Figure 4–6. Thick scar as a result of inappropriate surgery.

Webs

With care there should be only one type of surgical complication—anterior glottic web. Some webs are unavoidable and are so small that they are visible only when viewed with a telescope under general anesthesia; these webs do not cause significant symptoms. There may be persistent papillomas on or under larger webs, a situation that makes papilloma removal difficult and provides the potential for further iatrogenic trauma. A small number of patients have webs that occupy 20 to 30 per cent of the anterior glottic opening and that produce permanent voice disability.

Techniques to minimize web formation are important:

- Strict limitation of surgery to one side, especially at the anterior commissure.

- Use of small cup forceps to allow a "feel" of the underlying tissues, which is not obtained with laser surgery.

- Use of a laryngoscope to separate the false cords and to some extent the true cords to allow more precise surgical removal.

- External finger pressure on the neck to manipulate the papillomas into a direct line for laser treatment.

- Use of a metal mirror to bounce the laser beam into otherwise inaccessible anatomic areas.

- Use of metal "paddles" to protect tissues not being treated (e.g., the anterior edge of one vocal cord when treating papillomas at the anterior commissure).

- When the tumors cannot be completely removed at one operation, acceptance by the surgeon, the patient, and the parents of the need for repeated operations.

Large postsurgical webs that produce significant dysphonia should not be considered for treatment until there has been documented control of the papillomas for at least 1 year, and treatment should be undertaken only for serious dysphonia. It is possible that treatment of the webs might stimulate proliferation of further papillomas. If surgery is performed it should be endoscopic only. Laryngofissure with incision into the tissues of the larynx and web has the potential for stimulating the growth of more papillomas.

Airway Fire

Precautions are required when laser energy is used in the operating room. Combustible anesthetic gases are avoided if possible. If a combustible anesthetic tube is used, great care must be taken not to ignite it. *The cuff of the tube should be filled with saline. If there is any possibility that the tube has been burnt or is about to ignite **all laser treatment must be stopped and the tube removed immediately.*** An attempt can be made to protect the tube with aluminum foil, and so-called laser-sealed tubes are available, but the protection is not always reliable. Metal endotracheal tubes cannot, of course, be ignited.

Laser energy is absorbed by moisture, and when an endotracheal tube has been used saline-soaked surgical cottonoids can be placed around it to lessen the chance of inadvertent laser damage to the tube or to the surrounding tissues.

The surgeon must assume ultimate responsibility for safe use of laser energy.

The laser beam should not be allowed to reflect off shiny metal surfaces. A wet towel is used to protect the face and eyes of the patient. The eyes of all personnel in the operating room are safeguarded by having each person wear protective spectacles. The power switch of the laser is turned on only immediately before use, and it is turned off when the laser is no longer required.

Surgical vaporization with the laser and/or removal with cup forceps is palliative but remains the mainstay of treatment. The control rate is about 65 per cent for pediatric onset patients and 45 per cent for adult onset patients, with the pediatric patients requiring more frequent surgical treatment. The necessity for precise and comprehensive endoscopic evaluation of the upper aerodigestive tract using general anesthetic and a range of rigid telescopes and endoscopes must be recognized.

The benefits of a specialized treatment facility with the availability of skilled and experienced anesthetic and surgical personnel has become apparent. Equipment such as the CO_2 laser, pediatric endoscopes, and telescopes need to be available. Special anesthetic techniques are used frequently and consequently are safe and have better patient acceptance. The nursing staff and recovery ward personnel become experienced and more understanding of the patient's needs so that psychologic and emotional trauma is reduced. Outpatient treatment has become well accepted and minimizes hospitalization costs. A team approach gives patients a feeling of security in their continuing management. Repeated general anesthesia apparently has no ill effects when given expertly, indicating that the operations are relatively safe in a specialized facility.

When the tumors cannot be removed completely at one operation, the surgeon, the patient, and the parents should accept the need for repeated operations. There is less hesitation to perform further surgery when surgical trauma is minimal; scarring of the tissues and webbing of the anterior commissure is avoided; and the best long-term results are obtained with minimal morbidity.

References

1. Cohn AM, Kos JT, Taber LH, Adam E: Recurring laryngeal papilloma. Am J Otolaryngol 2:129, 1981.
2. Mackenzie M: A Manual of Disease of the Throat and Nose, Vol. 1, Diseases of the Pharynx, Larynx and Trachea. New York, William Wood & Company, 1880, p 305.
3. Batsakis JG, Raymond AK, Rice DH: The pathology of head and neck tumors: Papillomas of the upper aerodigestive tracts, part 18. Head Neck Surg. 5:332, 1983.
4. Simpson GT, Strong MS: Recurrent respiratory papillomatosis: The role of the carbon dioxide laser. Otolaryngol Clin North Am 16:887, 1983.
5. Strong MS, Vaughan CW, Healy GB, et al.: Recurrent respiratory papillomatosis. Management with the CO_2 laser. Ann Otol Rhinol Laryngol 85: 508, 1976.
6. Holinger PH, Johnston KC, Anison GC: Papilloma of the larynx: A review of 109 cases with a preliminary report of Aureomycin therapy. Ann Otol Rhinol Laryngol 59:547, 1950.
7. Benjamin B, Parsons D: Recurrent respiratory papillomatosis. J Laryngol Otol 102:1022, 1988.
8. Weiss MD, Kashima HK: Tracheal involvement in laryngeal papillomatosis. Laryngoscope 93:45, 1983.
9. Mounts P, Shah KV, Kashima H: Viral etiology of juvenile and adult onset squamous papilloma of the larynx. Proc Natl Acad Sci USA 79:5425, 1982.
10. Quick CA, Watts SL, Krzyzek RA, Faras AJ: Relationship between condylomata and laryngeal papillomata. Clinical and molecular virological evidence. Ann Otol Rhinol Laryngol 89:467, 1980.
11. Batsakis JG: Tumors of the head and neck. Baltimore, Williams & Wilkins Co, 1979, p 137.
12. Zehnder PR, Lyons GD: Carcinoma and juvenile papillomatosis. Ann Otol Rhinol Laryngol 84:614, 1975.
13. Cohen SR, Geller KA, Seltzer S, Thompson JW: Papilloma of the larynx and tracheobronchial tree in children. A retrospective study. Ann Otol Rhinol Laryngol 89:497, 1980.
14. Mehta P, Herold N: Regression of juvenile laryngobronchial papillomatosis with systemic bleomycin therapy. J Pediatr 97:479, 1980.
15. Abramson AL, Waner M, Brandsma J: The clinical treatment of laryngeal papillomas with hematoporphyrin therapy. Arch Otolaryngol Head Neck Surg 114:795, 1988.
16. Benjamin B: Techniques of endoscopy. *In* Benjamin B: Diagnostic Laryngology: Adults and Children. Philadelphia, WB Saunders, 1989.
17. Benjamin B: Anesthesia for laryngoscopy. Ann Otol Rhinol Laryngol 93:338, 1984.
18. McCabe BF, Clark KF: Interferon and laryngeal papillomatosis. The Iowa experience. Ann Otol Rhinol Laryngol 92:2, 1983.
19. Benjamin B, Gatenby P, Kitchen R, et al.: Alpha-interferon (Wellferon) as an adjunct to standard surgical therapy in recurrent respiratory papillomatosis. Ann Otol Rhinol Laryngol 97:376, 1988.

CHAPTER 5

ENDOSCOPIC LASER ARYTENOIDECTOMY

Robert H. Ossoff

James A. Duncavage

Glenn W. Knox

Most patients with bilateral vocal cord paralysis have good vocal quality, but their airways are usually unsatisfactory. The management of such patients presents a challenge to the otolaryngologist–head and neck surgeon. Numerous surgical procedures have been promoted in an attempt to improve the patient's airway insufficiency without leaving a breathy, weak voice or an incompetent larynx.[1,17]

HISTORICAL PERSPECTIVE

Tracheotomy was the only procedure available to the patient with bilateral vocal cord paralysis until 1922, when Jackson reported a surgical procedure that removed the entire vocal cord and ventricle.[5] This produced an excellent airway but also resulted in an extremely breathy voice.

Ten years later, Hoover introduced the concept of submucous resection of the vocal cord for the treatment of patients with bilateral vocal cord paralysis.[4] This procedure failed, however, because it produced severe dyspnea as a result of scar tissue formation that narrowed the glottis.

In 1939, King introduced a procedure that mobilized the arytenoid cartilage through a lateral, extralaryngeal approach.[7] He sutured the arytenoid to the cut end of the anterior belly of the omohyoid muscle. Initially, the success of this procedure was thought to be attributable to the restoration of vocal cord function by the muscle transfer. However, it was determined later that the mobilized arytenoid cartilage became fixed in the abducted position by fibrosis and the omohyoid muscle transfer was subsequently eliminated from the operation.

Kelly modified the King procedure in 1941 by dissecting and removing the arytenoid through a small window in the thyroid cartilage; the vocal cord became abducted as a result of the formation of scar tissue.[6] Because the placement of the vocal cord was not satisfactory in all cases, Kelly modified his own technique by fixing the vocal cord in the abducted position with a lateralizing suture. Orton, in 1944, introduced further minor modifications in the suture placement.[9]

In 1946, Woodman[19] introduced a technique that is still popular today. Through a posterolateral extralaryngeal approach, he exposed the arytenoid cartilage by separating the joint between the cricoid cartilage and the inferior cornu. After this exposure was accomplished, he removed the arytenoid but preserved the vocal process, which he lateralized. This was performed by placing a

44

submucosal suture around the vocal process and anchoring the suture to the inferior cornu of the thyroid cartilage.

Thornell, in 1948, reported on the first arytenoidectomy performed by an intralaryngeal approach.[14] This technique represented a significant advance in the treatment of bilateral vocal cord paralysis. After first performing a tracheotomy, Thornell removed the arytenoid cartilage using the Lynch suspension laryngoscope. Following removal of the arytenoid, he electrocoagulated the surgical bed to stimulate scar tissue formation, which, in turn, facilitated further vocal cord lateralization. Whicker and Devine presented their large series of patients treated by the Thornell technique in 1972.[18] These authors reported relief of airway obstruction in 82 per cent of 147 patients.

In 1972, Helmus introduced a microsurgical thyrotomy approach for the surgical correction of bilateral vocal cord paralysis.[3] This technique affords the surgeon direct visualization for the exact placement of the vocal cord.

The nerve-muscle transposition operation was introduced by Tucker in 1976.[15] He transposed a nerve-muscle pedicle composed of the branch of the ansa hypoglossi, which innervated the anterior belly of the omohyoid muscle, to the posterior cricoarytenoid via an approach similar to that used for the Woodman operation.[16]

ARYTENOIDECTOMY TECHNIQUES

At present, arytenoidectomy is the most reliable method of treatment of patients with bilateral vocal cord paralysis. Both endoscopic and external approaches have been described in the literature for performing an arytenoidectomy; however, the endoscopic technique is more desirable because it requires no external incision and theoretically allows for the immediate assessment of airway size.[2,12] Bleeding and edema associated with the intraoperative manipulation of microsurgical instruments through the operating microlaryngoscope make this technique difficult for many surgeons to master.

The addition of the carbon dioxide (CO_2) laser to the surgical armamentarium offers certain refinements to the technique of endoscopic arytenoidectomy. Use of the CO_2 laser allows the otolaryngologist–head and neck surgeon to perform a precise operation through the relatively narrow field of the microlaryngoscope without the need for tissue manipulation.[13] Additional advantages associated with the use of the laser include increased hemostasis and decreased intra- and postoperative edema.

The surgical procedure used is a major modification of the Thornell endoscopic arytenoidectomy. The larynx is exposed using the modified Dedo microlaryngoscope or the posterior commissure microlaryngoscope with bifurcated suction channels. The tip of the laryngoscope is positioned to engage the posterior aspect of the arytenoid, which facilitates exposure of the posterior commissure and interarytenoid cleft.

Procedures are performed using a fundamental mode CO_2 surgical laser coupled to a Zeiss operating microscope with a 400 mm objective lens.[10] After exposure of the posterior commissure, the mucoperichondrium overlying the corniculate cartilage is vaporized, exposing the underlying corniculate, using the laser in the repeat mode (0.1 second pulses) at 1990 watts/cm^2. The corniculate cartilage is ablated, exposing the apex of the arytenoid. Next, the mucoperiosteum overlying the apex and upper body of the arytenoid is vaporized (Fig. 5–1). Using the laser in the continuous mode at 3185 watts/cm^2, the upper body of the arytenoid is ablated. At this time, the laser is switched back to the repeat mode at 1990 watts/cm^2, and the mucoperichondrium overlying the lower body of the arytenoid is vaporized, exposing the underlying cartilage. Working still in the repeat mode at 1990 watts/cm^2, the body of the arytenoid is further ablated working in a lateral to medial direction. During this step of the operation, the lateral ligament is encountered and transected. Laterally, the arytenoid is vaporized down to the underlying cricoid cartilage; medially, the vocal and muscular processes remain. At this time, the mucoperichondrium overlying the vocal

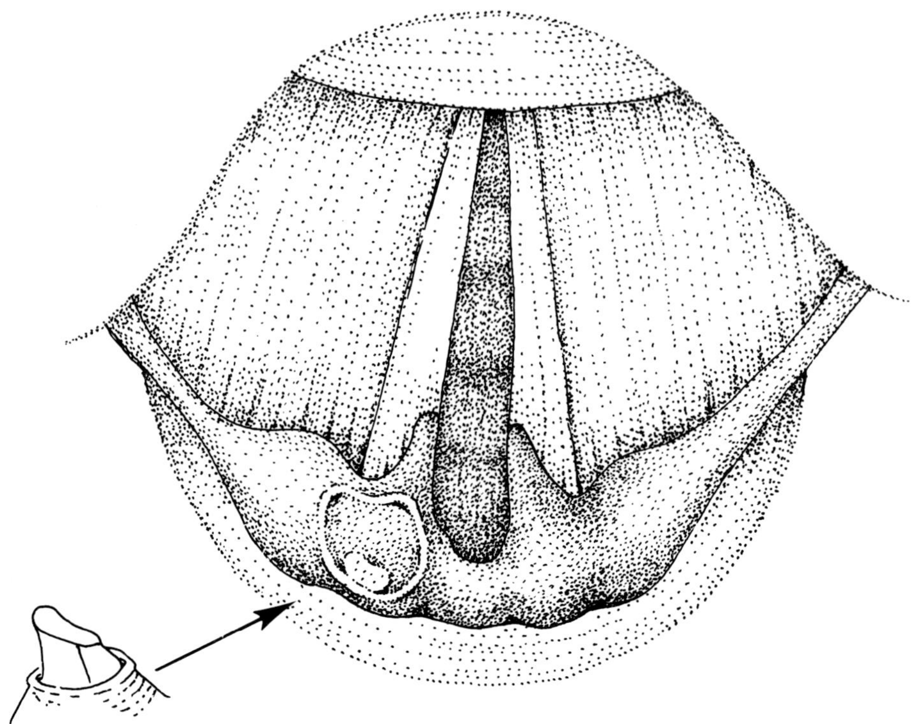

FIGURE 5–1. The mucoperichondrium overlying the upper body of the arytenoid cartilage has been vaporized.

process and most of the muscular process is ablated (Fig. 5–2). Next, the vocal process with an adjacent portion of vocalis muscle and the muscular process, up to but not including the attachment of the arytenoideus muscle, is vaporized. During this step, great care is exercised not to encroach on or vaporize the mucosa of the interarytenoid cleft. Following this step, a small area lateral to the vocalis muscle is vaporized to facilitate lateralization of the vocal cord during healing (Fig. 5–3). A remnant of the muscular process with the attached arytenoideus muscle remains. Further lateralization of the vocal cord occurs during healing; the wound is covered by a white coagulum from the second postoperative day through the second postoperative week. By the end of the third postoperative week, the wound is covered with healthy-appearing mucosa.

All of the patients are given a broad spectrum antibiotic (cefazolin sodium) for 5 postoperative days. Additionally, an intraoperative dose of corticosteroids (dexamethasone sodium phosphate) is given.

ADVANTAGES AND COMPLICATIONS

The utilization of the CO_2 laser for the treatment of bilateral vocal cord paralysis via the endoscopic route is a logical extension of the clinical application of this instrument. Use of the CO_2 laser attached to the operating microscope allows the otolaryngologist–head and neck surgeon to perform hands off endoscopic surgery in a relatively narrow operative field. Ablation rather than excision and delivery of the arytenoid cartilage represents the major difference between this operation and the Thornell endoscopic arytenoidectomy. The advantages of precision, hemostasis, decreased postoperative edema, and decreased scarring facilitate visualization and control over the final result of the operation. The minimal voice loss associated with this operation is an additional advantage.

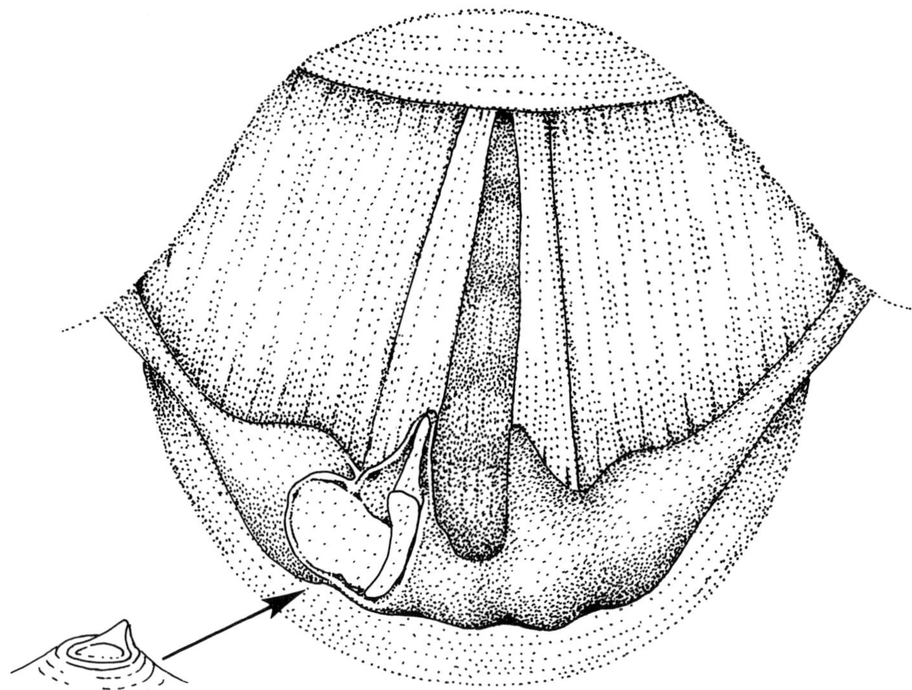

FIGURE 5–2. The mucoperichondrium overlying the vocal process has been vaporized, exposing the vocal process and vocalis muscle.

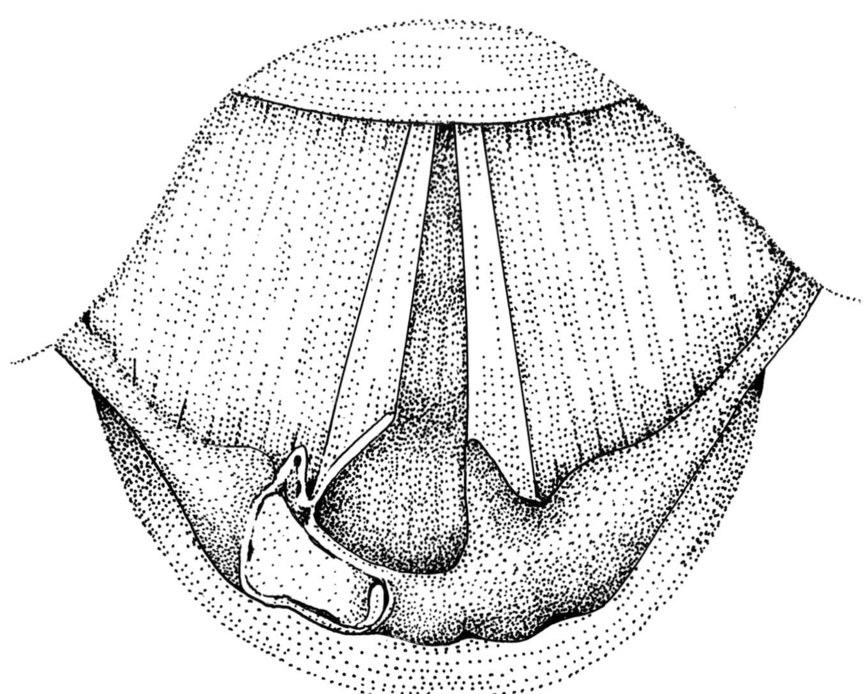

FIGURE 5–3. The completed operation. Note the remnant of muscular process with the attached arytenoideus muscle. The area of ablation lateral to the vocalis muscle (*arrow* in Figs. 5–1 and 5–2) facilitates lateralization of the vocal cord.

Prior to the use of the CO_2 laser for this surgical procedure, troublesome bleeding and poor visualization added to the technical difficulty of performing an endoscopic arytenoidectomy. Less control in the placement of the vocal cord than that obtained with external operations, the necessity for learning to use a relatively new surgical delivery system, and the risk of an explosion burn represent the major disadvantages associated with this operation. Potential complications include the formation of a granuloma, probably from retained carbonaceous debris caused by laser surgery, loss of adequate voice production, arytenoid perichondritis, aspiration, and endotracheal or tracheotomy tube ignition.[11] The postoperative complication of posterior laryngeal web associated with failure to gain an adequate airway experienced by one of the authors' patients most likely resulted from a submucosal thermal injury to the tissues of the interarytenoid cleft. This anatomic area of the larynx is vulnerable during laser arytenoidectomy and must be protected from any direct or submucosal laser irradiation to prevent the formation of posterior commissure webs or fibrosis, both of which can lead to further compromise of the airway.

Endotracheal or tracheotomy tube ignition is a potential catastrophic complication of laser surgery in the upper aerodigestive tract; it can be readily avoided with the appropriate precautions. Red rubber or silicone endotracheal tubes should be wrapped with reflective tape, and metal tracheotomy tubes should be used in place of plastic ones. Inflation of the cuff with methylene blue–colored saline further reduces this risk. The placement of saline-saturated neurosurgical cottonoids below the vocal cords to protect the cuff of the endotracheal tube and the use of the operating platform in the subglottic larynx can minimize the possibility of an airway fire even further.

During performance of an endoscopic laser arytenoidectomy, the surgeon must work slowly and deliberately at some stages of the procedure. Here, judicious use of the single or repeat pulse mode allows the otolaryngologist–head and neck surgeon to proceed with the great care that is necessary to avoid injuring adjacent tissues.

References

1. Applebaum EL, Allen GW, Sisson GA: Human laryngeal reinnervation: The Northwestern experience. Laryngoscope 89:1784, 1979.
2. Eskew JR, Bailey BJ: Laser arytenoidectomy for bilateral vocal cord paralysis. Otolaryngol Head Neck Surg 91:294, 1983.
3. Helmus C: Microsurgical thyrotomy and arytenoidectomy for bilateral recurrent laryngeal nerve paralysis. Laryngoscope 82:491, 1972.
4. Hoover WB: Bilateral abductor paralysis, operative treatment of submucous resection of the vocal cord. Arch Otolaryngol 15:337, 1932.
5. Jackson C: Ventriculocordectomy. A new operation for the cure of goitrous glottic stenosis. Arch Surg 4:257, 1922.
6. Kelly JD: Surgical treatment of bilateral paralysis of the abductor muscles. Arch Otolaryngol 33:293, 1941.
7. King BT: A new and function restoring operation for bilateral abductor cord paralysis. JAMA 112:814, 1939.
8. May M, Lavorato AS, Bleyaert AL: Rehabilitation of the crippled larynx: Application of the Tucker technique for muscle-nerve reinnervation. Laryngoscope 90:1, 1980.
9. Orton HB: Extralaryngeal surgical approach for arytenoidectomy: Bilateral abductor paralysis of the larynx. Ann Otol Rhinol Laryngol 53:303, 1944.
10. Ossoff RH, Duncavage JA, Gluckman JL, et al.: Universal endoscopic coupler for bronchoscopic CO_2 laser surgery: A multi-institutional clinical trial. Otolaryngol Head Neck Surg 93:824, 1985.
11. Ossoff RH, Hotaling AJ, Karlan MS, et al.: The carbon dioxide laser in otolaryngology–head and neck surgery: A retrospective analysis of complications. Laryngoscope 93:1287, 1983.
12. Ossoff RH, Karlan MS, Sisson GA: Endoscopic laser arytenoidectomy. Lasers Surg Med 2:293, 1983.
13. Strong MS, Jako GJ, Vaughan CW, et al.: The use of the CO_2 laser in otolaryngology: A progress report. Trans Am Acad Ophthalmol Otolaryngol 82:595, 1976.
14. Thornell WC: Intralaryngeal approach for arytenoidectomy in bilateral abductor vocal cord paralysis. Arch Otolaryngol 47:505, 1948.
15. Tucker HM: Human laryngeal reinnervation. Laryngoscope 86:769, 1976.
16. Tucker HM: Human laryngeal reinnervation. Long-term experience with the nerve-muscle pedicle technique. Laryngoscope 88:598, 1978.
17. Tucker HM: Vocal cord paralysis—1979: Etiology and management. Laryngoscope 90:585, 1980.
18. Whicker JH, Devine KD: Long-term results of Thornell arytenoidectomy in the surgical treatment of bilateral vocal cord paralysis. Laryngoscope 82:1331, 1972.
19. Woodman D: A modification of the extralaryngeal approach to arytenoidectomy for bilateral abductor paralysis. Arch Otolaryngol 43:63, 1946.

CHAPTER 6

Laryngeal Cancer: The Role of Laser Surgery

R. Kim Davis

Use of the carbon dioxide (CO_2) laser in the treatment of early laryngeal cancer has a fascinating history. When it first became apparent that the CO_2 laser could be used to incise tissue, and that such incisional surgery was possible with minimal postoperative edema or intraoperative bleeding, attention was quickly focused on the larynx. Techniques of surgery available at that time typically involved microsurgery with small knives or cup forceps. This technique was effective, but entailed moderately reduced visibility due to hemorrhage. If electrocautery was used to control this bleeding, the possibility of significant edema was present. If edema developed, airway obstruction was a postoperative threat, and the need to place an intraoperative tracheotomy had to be considered. Typically, such surgery could be done without tracheotomy, but the poor visualization caused by bleeding truly decreased the precision of the surgery. Thus, in general, only benign lesions were approached with microsurgery of the larynx. These lesions included vocal granulomas, vocal cord polyps, vocal cord nodules, and hypertrophic laryngitis. Carcinoma in situ was occasionally treated by vocal cord (stripping) techniques, but most frequently patients with these lesions were referred for irradiation therapy. As the CO_2 laser was quickly absorbed by tissue, resulting in little adjacent thermal effect, postoperative edema with this instrument was minimal. Moreover, as the laser was known to be able to control blood vessels less than 0.1 mm in diameter, it became clear in animal experiments that microsurgery of the benign lesions mentioned could be accomplished in the larynx with minimal bleeding.

Jako and Strong were pioneers in the introduction of the CO_2 laser into the armamentarium of otolaryngologists.[1,2] They initially treated benign lesions as mentioned above with excellent results. As their success in treating benign lesions increased, these researchers applied the same techniques to carcinoma in situ of the true vocal cord, as well as early malignant laryngeal lesions. This ultimately lead to surgical techniques of limited cordectomy and extended cordectomy, as well as anterior commissure excision with the CO_2 laser.[3] It is important to note that the work of these early pioneers was always done in highly selected circumstances, with great care taken to avoid extension of laser use beyond what truly was safe. This attention to detail and to safety has highlighted all of their work and indeed was the most important principle applied as their initial work was extended to more elaborate laser procedures in the larynx.

As new technologies are developed, it is always important to ask whether such technology truly confers an advantage over the currently accepted methods of treatment. When CO_2 laser excision of early vocal cord cancer was introduced, the most generally accepted method of treatment of this cancer was radiation therapy. Surgical techniques employed at that time usually involved open partial laryngectomy.[4] Endoscopic surgical techniques available at that time involved surgical (cold knife) techniques, using microcups, forceps, electrocautery, and cryosurgery. To best understand the cases in which these techniques were used, it is important to refer to a uniform system of cancer staging (Table 6–1). Radiation therapy was applied to all stages of laryngeal cancer, but was uniformly accepted as a preferred method of treatment for most patients with stage I cancer. Stage II cancer was also generally treated by radiation therapy alone, although open partial laryngectomy techniques were also employed with selected stage I and stage II glottic cancers.

The techniques of microendoscopic surgery were first applied to superficial stage I cancers. The difficulties with microsurgery, using instruments such as cup forceps and microscissors, were alluded to above. The main problem was poor visibility attributable to bleeding at the time of tumor excision. This caused potential uncertainty about tumor margins and, in general, led to the treatment of most patients by the nonsurgical option of radiation therapy. The techniques of microsurgery were used only to establish a diagnosis of cancer, and then the patient was referred for other treatment.

Endoscopic laryngeal surgery using electrocautery gained some acceptance. In this technique, the problems of poor hemostasis were circumvented by using instruments to deliver carefully applied electrical current as a cutting device. The problem with acceptance of this technique generally involved the threat of postoperative swelling or subsequent scar tissue formation because of the wide field effect of the electrical current. Although cutting was effective, damage to residual tissue was significant. Thus this technique also was never widely used.

The technique of cryosurgery was successfully applied to stage I laryngeal cancer by Miller[5] and others. In this technique, biopsy of the cancer was obtained initially to prove its histologic type, and the specimen then was selectively frozen. This was successfully used by Miller, but was not widely adopted for two reasons. One of the potential side effects of cryosurgery is postoperative edema, which can lead to airway compromise. Second, when a lesion is destroyed by freezing, it is not possible to know the true original extent of the lesion. Although recurrence rates were not unduly high with this technique, the potential for deeply invasive cancer not to be fully controlled by cryotherapy and the possibility for cartilage invasion to be unknown and not assessed at surgery existed.

Table 6–1. TUMOR CLASSIFICATION FOR CANCER STAGING

Supraglottis

T1S	Carcinoma in situ
T1	Tumor confined to site of origin with normal mobility
T2	Tumor involves adjacent supraglottic site(s) or glottis without fixation
T3	Tumor limited to larynx with fixation and/or extension to involve postcricoid area, medial wall of piriform sinus, or preepiglottic space
T4	Massive tumor extending beyond the larynx to involve oropharynx, soft tissues of neck, or destruction of thyroid cartilage

Glottis

T1S	Carcinoma in situ
T1	Tumor confined to vocal cord(s) with normal mobility (includes involvement of anterior or posterior commissures)
T2	Supraglottic and/or subglottic extension of tumor with normal or impaired cord mobility
T3	Tumor confined to larynx with cord fixation
T4	Massive tumor with thyroid cartilage destruction and/or extension beyond confines of larynx

Open partial laryngectomy was successfully accomplished by a number of investigators. This technique remains highly effective and leads to cure rates at least equal to if not greater than those with any other technique involving stage I laryngeal cancer.[6] This technique, however, does result in significant morbidity. It requires tracheotomy at the time of definitive tumor resection, as well as an external approach that involves thyrotomy and reconstruction of the removed hemilarynx. Almost all patients are hospitalized for at least 1 week, and most usually for at least 10 to 14 days. Almost all patients experience some postoperative aspiration, and all patients have significant change in vocal function. Although many people can speak somewhat normally in a relaxed, quiet voice, all patients have decreased vocal volume and elements of hoarseness and breathiness. In addition, many patients must tolerate mild degrees of aspiration indefinitely after this procedure. These problems are generally tolerated by patients, and indeed seem more acceptable in cases of stage II cancer in which surgery may have a greater curative effect than irradiation. In stage I cancer, on the other hand, for which cure rates are similar, patients, when given the choice, usually elect to undergo irradiation instead of surgery. Irradiation usually causes less morbidity, as these patients rarely face problems of aspiration unless severe postirradiation changes lead to vocal cord immobility. Voice is clearly better after irradiation than after vertical partial laryngectomy.

Thus, a reasonable question to be asked is whether all patients with stage I cancer should not simply have irradiation therapy. Although there are several good answers to this question, one of the most compelling arguments against irradiating all patients came from a study by Lillie and Desanto.[7] In this study, more than 100 patients underwent cordectomy for stage I cancer. Most of these patients had undergone staging endoscopy and biopsy prior to the definitive cordectomy. Interestingly, approximately 22 per cent of these patients were found to have no residual cancer in the cordectomy specimen; these patients had been cured by the biopsy procedure itself. This observation occasioned a study by the author to verify these results. In this more limited study, nearly 30 per cent of patients had no residual cancer after cordectomy in which earlier biopsy established the diagnosis of cancer. It became apparent that a certain number of patients (approximately 20 to 30 per cent), who are referred for definitive treatment of early laryngeal cancer, may have been cured by the biopsy procedure alone. If this group of patients goes on to definitive radiotherapy, they are being overtreated. These patients need careful observation only. The problem in this regard is to determine which patients truly have been treated by biopsy alone and which patients need further therapy. Additional therapy would need to be less morbid than irradiation if the small number of patients who require no further treatment were not to be unduly treated. This subset of patients became one of the first groups best treated by laser therapy.

To appreciate which patients are best treated by laser surgery, attention must be directed to the classification of glottic cancer in Table 6–1. When open partial laryngectomy was first described by Ogura, careful attention was applied to defining which patients could be treated by this technique versus patients who needed total larynectomy. These limitations of open partial laryngectomy are referred to in Table 6–2. The statements concerning inferior extent of tumor need particular comment. The criterion of anteroinferior tumor extension of less than 10 mm was established because tumors that extend beyond 10 mm can escape the confines of the larynx through the cricothyroid membrane. Such tumor extension is not encompassed with open vertical partial laryngectomy. Posteriorly, tumor that extended more than 7 mm inferiorly had the potential to invade

Table 6–2. CLASSIC LIMITATIONS OF OPEN PARTIAL LARYNGECTOMY IN GLOTTIC CANCER

1. Cancer must be stage T1 or T2 (or highly selected stage T3 lesions)
2. Cancer can extend to the anterior commissure soft tissues (with no cartilage involvement)
3. Subglottic extension must be less than 10 mm anteriorly, 7 mm posteriorly
4. Contralateral true vocal cord involvement must not extend beyond the anterior third

the cricoid cartilage, again escaping the bounds of open partial laryngectomy. Tumors that extended beyond the midline for more than one third of the anterior aspect of the opposite true vocal cord mandated tumor excisions that left almost no functioning opposite true vocal cord. Clearly these limitations of open partial laryngectomy were critical, and remain so. Although some procedures extending open partial laryngectomy to include cricoid resection have been successful, this remains a difficult procedure for most surgeons.[8] Second, the test of time will need to be applied to determine if recurrence rates are acceptable if more extensive lesions are treated by open partial procedures beyond what Ogura described.

With the open partial laryngectomy techniques, the risk of postoperative aspiration is greatly decreased by the ability to reconstruct intraoperatively the portion of the larynx removed. Such reconstruction places muscle, fat, or mucosa near the midline where the removed vocal cord would have moved for vocal cord approximation. This allows the remaining vocal cord to approximate against a buttress for voice and airway protection.

When any endoscopic procedure is contemplated, it is possible to remove the full true vocal cord and the associated arytenoid cartilage, as is accomplished in open partial procedures. The problem with doing this endoscopically is that it is not possible to adequately reconstruct this area and prevent aspiration. Early experiments by Vaughan and others in using the CO_2 laser showed that, whereas arytenoidectomy was easily technically possible coupled with cordectomy, the resultant laryngeal dysfunction led to intolerable aspiration.[9] In this regard, the limitation to all endoscopic techniques clearly involved leaving the arytenoid cartilage present when the true vocal cord was removed. In other words, all limitations of endoscopic laryngeal surgery for cancer clearly fall well within the limitations of open partial laryngectomy originally described by Ogura. In none of the endoscopic techniques can the arytenoid cartilage be removed without resulting in intolerable aspiration, pulmonary morbidity, and possible mortality.

ANATOMIC LIMITATIONS

Early work with the CO_2 laser clearly showed that superficial limited stage I laryngeal cancer could be treated effectively with the laser.[9] The operative approach advocated by these surgeons involved excision of the lesion with frozen section analysis of margins. Additionally, biopsies taken with standard microinstrument technique in the residual vocal cord after excisional biopsy were also undertaken. If the lateral and deep margins of biopsy specimens were clear, endoscopic surgery was believed to be adequate. In an attempt to determine how far this type of approach could be carried, a cadaver study was undertaken to establish the true anatomic limits of laser cordectomy.[10] In this study cadaver larynges were suspended in a special holder developed by the Rontals. A large bore laryngoscope was then positioned and laser surgery undertaken in this idealized situation. As it was well established that the arytenoid cartilage could not be removed without intolerable aspiration, this study involved transection of the vocal process of the arytenoid posteriorly, with resection then carried into the paraglottic deep tissues as far as possible. This approach is shown in Figures 6–1 through 6–3.

Figure 6–1 shows a whole mount sagittal section of a paraffin embedded laryngeal specimen. This section represents the normal true vocal cord before surgery and defines the vocal process of the arytenoid cartilage, as well as the soft tissues of the true cord, and the outer lying thyroid cartilage.

Figure 6–2 shows a similar section after a limited cordectomy has been accomplished. Attention should be directed to the posterior line of excision, which crosses the vocal process of the arytenoid tissue and extends partially into paraglottic musculature. Anteriorly, this excision has removed much of the vocalis muscle, but leaves intact the anterior commissure tendon.

Figure 6–3 shows the full extent of cordectomy possible in this model. The vocal process of the arytenoid cartilage is transsected, and a surgical angle at approximately 90 degrees to this

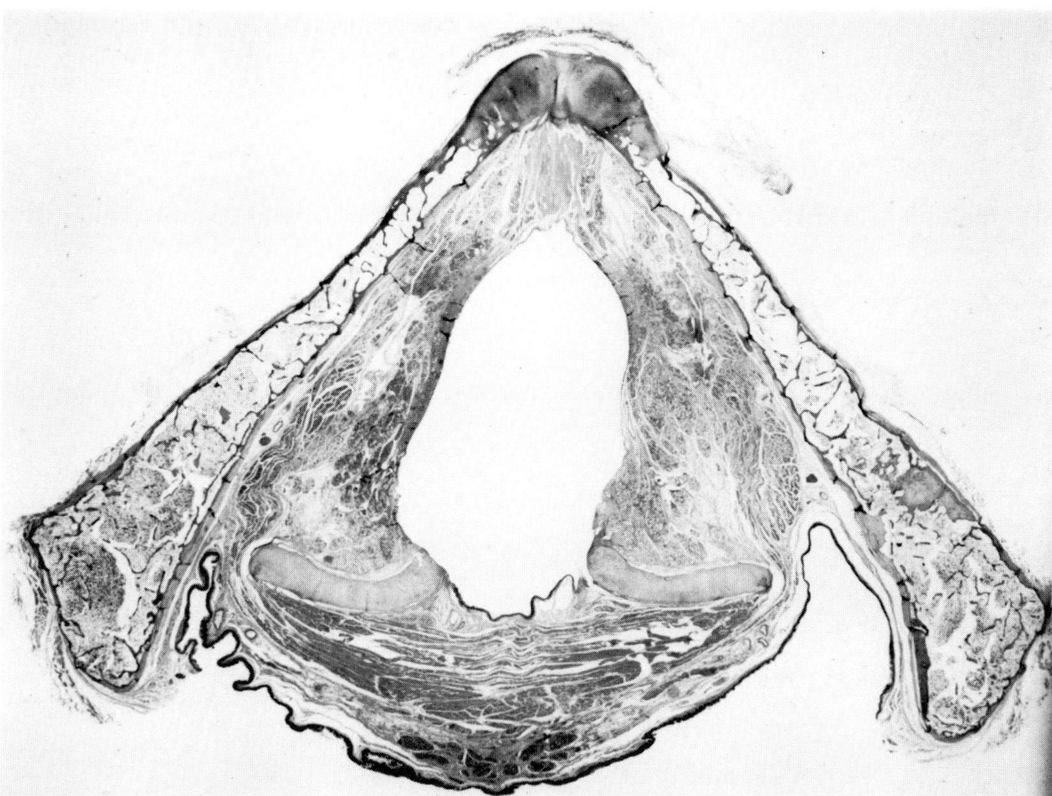

FIGURE 6–1. A whole mount serial section of the larynx. Notice the width of the posterior aspect of the true vocal cord compared with the width at the anterior commissure.

process is extended all the way to the thyroid cartilage. Anteriorly the excision is carried to the vocal tendon.

Anatomic limitations were also established for excision of the anterior commissure and the anterior aspect of both true vocal cords (Figs. 6–4 and 6–5). In Figure 6–4, the laser excision has been carried across both true vocal cords and directed toward the anterior commissure; the anterior commissure tendon is still present. In Figure 6–5, the excision has been carried all the way to the thyroid cartilage, which is readily accomplished.

The ability to perform any surgical technique satisfactorily from safety and oncologic perspectives depends on adequate visualization. The study of the anatomic limitations of CO_2 laser cordectomy shows that surgery can be performed across the vocal process of the arytenoid cartilage at a right angle out into the paraglottic space. The ability to do this, however, depends on having a patient who will accept a large bore laryngoscope to allow visualization of this area. As excision is carried out into the paraglottic space, the degree of carbonization of the remaining tissue increases as the excision approaches the thyroid cartilage. This increase in carbonization in essence absorbs light and makes visibility progressively worse as tumor excision is carried to this deep level. Because of this, it clearly is not advisable to attempt to proceed more posteriorly in the paraglottic space.

Two further reasons make such extended posterior dissection unwise. The first consideration is that tumor that gets into the deep paraglottic space is well beyond the confines of stage I or potentially even stage II cancer. Kirchner has elegantly shown that this deep paraglottic space is the avenue of transglottic cancer spread.[11] Tumor in this location is clearly beyond the confines of endoscopic laser surgery and probably beyond the confines of open partial laryngectomy. Second,

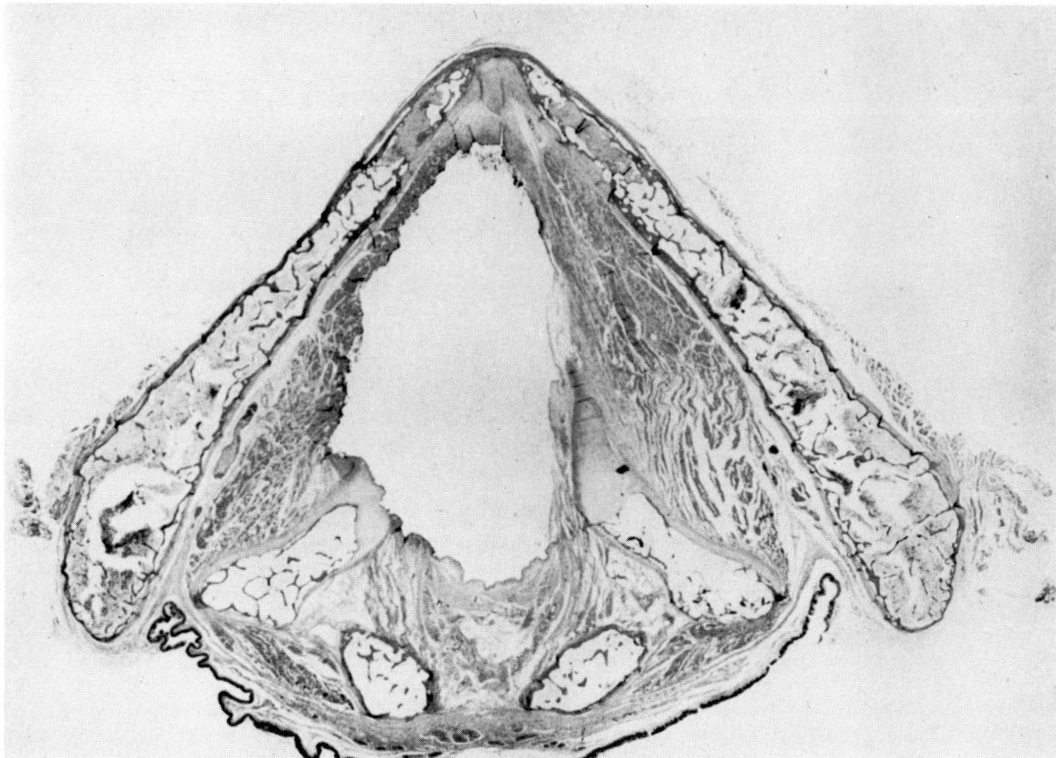

FIGURE 6–2. The first step of laser cordectomy. Notice that the vocal process of the arytenoid cartilage *(posterior left)* has been transected, and much of the vocalis muscle has been removed.

blood vessels larger than 0.1 mm in diameter exist in the deep paraglottic space and are larger than those readily controlled with the CO_2 laser. Bleeding in this area, therefore, becomes difficult to control, owing to the size of the vessels and the poor visualization at this deep level.

When CO_2 laser excision extends to the thyroid cartilage, this cartilage almost always can be easily identified. The cartilage itself is white and reflects a greater degree of carbonization and burn as the laser has impact on it. Second, as laser energy has impact on cartilage, it produces a fluorescence that is easily seen. The problem in approaching cartilage with laser excision is that, although the cartilage may be readily seen, cartilage destroyed by tumor will not be readily appreciated. If tumor extends deeply into the vocalis, it has escaped the confines of laser surgery and should not be pursued.

Excision in the anterior commissure area can be readily done. This again depends on adequate visualization of the anterior aspect of the larynx. This is sometimes not possible with the large bore laryngoscopes, such as the Jako laryngoscope. Large bore laryngoscopes with an anterior commissure bend allow work to be done here safely. Again, visualization must be excellent. When this area can be visualized it is easy to proceed to the thyroid cartilage. Cartilage is identified as described above. If tumor extends all the way to the cartilage, such tumor has truly escaped the reach of laser surgery. As tumors extend for a greater distance inferiorly in the anterior commissure, they approach the cricothyroid membrane. Obviously tumor that extends through the cartilage or extends through the cricothyroid membrane has become stage IV cancer and is well beyond the confines of laser surgery. If tumor extends more than 5 mm anteroinferiorly, the possibility of extension through the crythyroid membrane becomes significant. Laser surgery cannot control such tumor spread. Moreover, if the laser excision extends toward the cricothyroid membrane, there is a chance that large vessels in this area will be penetrated by the laser, but not controlled. As this again is at an inferior limit of visualization, such laser surgery is dangerous.

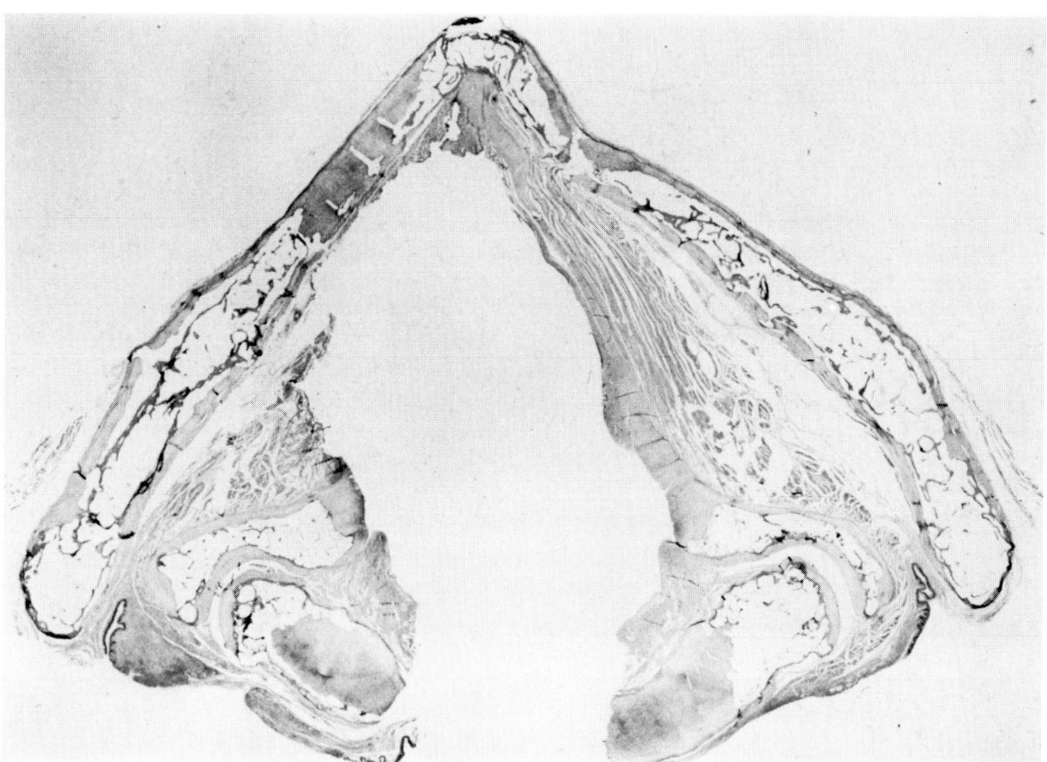

Figure 6–3. The completed total cordectomy. The posterior line of excision is at a right angle across the vocal process of the arytenoid, with excision carried all the way to thyroid cartilage.

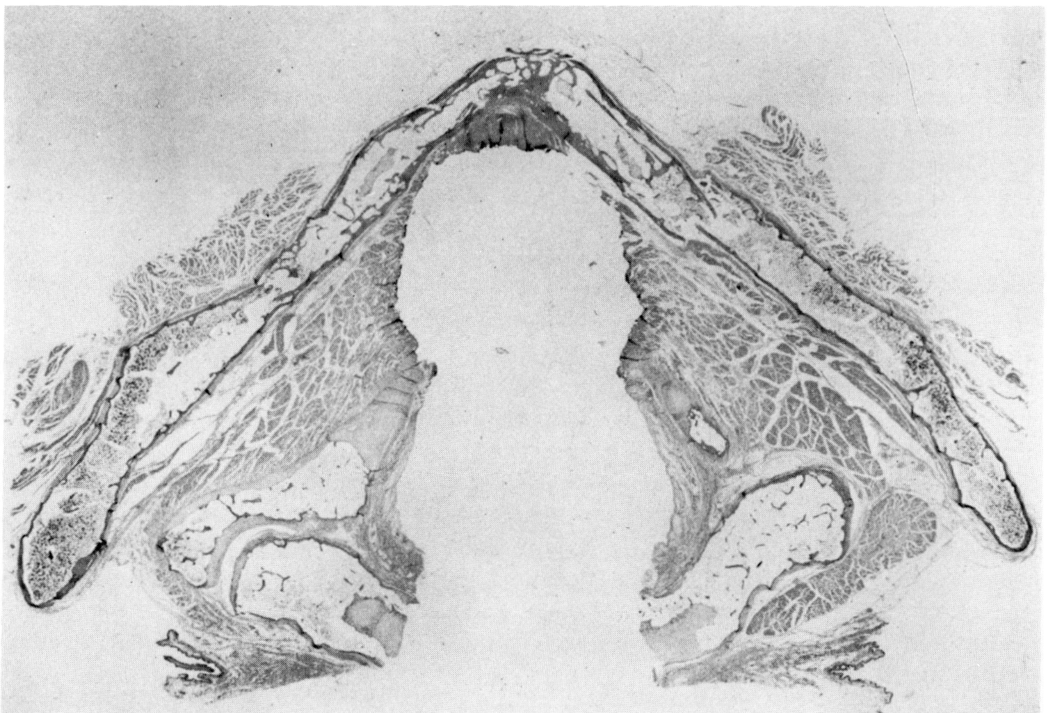

Figure 6–4. This whole mount serial section shows the first step in a vigorous anterior commissure excision. Notice that the true vocal cords have been transected at right angles to the free edge of the cord, with the excision carried toward the thyroid cartilage. The anterior commissure tendon is yet present.

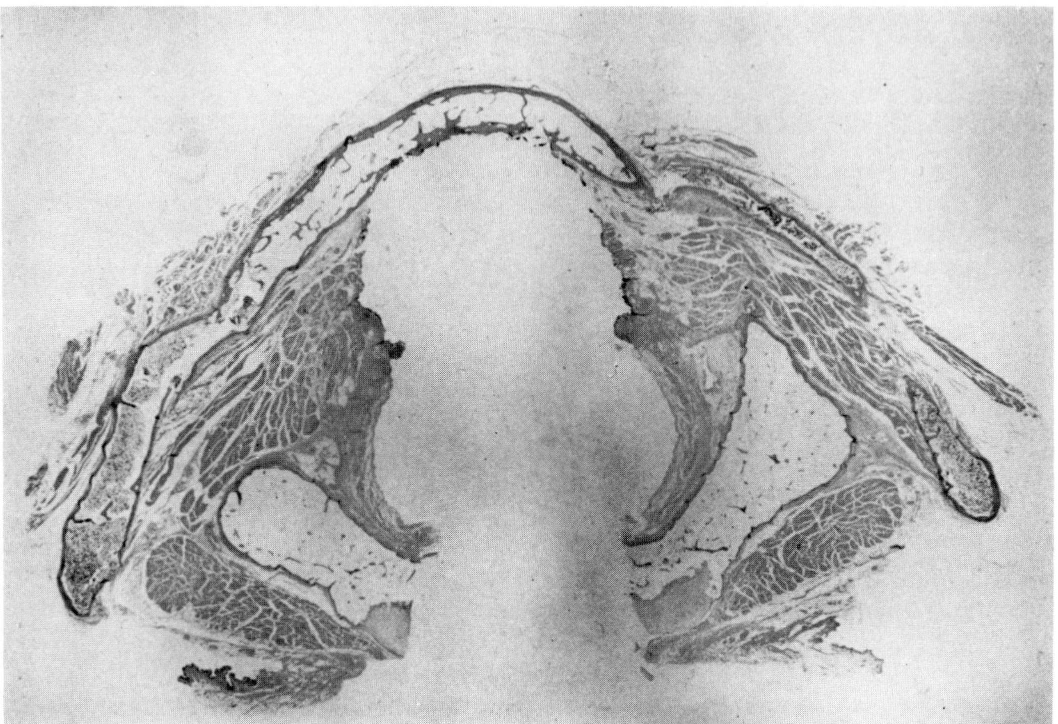

FIGURE 6–5. Full anterior commissure excision has been carried to the cartilage.

The limitations of cordectomy as described above must be carefully adhered to in T1 glottic cancer tumor excision. In summary, these limitations include (1) posterolaterally, excision across the vocal process of the arytenoid at a right angle; (2) laterally, the thyroid cartilage; (3) anteriorly, the thyroid cartilage; and (4) anteroinferiorly, 5 mm below the anterior commissure where the superior surface of the true cords meet.

LASER CORDECTOMY TECHNIQUES

This section considers the basic principles involved in laser cordectomy. Certainly the overriding first principle is that the lesion to be excised must be adequately visualized. The second principle needing special emphasis is that the lesion must be excised, and not vaporized. There is a temptation in using the CO_2 laser to perform a biopsy initially and define a lesion and then simply to vaporize the lesion in a ''no touch'' technique. This approach is reasonable for benign lesions, for which knowledge of exact margins is less critical. In the case of malignancy, however, strict adherence to principles of surgical oncology must be maintained. This includes the ability to excise a lesion and know pathologically the margins of the excision. Vaporization does not allow this. As stated above, techniques that have not allowed analysis of margins have basically never gained great acceptance. These approaches include cryosurgery and electrocautery used to fulgurate a lesion. Safety with laser excision depends on the ability to determine surgical margins.

Another general surgical principle is that traction and countertraction on a lesion greatly facilitate the ability to cut. This principle is well accepted with sharp knife dissection in the neck and also pertains to laser excision.

Figures 6–6 through 6–11 illustrate laser cordectomy of a small lesion on the left true vocal cord. This lesion is well visualized with the endoscope and is situated anteriorly far enough to allow easy excision (Fig. 6–6). The lesion is approached by first grasping the edge of the vocal

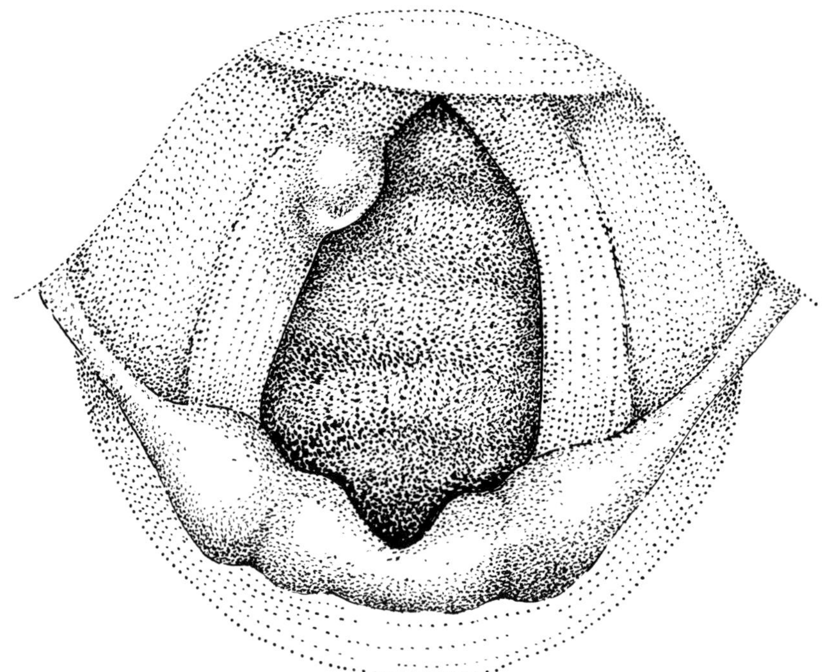

Figure 6–6. A neoplasm of the left true vocal cord on the anterior aspect.

cord with the cup forceps, as shown in Figure 6–7. This places tension on the lesion and greatly facilitates cutting with the laser. The lesion is carefully outlined by dots placed with the CO_2 laser using a 0.5 to 1 mm spot size. If the laser cannot be focused more precisely than at 1 mm, it is more difficult to determine margins and also more likely for charring of the incision line to occur. It usually is best to deepen the incision around the lesion by starting posteriorly and carrying the incision through the mucosa into the submucosa. With the lesion under tension, this incisional area can be defined to the limits of easy visibility. This work is best accomplished using a laryngoscope with a separate channel that can be hooked up to suction apparatus to allow evacuation of smoke. If bleeding occurs during the initial incision, the laser can be defocused slightly, or the power can be decreased to better photocoagulate the bleeding sites. Rarely are troublesome bleeding sites found in the early phases of excision as currently performed. The depth of excision is extended to the underlying vocalis muscle without greatly entering into this muscle. This is easily visualized under the microscope.

Figure 6–8 shows the specimen freed in the posterior aspect, with the cup forceps yet providing traction to allow anterolateral and direct anterior excision. Figure 6–9 shows the specimen removed and the underlying surgical bed exposed. Usually a small amount of carbonization is present at this time. This can be removed by gently irrigating with normal saline and suctioning the area. It also should be noted that the excision was carried toward the cartilage at the anterior commissure (Fig. 6–9). Excision involved the anterior commissure on the left side and was adjacent to the attachment of the right true vocal cord. If the right true cord is not damaged, and the mucosa is intact to this level, minimal webbing occurs.

The excised specimen is submitted for pathologic analysis. It can be pinned to a small piece of Telfa, with the orientation identified for the pathologists. Commonly, the margins of tumor approximate the edges of the surgical resection, as this is a small specimen. To ensure that the lesion has been successfully excised, standard biopsies are taken at several sites in the excision bed. This is demonstrated in Figure 6–10.

When a patient is initially treated in this manner, the deep biopsy specimens taken are sent for routine pathologic examination and rarely for frozen section analysis. This is because, if cancer is

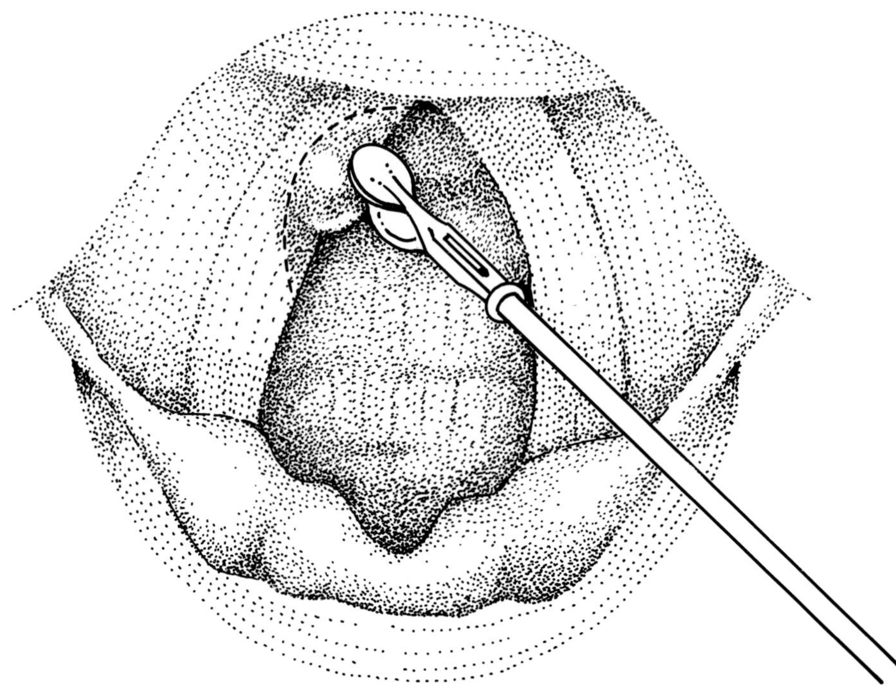

FIGURE 6–7. The area of the actual lesion has been outlined, and the lesion is placed under tension with a cup forceps.

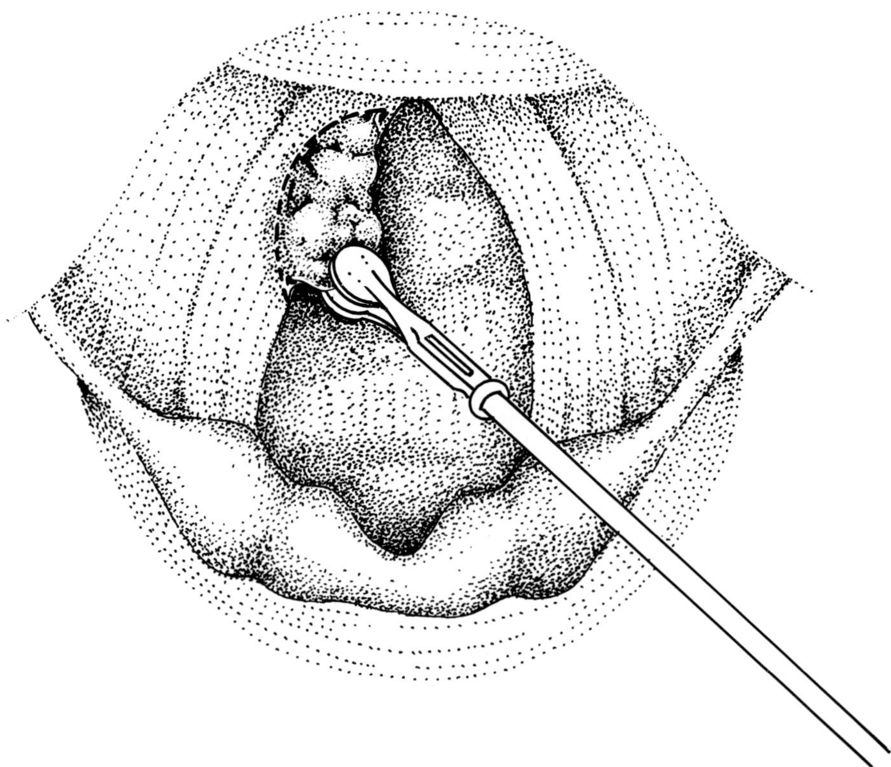

FIGURE 6–8. The neoplasm has been partially excised. Notice that the cup forceps is applying tension on the lesion to allow excision with less thermal damage.

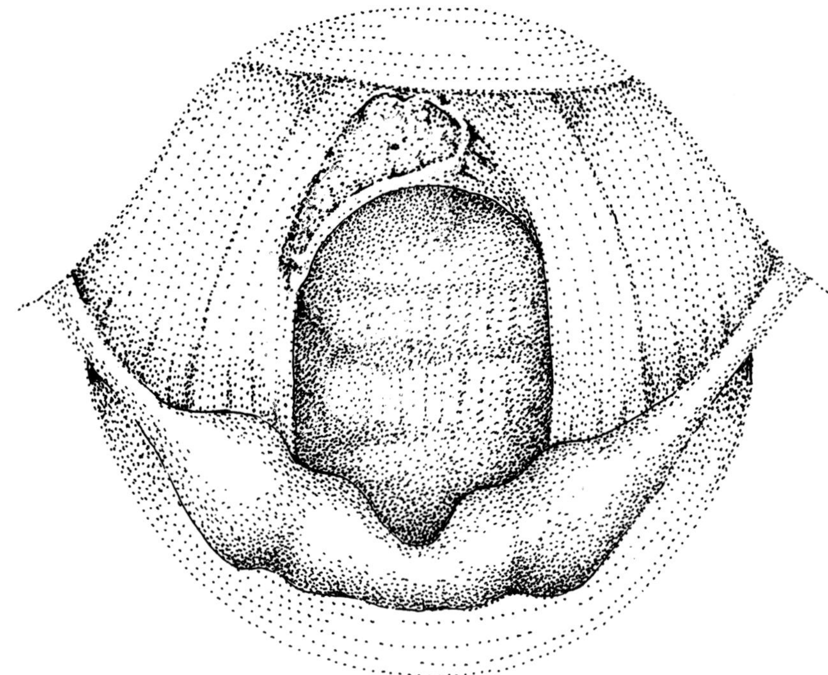

FIGURE 6–9. The defect after limited cordectomy.

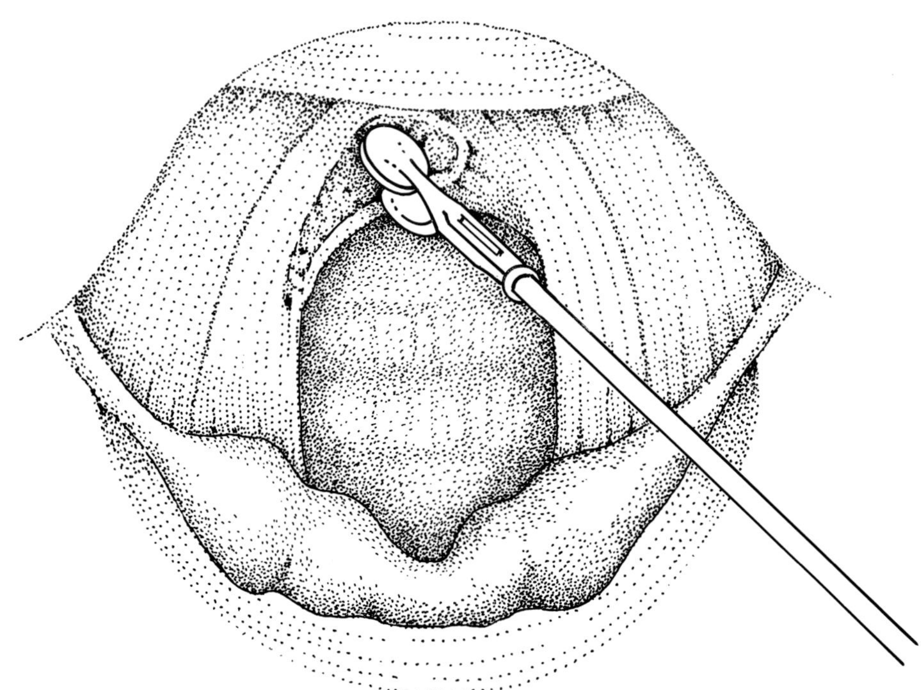

FIGURE 6–10. A cup forceps is used for conventional biopsies in the surgical bed after laser excision.

indeed present in the deep biopsy specimens, by definition it is present in the vocalis muscle. Cancers that invade this deeply into muscle are not best treated by initial full laser excision. Although this potentially could be successfully done, the risk of damage to the voice is significantly higher than with more limited excisions. Second, tumors that have invaded to the area of the vocalis muscle are biologically much more active than tumors that have not invaded this far. Laser excision for such lesions may not be fully effective. If permanent sections show the presence of cancer in deep biopsy specimens, most patients are referred for radiation therapy. If patients do not wish to undergo irradiation therapy, a decision must be made between open partial laryngectomy and an extended laser excision to the limits of cordectomy (as described above). This decision is usually determined preoperatively so that extension of the laser procedure can be accomplished at the initial surgical procedure. In these patients a further excision is accomplished, and the specimen is sent for frozen section examination. If frozen section analysis reveals invasion deep into the vocalis muscle, these patients will need an open laryngectomy process (usually partial laryngectomy). Figure 6–11 shows a side view of the excision bed. It should be noted that the inferior limit of excision encompasses the full true vocal cord. It is easy to extend excision farther than one realizes if one does not have adequate laboratory or clinical experience.

Anterior commissure excision is represented in Figures 6–12 through 6–15. Figure 6–12 shows a bulky lesion at the anterior commissure. This lesion is approached by placing tension on one side of the lesion. The laser is used to outline the lesion on both sides (Fig. 6–13). As many tumors are somewhat friable, care is taken to avoid grasping the lesion more than once if possible. The excision is started by carrying the outlined area of excision to the underlying vocalis muscle. This is done on one side of the lesion with tension applied. As this area becomes free, the cup

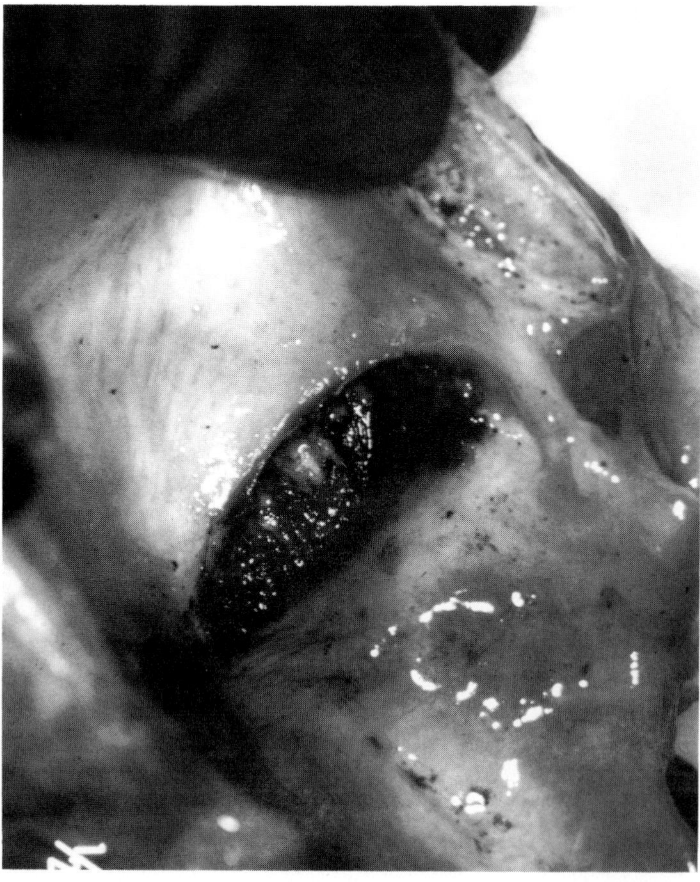

FIGURE 6–11. An open cadaver larynx after true cordectomy. It should be noted that the cranial caudal extent of the excision in this case is appropriate. It is easy to carry the excision more deeply than anticipated. Caution must be exercised in this regard.

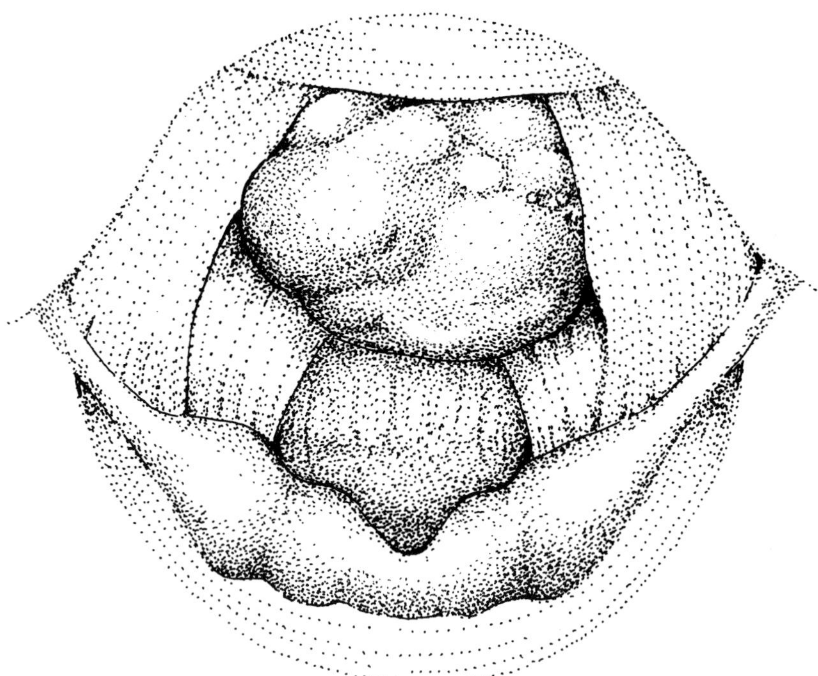

Figure 6–12. A large mass that obscures the anterior commissure, making identification of the true mucosal extent of the tumor almost impossible to ascertain.

forceps can be shifted more to the anterior position, and the lesion is pulled posteriorly to expose the full extent of the anterior commissure. Usually it is possible to define a line of excision around the tumor without violating the tumor. The cup forceps is then used to grasp the opposite side, and the same procedure is accomplished on the opposite side. When the lesion is carefully freed on both sides, attention is focused directly anteriorly where the lesion is carefully excised. Care must be taken not to extend the laser excision beyond 5 mm inferiorly. If the tumor clearly goes beyond 5 mm, excisional biopsy should not be attempted.

After the bulk of the specimen has been removed, the actual extent of primary mucosal involvement can be determined (Fig. 6–14). If the lesion cannot be fully removed in the anterior aspect, the specimen can be grasped and the laser excision carried farther around the lesion to the point of exposing the anterior commissure thyroid cartilage. If the lesion extends to the cartilage, it has progressed beyond the T1 stage and must be treated by conventional therapy. Laser therapy in this case will not be adequate. If the lesion can be freed from the soft tissue prior to arriving at the thyroid cartilage, deep biopsies are taken to fully stage the lesion. Figure 6–15 shows the tumor bed after excision.

When the anterior commissure is excised in this manner, a small degree of webbing is usually found as the area heals. This rarely is clinically symptomatic for a patient if care has been taken to preserve the true vocal cords distal to the area of excision. Moreover, when excision is carried all the way to the thyroid cartilage, this removes all soft tissue in the area and allows space for a neocord to form without undue webbing.

With both laser excision techniques, the airway must be maintained and anesthesia safely administered. In the case of anterior commissure excision, it almost always is possible to use an appropriate endotracheal tube, which is positioned in the posterior glottis and does not interfere with visualization. These tubes include the aluminum metal–taped Rusch tube, the Norton stainless steel tube, or one of the newer tubes that have been specifically designed for laser therapy. Clearly, polyvinyl chloride tubes are never appropriate, even when protected by aluminum tape. These tubes are highly explosive and are contraindicated in any laser procedure.

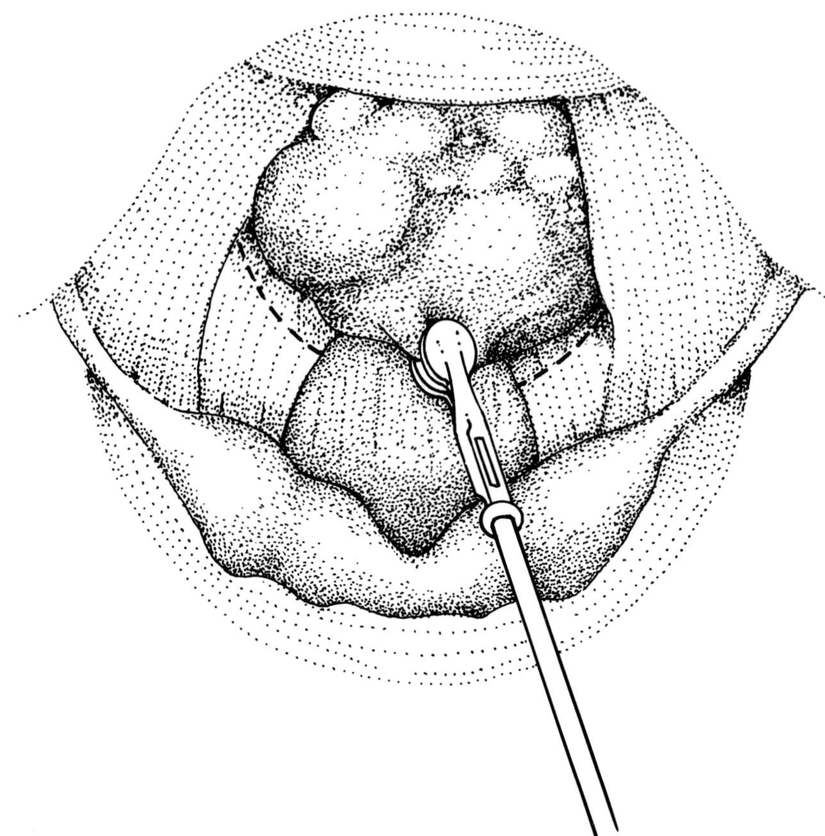

FIGURE 6–13. The mass has been placed under tension, and the lines of later laser excision have been outlined.

When limited anterior commissure lesions are approached with this technique, the author's preference is to use a metal-taped Rusch tube. The endotracheal tube itself often helps to separate the cords and does not interfere with visualization.

When larger lesions extend back toward the vocal process of the arytenoid cartilage, different techniques must be used. The two most commonly used techniques in this circumstance are the Venturi jet ventilation technique and the apneic technique. The Venturi system involves placement of a small clip with a jet ventilator attached to the laryngoscope. When the laryngoscope can be positioned to allow the glottis to remain open, and when the lesion has no ball valve effect on the glottis, the Venturi system can safely be used. Obviously great coordination is needed between the surgeon and the anesthesiologist to ensure that at no time is the glottis closed immediately after delivery of pressurized air, leading to potential pneumothorax. The technique developed by Benjamin can also be utilized (see Chapter 4).

The apneic technique is preferred in lesions that extend more posteriorly in the larynx in a patient who can easily be ventilated. This technique involves initial intubation of the patient with a small regular endotracheal tube. The suspension system used for laser laryngoscopy is then placed, and a large bore laryngoscope is positioned and suspended. The endotracheal tube is then withdrawn, allowing full visualization of the endolarynx and the associated lesion. The patient is monitored by pedal oximetry to follow oxygen saturation. In adults, usually at least 1 to 2 minutes of laser application time is allowed before the patient must be reintubated. As the oxygen saturation decreases, the patient is reintubated through the large bore laryngoscope. Full oxygen saturation is restored as well as carbon dioxide blown off by hyperventilation techniques. When the patient is

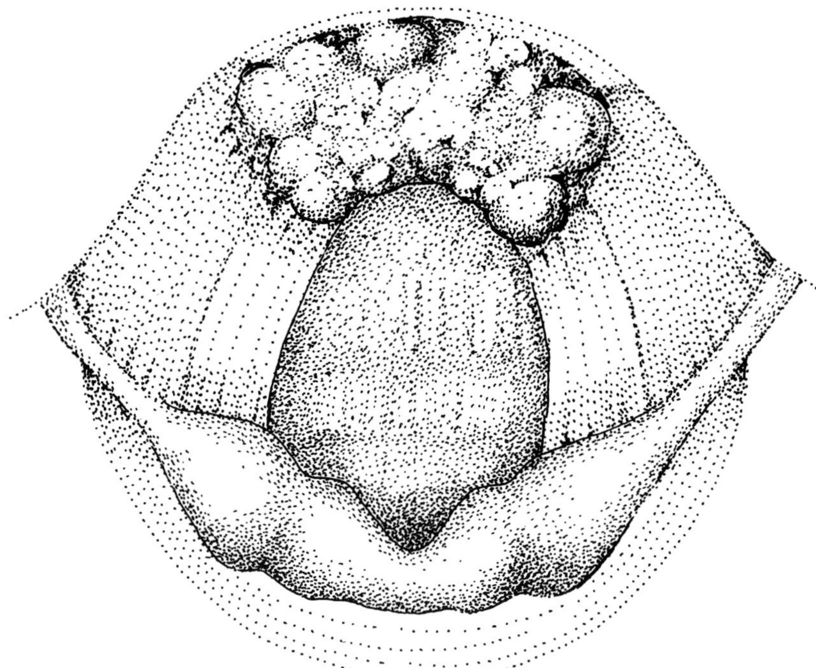

FIGURE 6–14. The actual attachment of the tumor involved the anterior commissure, but was considerably smaller than the mass of tumor itself.
Additionally, the mucosa and submucosa have been removed from the anterior aspect of both vocal cords up to the point of tumor attachment.

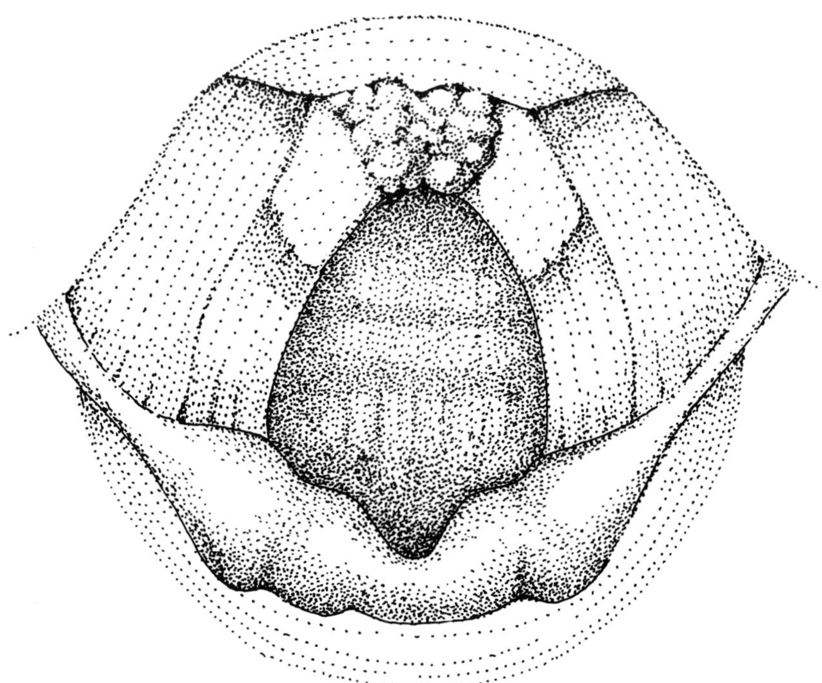

FIGURE 6–15. The surgical bed after full anterior commissure excision. Even with extensive defects of this nature, a neocord will form, usually with minimal anterior webbing.

reintubated, end tidal CO_2 level measurements are obtained. When levels are acceptably low, the endotracheal tube is removed and the laser application again commences. If end tidal CO_2 monitoring is not available, periods of laser excision should be kept under 2 minutes to prevent undue build-up of carbon dioxide. The process of laser excision alternated with reintubation is continued until the lesion can be successfully removed and deep biopsies taken.

SURGICAL INDICATIONS

One of the best uses of laser surgery is in the case of severe true vocal cord dysplasia or carcinoma in situ.

Treatment of severe vocal cord dysplasia is illustrated in Figures 6–16 and 6–17. In Figure 6–16 only the anterior aspect of the left true vocal cord appears visually normal. The remainder of the left cord and the full right cord show irregularity, thickening, and areas of erythroplasia. This type of lesion is well approached using the apneic technique. With the large bore laryngoscope carefully placed to allow visualization, as shown in Figure 6–16, the endotracheal tube is removed and the posterior aspect of the one true vocal cord is grasped. The laser is then used to make a small incision in the mucosa at the posterior aspect of the cord while the area to be excised is being held under tension with the cup forceps. This incision is carried through the mucosa and submucosa to the area of the vocalis muscle. Tension is then placed to draw the specimen anteromedially, and the laser is used to ''paint'' along the interface between the submucosa and the vocalis muscle. This excision is carried all the way toward the anterior commissure on the right where the cup forceps is then used to grasp the lesion in the anterior aspect and pull it up posteriorly, thereby allowing the anterior incision line to be placed. This specimen is removed and sent for pathologic examination. The postexcision bed is shown in Figure 6–17. Deep biopsies are taken to ensure complete removal. If the anterior commissure is violated in this approach, some vocalis muscle is excised in the excision bed anteriorly to create a small deficit of soft tissue at this site. This excision can be extended in the anterolateral aspect of the involved cord almost to the thyroid cartilage. Caution is taken not to damage the opposite true vocal cord at the anterior commissure. This removal of additional soft tissue allows the neocord to form with minimal webbing.

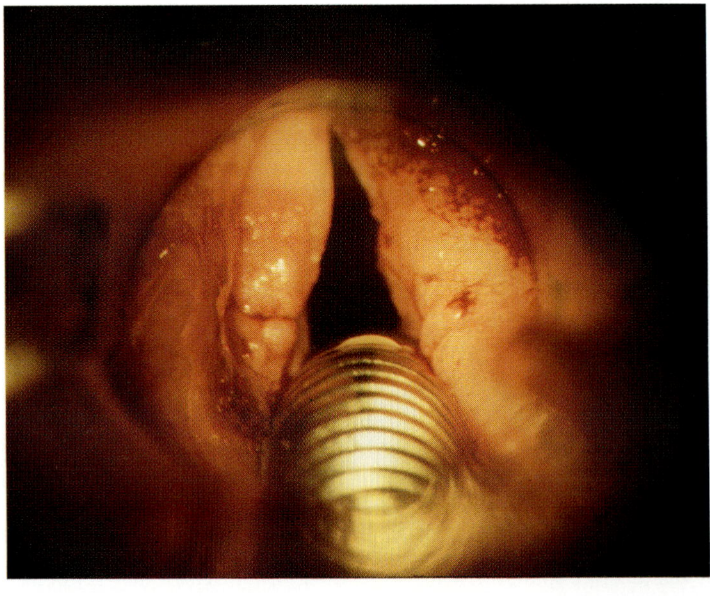

FIGURE 6–16. Severe dysplasia of the total right true vocal cord and the posterior aspect of the left true vocal cord.

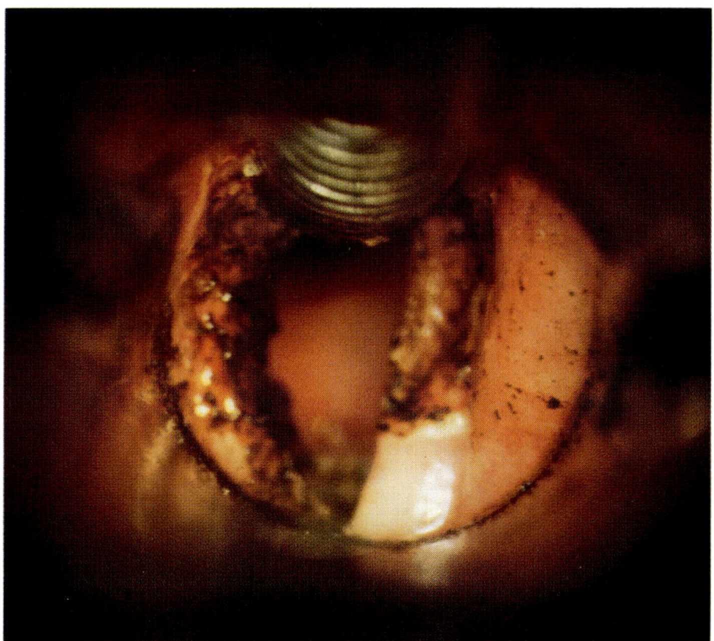

Figure 6–17. Excisional biopsy of the areas of dysplasia has been accomplished, leaving only the normal-appearing mucosa of the anterior aspect of the left true vocal cord.

Carcinoma in situ is effectively treated in this manner. Occasionally, the excision proceeds well, with apparently clear margins encountered. If examination of one of the deep margins shows severe dysplasia or possible cancer, a difficult decision must be made as to how to further treat the patient. In reliable patients, an acceptable approach is to carefully watch the patient through 3 months postoperatively as the patient heals. The patient can then be taken back to surgery and a second (cord stripping) procedure accomplished. If any cancer is found in the second resected specimen, the patient must undergo standard therapy, either irradiation or open partial laryngectomy. If the second resected specimen contains no residual tumor, the patient can be safely managed by observation only. This principle pertains also to superficially invasive cancers with the same question of residual cancer. In this case, it is appropriate simply to treat the patient by full course irradiation. Many patients, however, choose not to undergo the irradiation therapy and, therefore, definitely should undergo a second endoscopic procedure.

Figure 6–18 shows a verrucous-appearing lesion in the anterior true cord, which approaches the anterior commissure. Figure 6–19 shows that this area easily excised with minimal interference with the anterior commissure. Figures 6–20 and 6–21 show a somewhat more bulky lesion, which also was only superficially invasive. Cancers of this type that occur in the anterior aspect of the true vocal cord are well treated by laser cordectomy as well as by full course irradiation. A classic paper by Wang reported that patients with limited cancers of the anterior true cord were cured more than 94 per cent of the time.[12] In this same paper, 82 per cent of patients who had involvement of both vocal cords or the anterior commissure exhibited no evidence of disease (NED) after 3 years. Patients with tumors that involved the entire true vocal cord or the posterior third of the vocal cord had only a 75 per cent 3 year survival. Although Wang's study represents one of the most satisfactory results with irradiation, it certainly is clear that anteriorly placed lesions have the best prognosis. Lesions that extend posteriorly to a point where they cannot be encompassed by transsection of the vocal process of the arytenoid cartilage should not be approached by laser surgery. In light of the lower radiation cure rates achieved when posterior cord involvement is present, it seems reasonable that these lesions could be approached by open partial laryngectomy. On the other hand, the number of patients with small anterior commissure lesions that were cured by the initial biopsy only is not known in this study. As mentioned above, between 20 and 30 per cent of patients

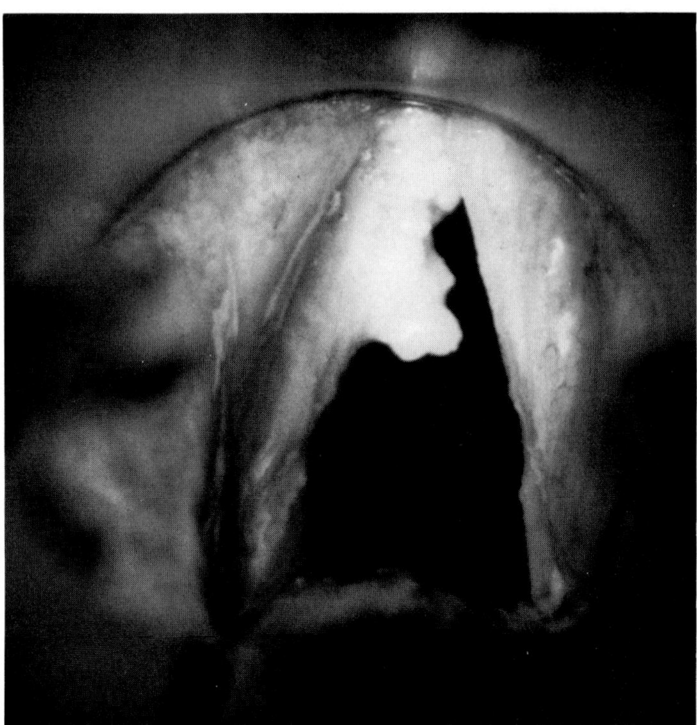

FIGURE 6–18. A prominent mass in the anterior aspect of the left true vocal cord.

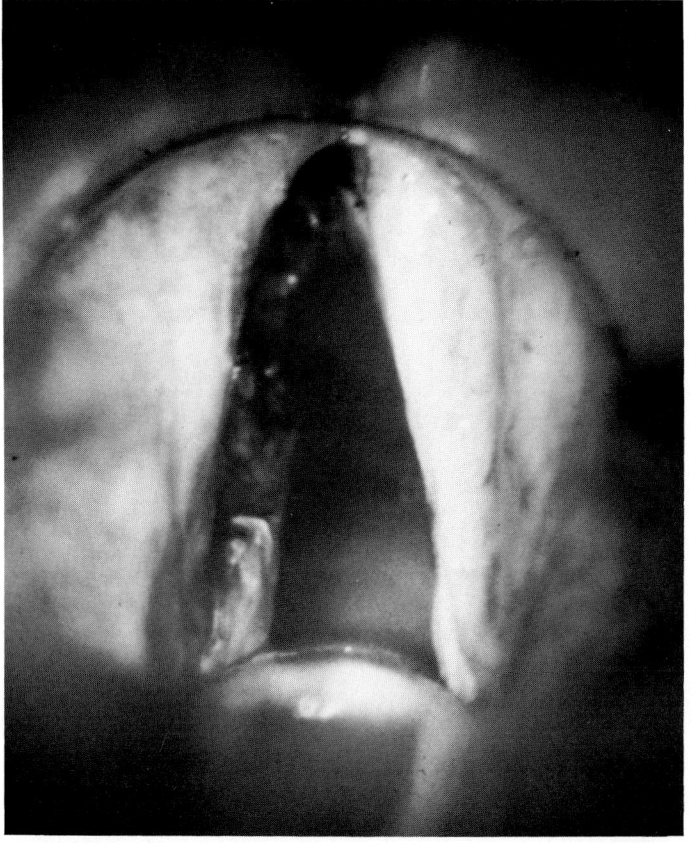

FIGURE 6–19. The small post-excision bed after removal of the anterior commissure lesion in Figure 6–18. This lesion did not extend into the vocalis muscle.

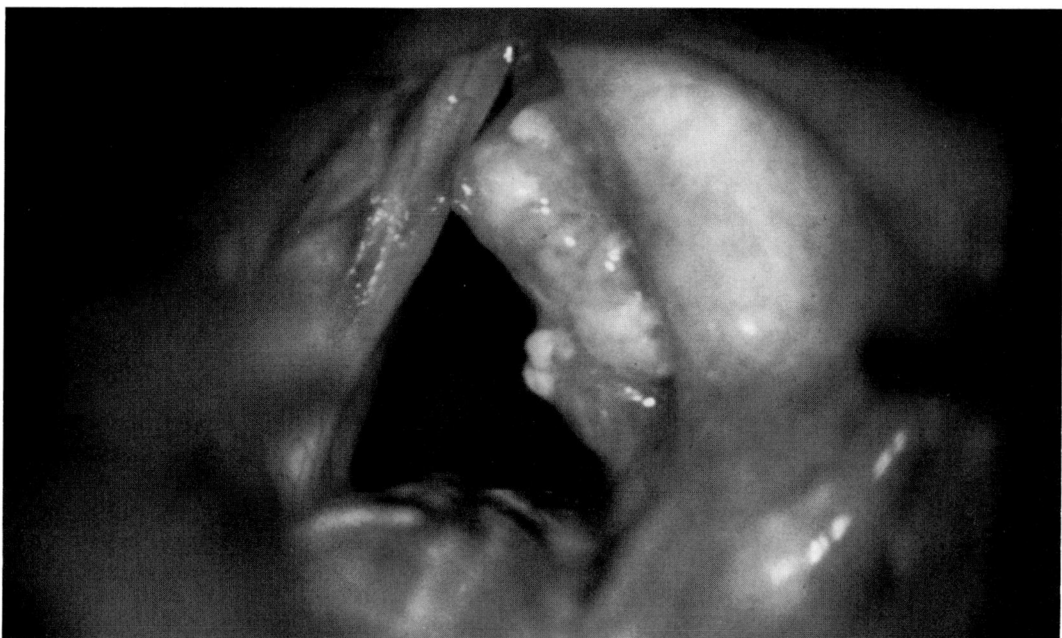

FIGURE 6–20. A large left anterior commissure mass.

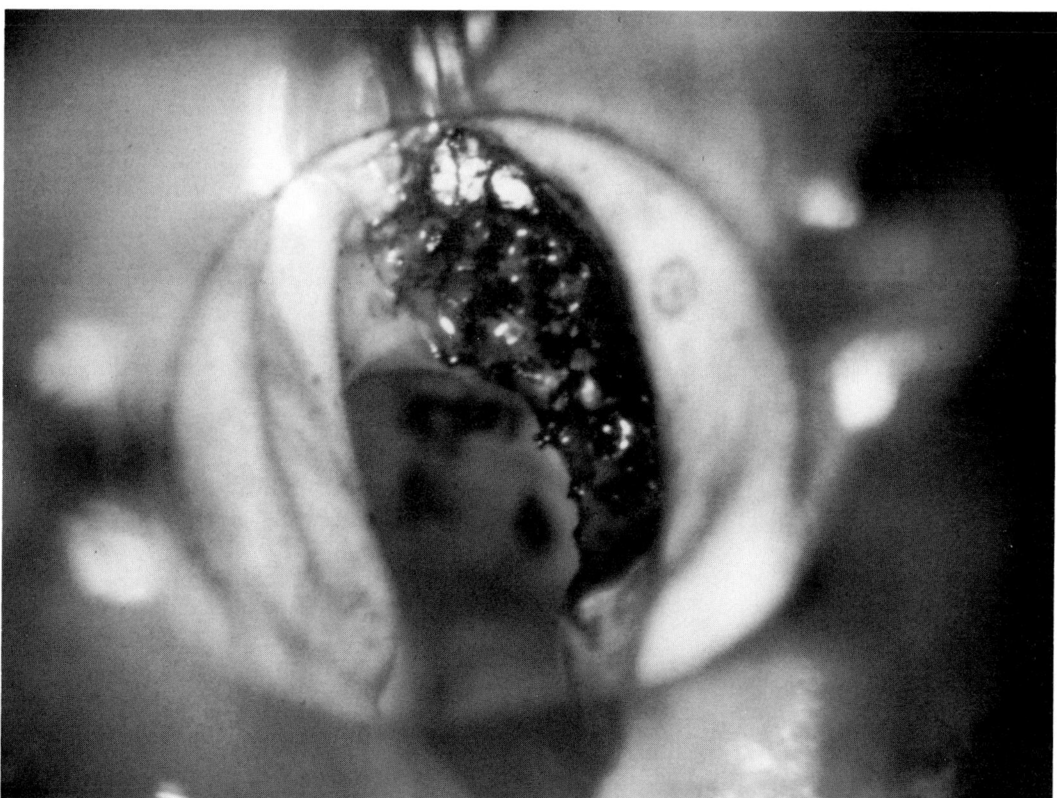

FIGURE 6–21. The postexcision surgical bed of the mass in Figure 6–20. This mass extended slightly into the vocalis muscle. Results of deep biopsies of this bed were normal.

referred for further therapy can have been cured by biopsy alone. If this group were excluded from Wang's data, the overall rates of successful radiation therapy results may be lower. To offer patients the option of laser excision for anterior lesions certainly seems reasonable.

Figure 6–22 presents a typical verrucous carcinoma. This extends to the vocal process posteriorly, as well as across the anterior commissure. These lesions present a special challenge, as they have in the past been thought to be somewhat resistant to irradiation. With current radiotherapeutic technique, it is probably better stated that these lesions are radiosensitive and possibly radiocurable.[12] A problem with radiotherapy in these lesions is the possibility of later dedifferentiation of tumor to a highly anaplastic type.[13] In light of both concerns, surgical excision of these lesions, if this can be done without morbidity, remains the treatment of choice. The lesion in Figure 6–22 certainly approaches the limits of resectability.

Figure 6–23 shows the lesion in Figure 6–22 fully excised, with the excision necessarily carried to cartilage in the anterior commissure. If the biopsy results are normal, such a lesion can be carefully followed by observation only. The reported cure rate of verrucous lesions using these principles of laser surgery has been high.[14]

Figure 6–24 shows a well-differentiated squamous cell carcinoma of a nonverrucous type. This lesion extended toward the vocal process of the arytenoid cartilage and toward the anterior commissure. Figure 6–25 shows the excision bed of this tumor. In this case, results of deep biopsies still indicated the presence of cancer, and the patient was referred for radiation therapy.

Anterior commissure cancer carries a special challenge, as it is often difficult to precisely define the full extent of these lesions. Such a lesion is shown in Figure 6–26. Clinical evaluation of the lesion with mirror technique, with Hopkins rod technique, or via the flexible nasopharyngoscope fails to give full information about the extent of tumor attachment anteriorly. In these cases, preoperative computed tomography (CT) or magnetic resonance imaging (MRI) can be helpful.

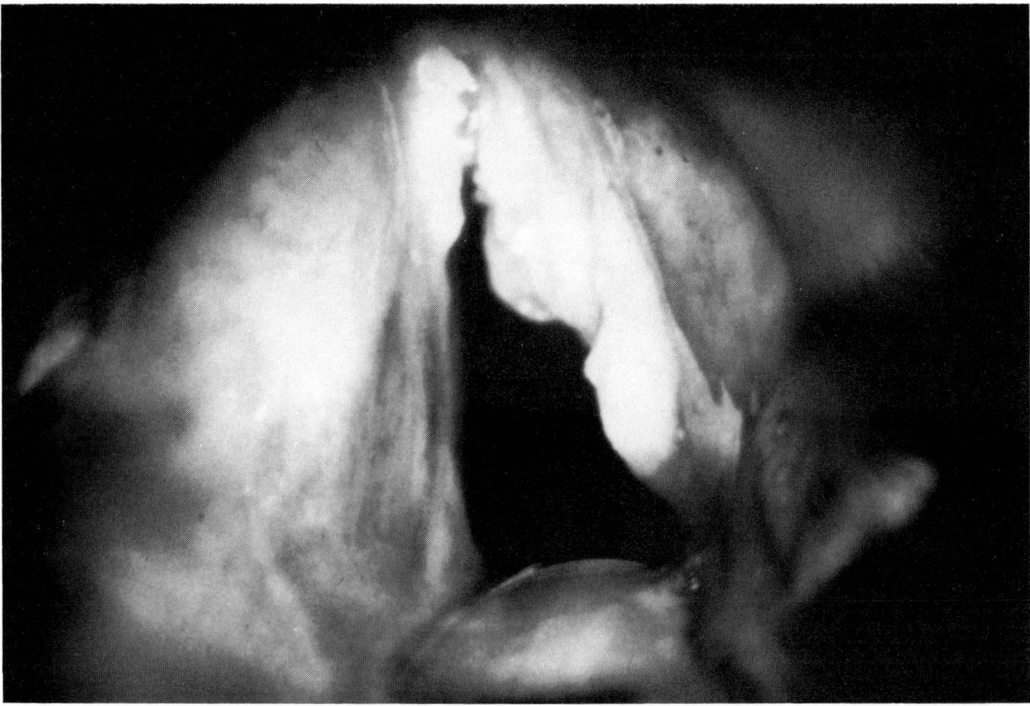

FIGURE 6–22. A large verrucous carcinoma of the full right true vocal cord, anterior commissure, and anterior aspect of the left true vocal cord.

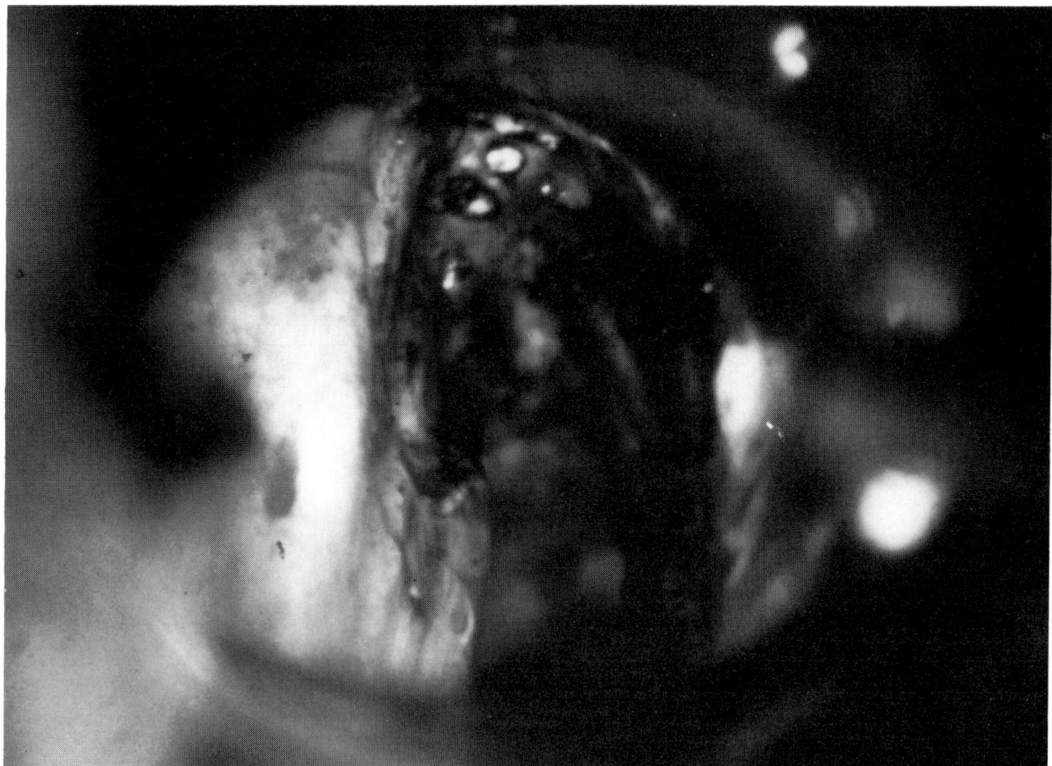

FIGURE 6–23. The verrucous cancer in Figure 6–22 has been widely excised, with the dissection carried all the way to thyroid cartilage, which shows as the white spot anteriorly.

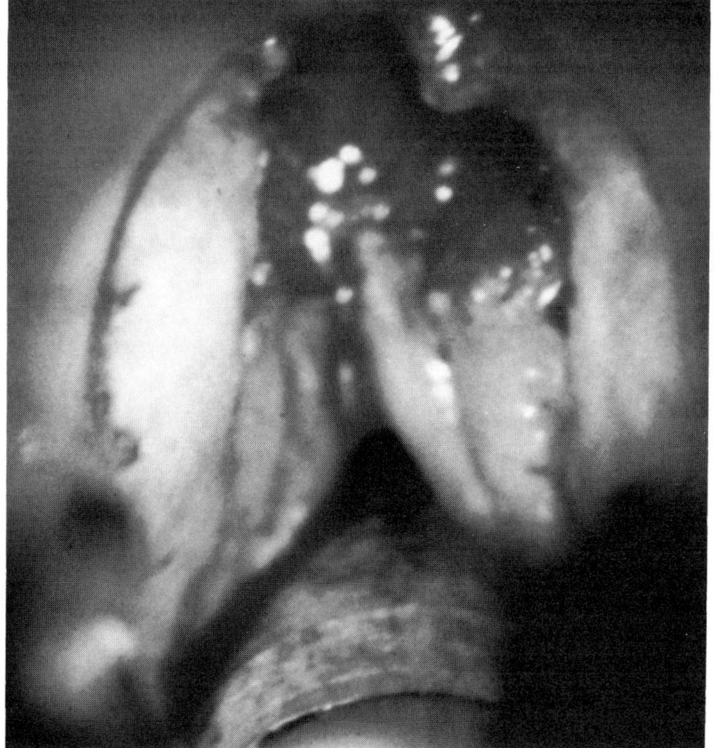

FIGURE 6–24. A large carcinoma involving the full right true vocal cord.

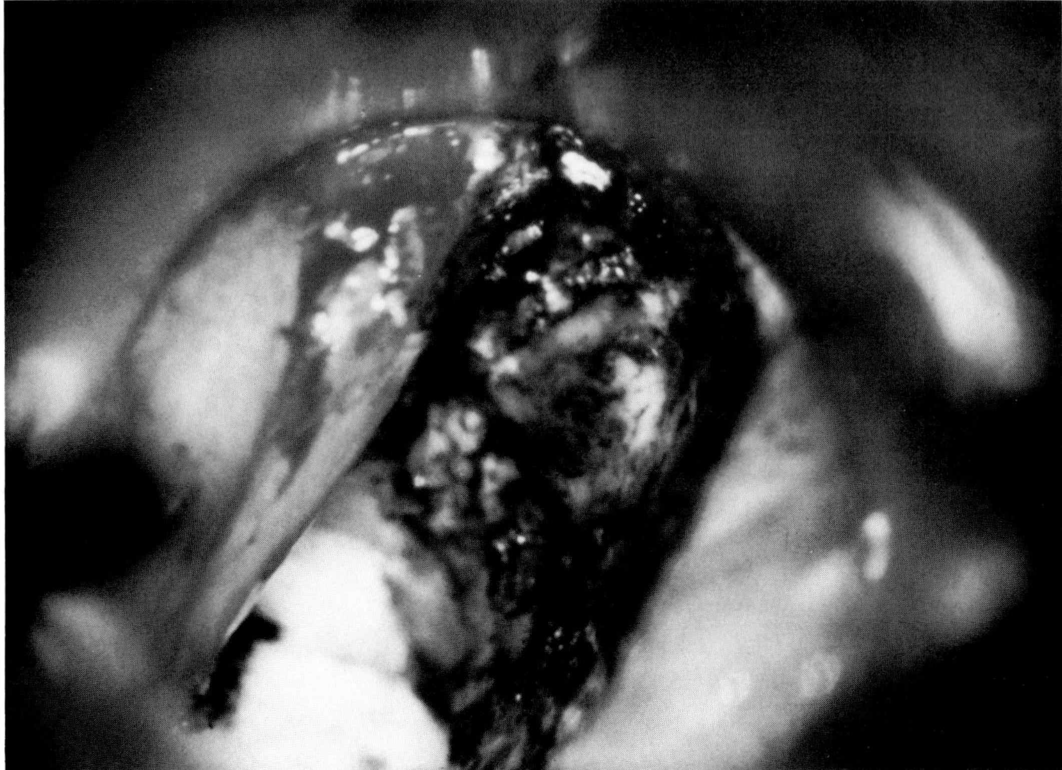

FIGURE 6–25. The postexcision bed of the tumor in Figure 6–24. Cartilage has been bared anteriorly, and the vocal process of the arytenoid cartilage has been transected posteriorly.

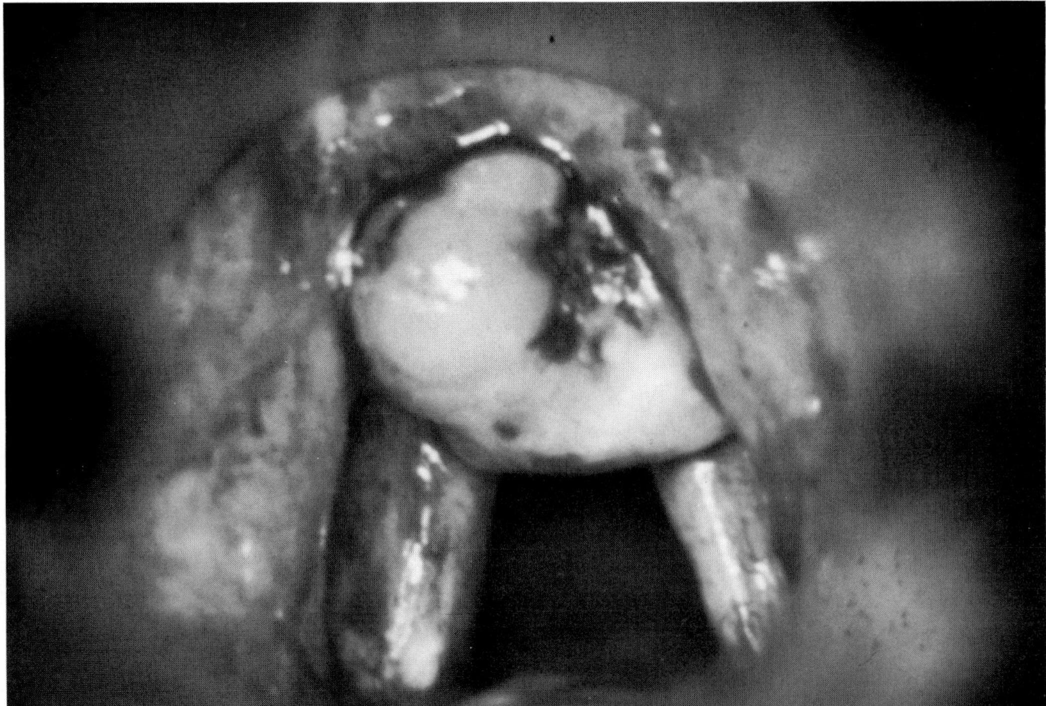

FIGURE 6–26. A large anterior commissure mass. (Patient of Dr. Geza Jako.)

The CT scan in Figure 6–27 presents an example of a lesion with extensive involvement of the anterior commissure thyroid cartilage. In such cases, laser excision has no role. Simple biopsy techniques using standard approaches are adequate to define the lesion. The laser can be used to incisionally perform a biopsy of such a lesion to help decrease bleeding and clear the airway of the lesion. Extended anterior commissure resection is obviously not indicated in light of tumor extent.

For lesions such as the one shown in Figure 6–26, CT scanning will not always be helpful. Figure 6–28 shows a CT scan obtained in a patient with a lesion similar to that in Figure 6–26. In this case, clear-cut cartilaginous invasion could not be determined. This often occurs because the variable ossification of the thyroid cartilage makes interpretation of cartilaginous invasion almost impossible. In these circumstances, anterior commissure tumor excision with direct visualization of excision to the thyroid cartilage remains a valuable mapping technique. Owing to the problem with variable ossification, CT or MRI scans remain of limited value in this circumstance. Anterior commissure excision for staging remains a viable approach.

Figures 6–29 through 6–32 present treatment of an extensive laryngeal lesion with anterior commissure extension that would almost certainly cause significant airway distress, leading to tracheotomy. Computed tomography scanning of such a lesion may not show obvious anterior thyroid cartilage invasion. In this circumstance, the lesion (Fig. 6–29) can be divided into quadrants to allow excision before the anterior commissure can be explored. Figure 6–30 shows the quadrants of laser excision outlined.

Figure 6–31 shows the posterior half of the lesion removed, and Figure 6–32 shows the actual small area of attachment of the lesion after the bulk of the lesion was removed. Figure 6–33 is of an actual surgical procedure in which the anterior commissure excision was taken to the thyroid cartilage, which was clear. In this case, the patient was able to be decannulated while further evaluation of the lesion was accomplished.

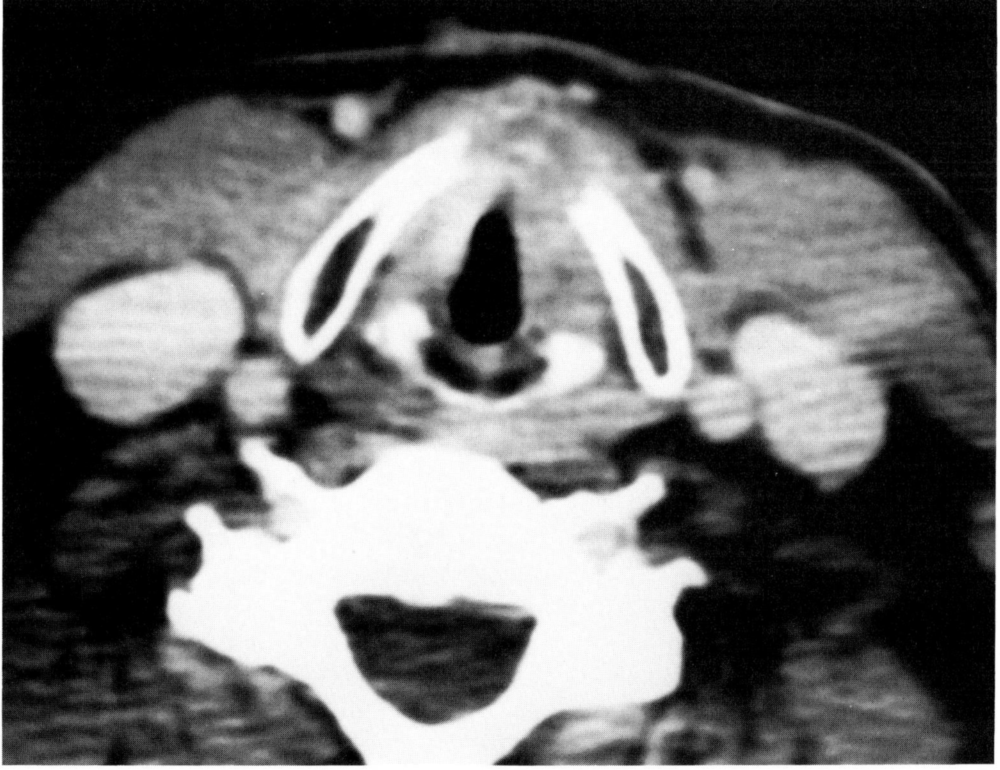

FIGURE 6–27. A CT scan shows extensive involvement of the thyroid cartilage from an endolaryngeal lesion.

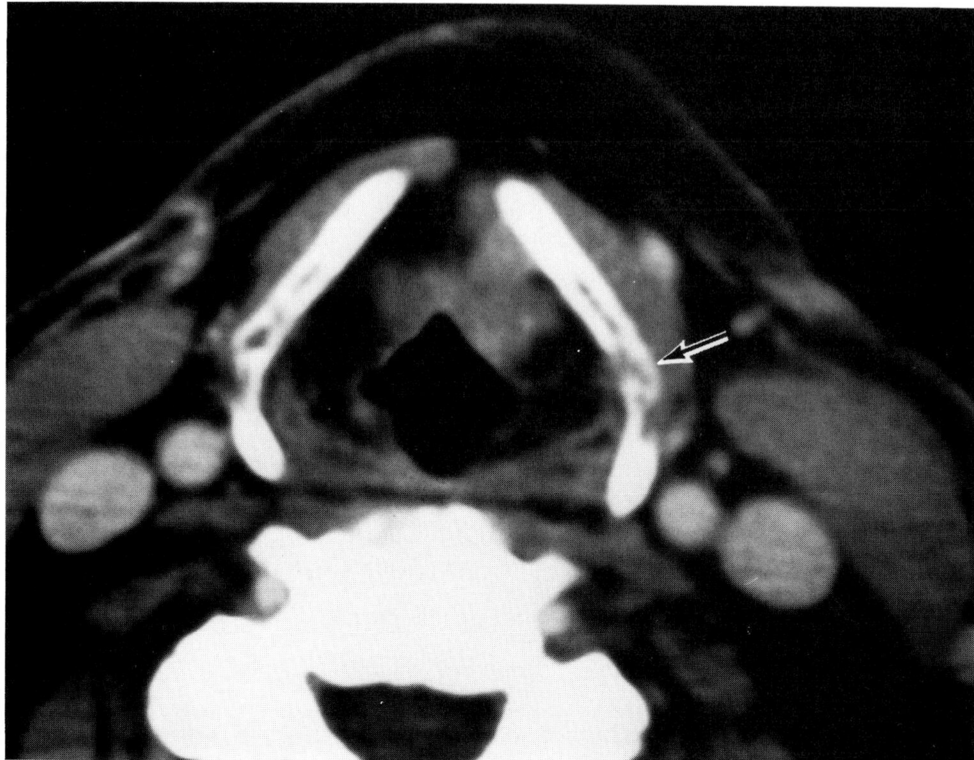

FIGURE 6–28. This patient had cancer of the right true vocal cord, but CT scanning fails to clearly determine whether the thyroid cartilage *(arrow)* is involved. In patients with variable ossification, it often is difficult to determine the presence or absence of cartilage involvement.

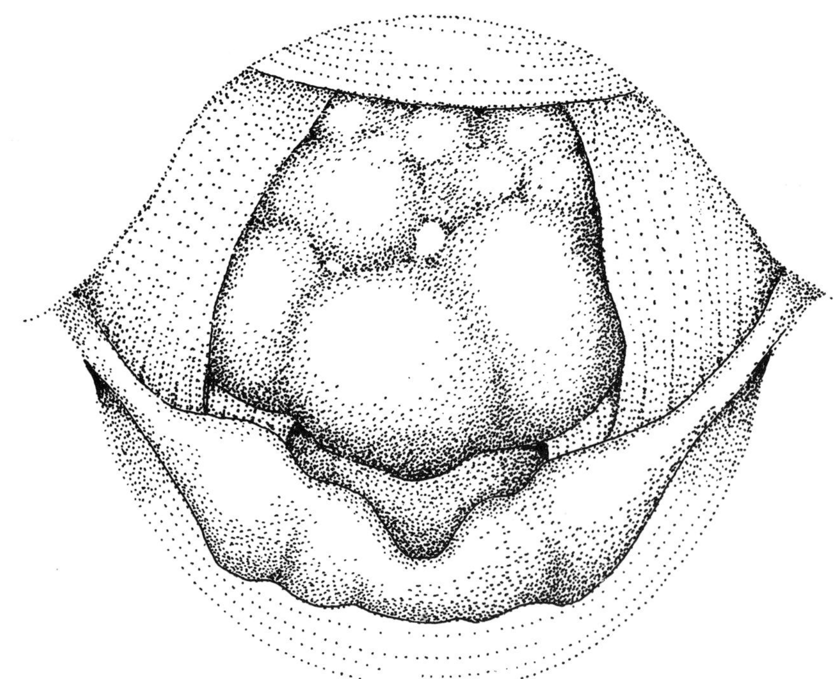

FIGURE 6–29. An extensive laryngeal cancer with anterior commissure extension.

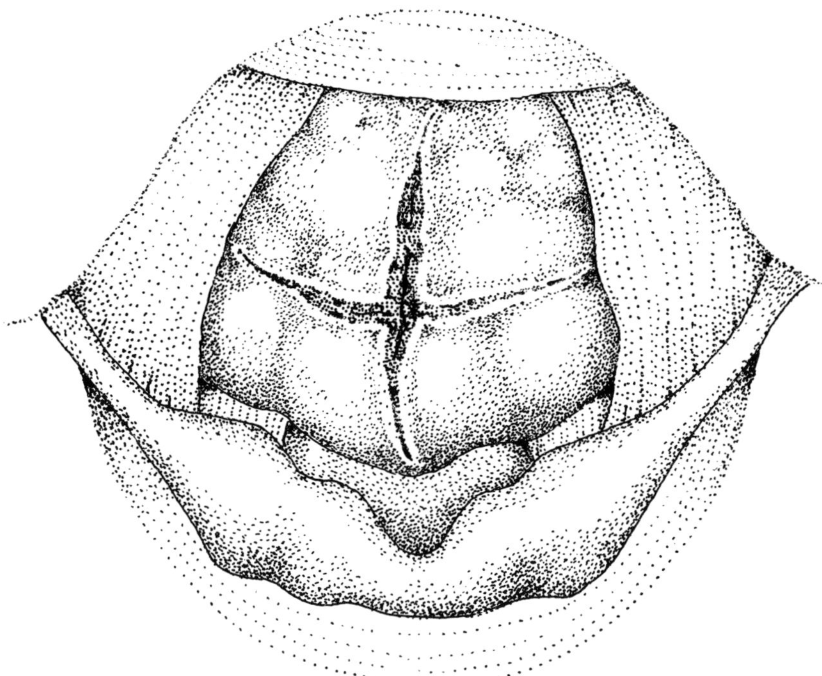

FIGURE 6–30. Division of the specimen into four quadrants (i.e., laser outlining of the excision lines in four quadrants).

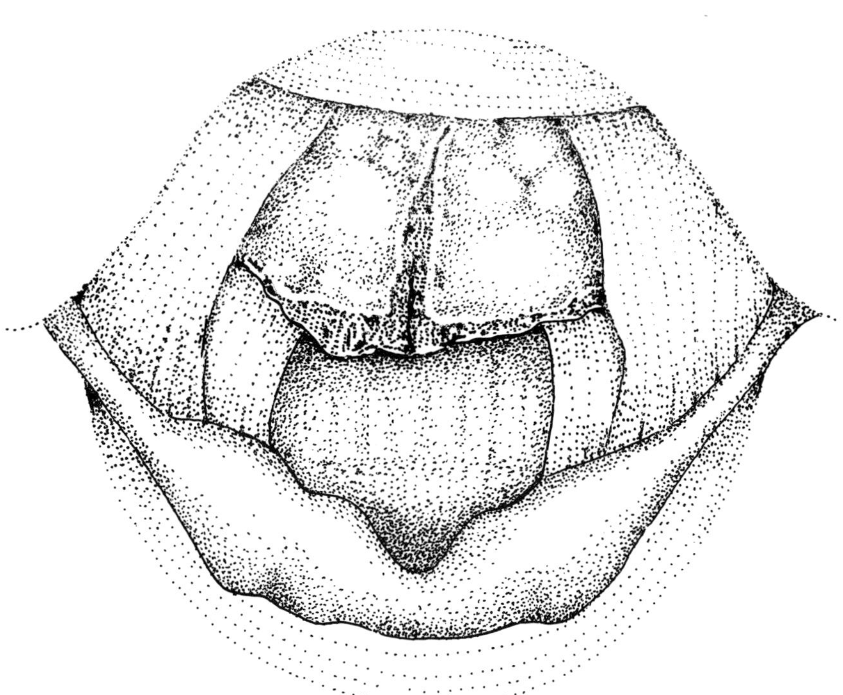

FIGURE 6–31. The specimen after the posterior one half has been removed.

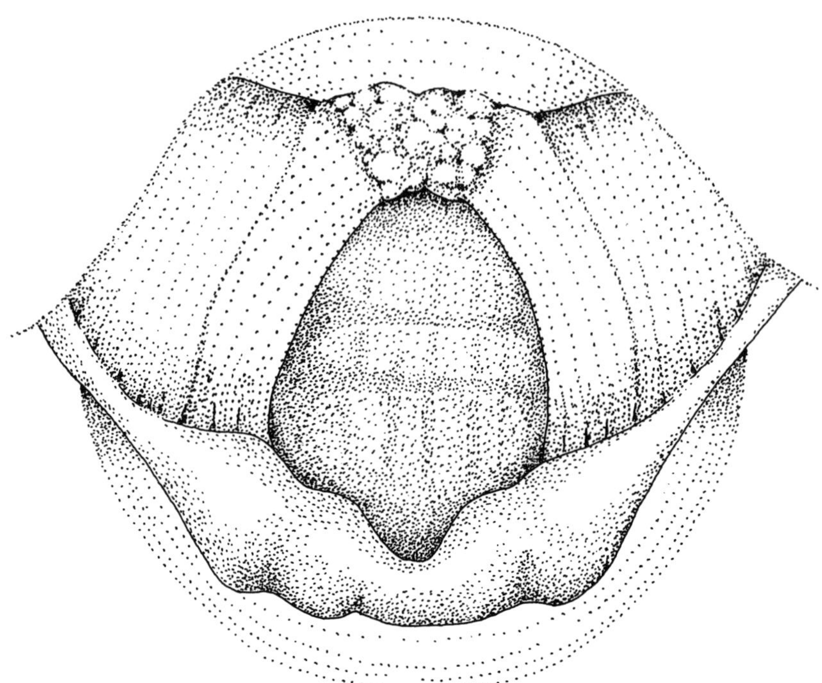

FIGURE 6–32. The small anterior commissure attachment, which was the base of the large tumor.

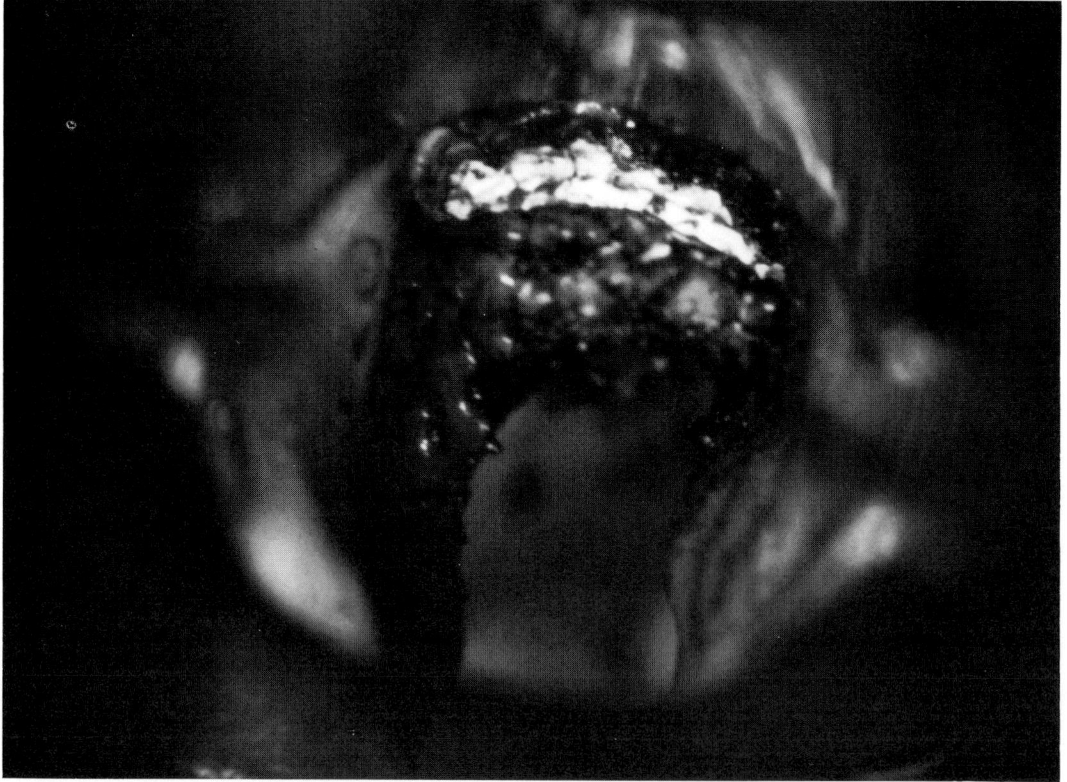

FIGURE 6–33. The next step in surgical excision in which the area of attachment is removed, with the excision carried to thyroid cartilage, which appears white in the illustration.

Laser excision has a limited role for patients who have been irradiated previously. In this situation, tumor may be suspected in one small area. Biopsy can be done as described above, using the laser to "strip" the involved cord. When tumor is found to be superficial and limited, a difficult question is faced by the clinician. As the patient has been previously irradiated, is it reasonable to subject the patient to an open partial laryngectomy with the risks of poor healing due to irradiation, or worse to subject the patient to total laryngectomy? The standard approach would usually be one of these two modalities. An alternative is to perform further biopsy of the cord in the area of the limited tumor. If results of these deep biopsies are normal, the patient could be managed by careful observation. Clearly, if biopsy results were abnormal in the vocalis muscle deep to the excision, open partial laryngectomy or total laryngectomy must be considered. Such extended laser excision must encompass the whole area of original tumor presentation, or it should not be used.

In patients with limited cancer of the anterior true vocal cord that recurs after irradiation therapy in the same limited area, total cordectomy done endoscopically with the laser is a reasonable approach. In this case the cordectomy is carried all the way to thyroid cartilage laterally and anteriorly. There is no reason to save the underlying vocalis muscle in this context. The patient cannot be reirradiated, and the risk of cancer within the muscle is too high not to remove it. In addition, the neocord that forms in this circumstance allows an adequate voice and glottic closure. Voice in this context is uniformly superior to that obtained using open partial laryngectomy techniques. Moreover, the risk of aspiration and poor phonation related to open partial techniques in an irradiated patient can often be avoided.

Full cordectomy can also be accomplished in patients who develop a second primary cancer that is limited to the true vocal cord area and who have been irradiated for other head and neck cancers. When these portals of previous radiation have involved the larynx, irradiation therapy alone cannot be given. Cordectomy with the laser in this case is appropriate. In patients who have had previous irradiation of extensive T1 cancers, and certainly any cancers greater than T1 staging, that recur, laser cordectomy is not appropriate.

CONTRAINDICATIONS TO LASER CORDECTOMY AND ANTERIOR COMMISSURE EXCISION

Carbon dioxide laser cordectomy is contraindicated in any lesion of T2 stage or greater. In these cases, endoscopic surgery with the laser could theoretically remove the lesion, but would leave a defect resulting in glottic incompetence that could not be treated endoscopically. In general, T2 glottic lesions are rarely bulky enough to be obstructive to the airway, and the laser debulking of such lesions is not necessary. The laser can be used as a biopsy instrument in obtaining small incisional biopsies. This can be adequately done using standard microsurgical techniques without the laser. Clearly, any lesion causing true vocal cord fixation (which is a T3 lesion) should not be approached with laser surgery. T1 lesions that involve the posterior one third of the vocal cord also are not suitable for laser excision. Such excision would necessarily involve removal of major portions of the arytenoid cartilage, which likely would lead to arytenoid fixation with airway incompetence and speech dysfunction. As noted above, such lesions may not be best treated by radiation therapy and probably should be treated by open partial laryngectomy.

When tumors extend beyond 5 mm below the free edge of the cords in the anterior commissure, such lesions also should not be excised with the laser. The chance of such laser excision's extending through the cricothyroid membrane would be high. More important, tumors that escape through this area are T4 lesions, which cannot be treated endoscopically. Any lesion with known cartilage invasion also should not be approached with laser excision. As mentioned above, cartilaginous invasion by tumor can be documented in some cases by prebiopsy CT or MRI scanning.

SUPRAGLOTTIC EXCISION
WITH CARBON DIOXIDE LASER

Supraglottic cancer is considered separately, as this is different biologically from true cord endolaryngeal T1 lesions. The main difference in biology is the relative lack of lymphatics on the true vocal cord versus the heavy lymphatic drainage of the supraglottic larynx. Related to this difference in lymphatic distribution is the great propensity for spread to regional lymph nodes of even T1 supraglottic lesions, making these lesions clearly not curable by limited resection. Treatment of most stage I suprahyoid lesions therefore requires treatment of the primary lesion as well as treatment of the regional lymphatics. Laser surgery does have some application in the treatment of the primary tumor, but has no role in regional therapy.

Figure 6–34 shows a cross section of the larynx. Particular attention should be given to the placement of the hyoid bone, which separates the supraglottic larynx into two compartments: (1) the suprahyoid supraglottis and (2) the infrahyoid supraglottis. Limited lesions of the suprahyoid supraglottis may be appropriately treated by local resection alone. Lesions of the infrahyoid supraglottis are almost never effectively treated by local resection alone. The one circumstance in which excision alone may be appropriate is illustrated in Figures 6–35 through 6–37.

Figure 6–35 shows a small T1 suprahyoid supraglottic carcinoma. The propensity for regional neck spread from such a lesion is less than 20 per cent. Such lesions have traditionally been treated either by irradiation therapy, which also would include the first echelon of lymph nodes, or by a

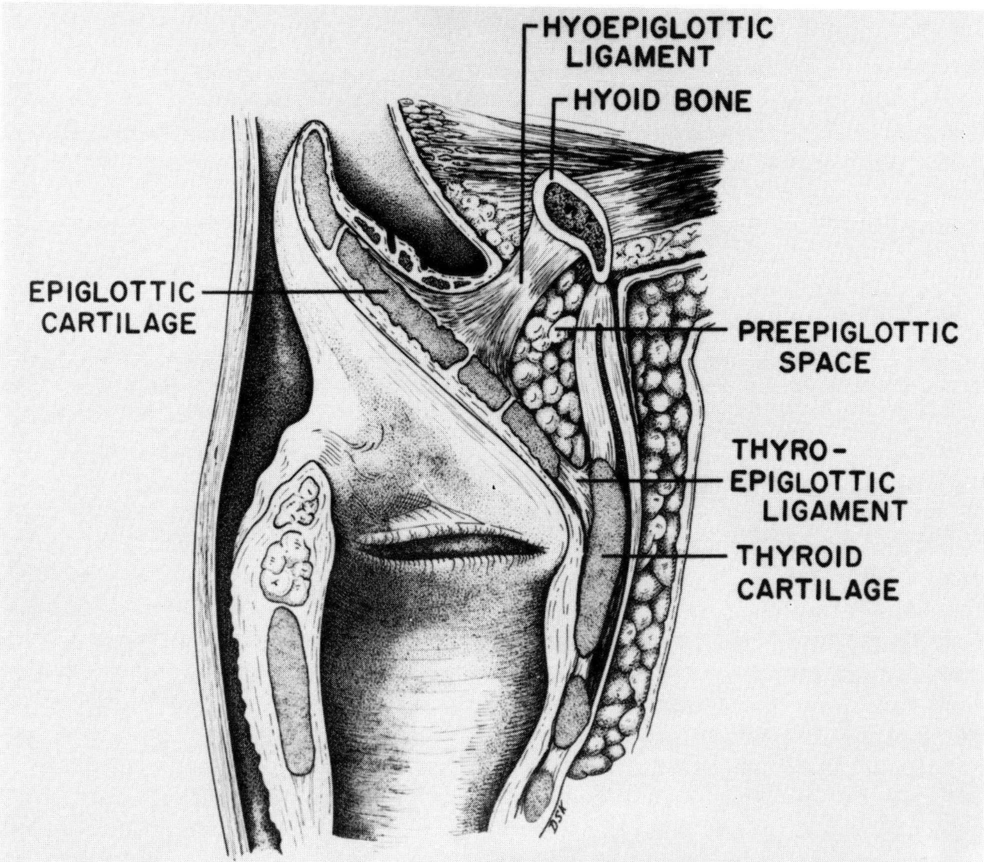

FIGURE 6–34. A sagittal section of the larynx. The hyoid bone separates the supraglottic larynx into the suprahyoid supraglottis and the infrahyoid supraglottis.

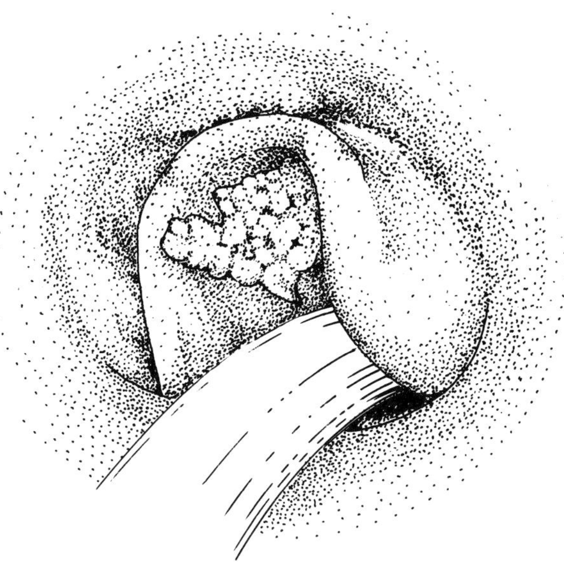

Figure 6–35. A small T1 suprahyoid supraglottic cancer.

supraglottic laryngectomy. The use of irradiation therapy in these lesions is appropriate, as potential microscopic disease is treated. The question is whether this is necessary in all limited cases. In general, lesions with greater than a 30 per cent propensity for microscopic spread should be treated. Surgeons advocating local excision alone would point to the lower incidence of such spread from this specific lesion.

Supraglottic laryngectomy by standard techniques requires an open approach. In almost every circumstance following even limited supraglottic excision such as epiglottectomy, a tracheotomy is necessary to ensure airway competence in the immediate postoperative period. An alternative to supraglottic resection (i.e., epiglottectomy) is endoscopic CO_2 laser epiglottectomy. The lesion shown in Figure 6–36 can be removed endoscopically by gaining visualization through a large bore laryngoscope. The standard microlaryngeal suspension system is used, and the lesion is surveyed. Attention is then directed to either side of the epiglottis near the pharyngoepiglottic fold. Laser excision is started near the pharyngoepiglottic fold by grasping the epiglottis and making an incision in the lingual mucosa (mucosa on the vallecular side). This incision can be carried down to epiglottic cartilage readily. This is shown in Figure 6–36. The epiglottis is then grasped at the opposite pharyngoepiglottic fold area, and a similar incision is done at this area. This usually requires repositioning of the laryngoscope to allow adequate visualization. When both sides have been excised down to cartilage, attention is directed to the epiglottic cartilage. The epiglottis is pulled forward (i.e., away from the larynx) so that the edge of the excision area near the laryngeal surface of the epiglottis can be visualized. Excision is then carried across this area. This also needs to be accomplished on both sides, which then should allow the specimen to be delivered. Figure 6–37 shows the cut edge of the epiglottis after removal of the specimen. Such excision for limited lesions (as shown in Figures 6–35 to 6–37) results in wide surgical margin around the tumor.

Patients treated in this manner do not require tracheotomy or overnight intubation. Intraoperative steroids are typically given to decrease any likelihood for laryngeal edema from the instrumentation. Patients are usually discharged the day following surgery. In a series by Davis and associates, no patient required hospitalization beyond 3 days postoperatively.[16] This is in great distinction to recovery from the open partial epiglottectomy procedures, which requires significantly longer hospitalization with tracheotomy placed (as noted above). Most patients aspirate mildly in the first day postoperatively, but rarely beyond 2 or 3 days postoperatively. No patient in the author's experience has developed significant problems with aspiration after epiglottectomy done in this manner.

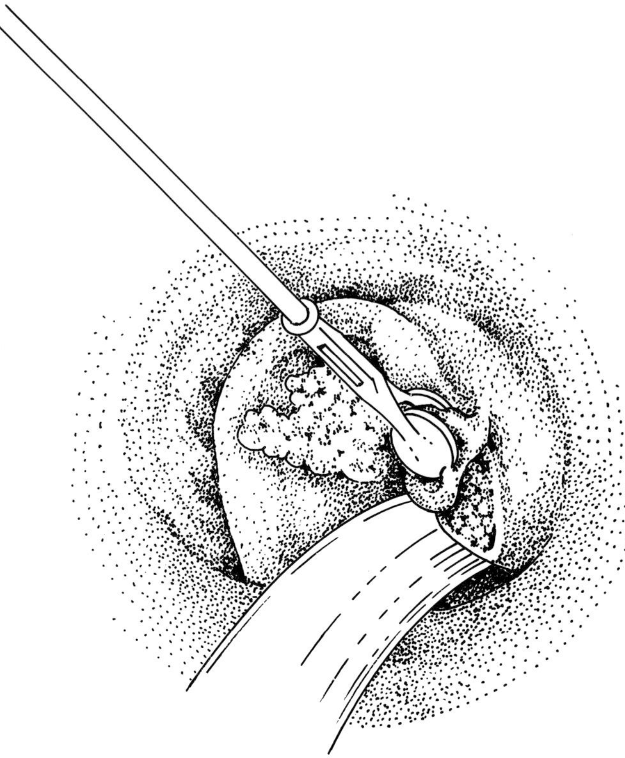

FIGURE 6–36. Excision of the epiglottis is accomplished by first starting a line of excision in the pharyngoepiglottic fold. This excision line is carried from lateral to medial. This is accomplished on both sides. When a large bore laryngoscope is used, it is often necessary to reposition the scope for each side. Caution is taken to protect the endotracheal tube and keep this out of the lines of laser excision.

When patients have a T2 N0 epiglottic lesion, treatment of the primary site and neck must be given. Standard approaches to this lesion include full course irradiation therapy to the primary lesion and the neck following endoscopic biopsy of the primary lesion. The second alternative is open partial supraglottic laryngectomy with bilateral neck dissection. Both of these techniques, if performed appropriately, lead to acceptable control and cure rates. Combined therapy for these lesions has been occasionally advocated and can be justified by the generally aggressive nature of these lesions. When such lesions extend to involve the aryepiglottic fold at the junction with the epiglottis, they can technically be resected by laser surgery as a preradiation therapy cytoreduction technique. If this is accomplished, biopsies must be taken after the lesion is excised, and this approach considered simply an excisional biopsy. Full course irradiation therapy to this area, as

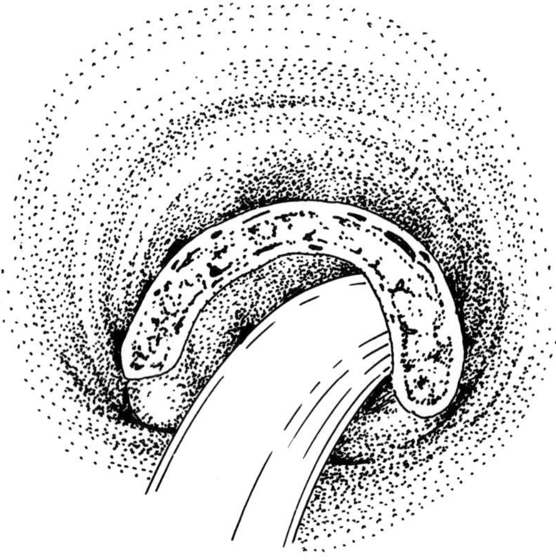

FIGURE 6–37. The transected base of the epiglottis with the indwelling endotracheal tube.

well as the neck, must then be given. Whether such an approach confers any advantage to a patient is not known. The role of the laser in this regard would be that of cytoreduction, with full course irradiation therapy supplied subsequently. As no large series have been reported using this technique, comments regarding efficacy of such treatment are at best anecdotal.

Patients with large obstructing supraglottic lesions (typically T2, T3, or T4 lesions) present significant challenges to the head and neck surgeon. Often these lesions are friable, bleed easily, and become swollen with any manipulation. With extensive lesions, intubation is difficult. Many of these patients have traditionally been treated by tracheotomy under local anesthesia followed by standard endoscopy with biopsies. Although this may be necessary in some cases, the placement of tracheotomy in this circumstance leads to a higher incidence of peristomal recurrence, and certainly leads to greater difficulty in subsequent total laryngectomy if this is appropriate.[16] Additionally, it results in all the morbidity of tracheotomy. In an earlier study by Davis and colleagues the concept of CO_2 laser debulking of such lesions for airway control was addressed.[17] This approach depends on the ability to gain airway control by intubation without tracheotomy. Airway control in this circumstance almost always requires awake intubation via either nasotracheal or orotracheal approach. Such intubation must be accomplished with a tube appropriate for laser surgery and usually requires the skills of the best trained anesthesiologist or the attending head and neck surgeon. When airway control can be gained in this manner, the laser can be used to remove enough of the obstructing neoplasm in repeated excisions to open the airway and allow safe extubation.

When patients have T1 N0 M0 lesions of the false vocal cord, these can be excised using the CO_2 laser. In great contrast to the case with T1 glottic lesions, in these lesions such excisional biopsy is not appropriate complete therapy. These lesions are in the infrahyoid portion of the supraglottis and have high propensity for regional lymphatic spread. Laser excision in this context is at best an excisional biopsy, which should lead to further therapy. Such therapy again can be either open supraglottic laryngectomy with appropriate neck dissection or, more commonly, full course irradiation therapy.

A suspicious area in the left false cord is shown in Figure 6–38. In Figure 6–39 the lines of proposed laser excision are outlined on the lesion. Figure 6–40 illustrates the lesion partially excised, with the cup forceps providing tension. Figure 6–41 shows the lesion fully excised and the true vocal cord visualized below this.

Excisional biopsies can also be performed for T1 N0 M0 lesions of the aryepiglottic fold. These lesions cannot extend more than 2 to 3 mm over the lateral edge of the aryepiglottic fold (or the medial wall of the piriform sinus). Lesions that extend beyond 5 cm in this regard actually act as hypopharyngeal tumors. Excision of aryepiglottic fold lesions can be accomplished without injury to the arytenoid cartilage when these are superficial. Any aryepiglottic fold lesion with vocal cord fixation clearly should not undergo excisional biopsy. Such cancers almost certainly escape in the lateral paraglottic space to the level of the true cord, leading to fixation, or exhibit direct arytenoid cartilage extension, which also leads to fixation. Any attempt to perform excisional biopsy of such a lesion causes glottic incompetence. Such excision also greatly oversteps the bounds of laser therapy and confers no advantage to the patient who will need to be treated by radiation or open surgery.

CONTRAINDICATIONS TO EXCISIONAL BIOPSY IN SUPRAGLOTTIS

Any supraglottic cancer with extension to the vallecula has extended beyond the realm of any laser excisional biopsy. Further, any tumor with tongue base involvement is clearly beyond benefiting from laser excision, with the exception of airway debulking. Preoperative evaluation of a clinical T2 supraglottic cancer by CT scanning is recommended. The CT scan in Figure 6–42 shows such a

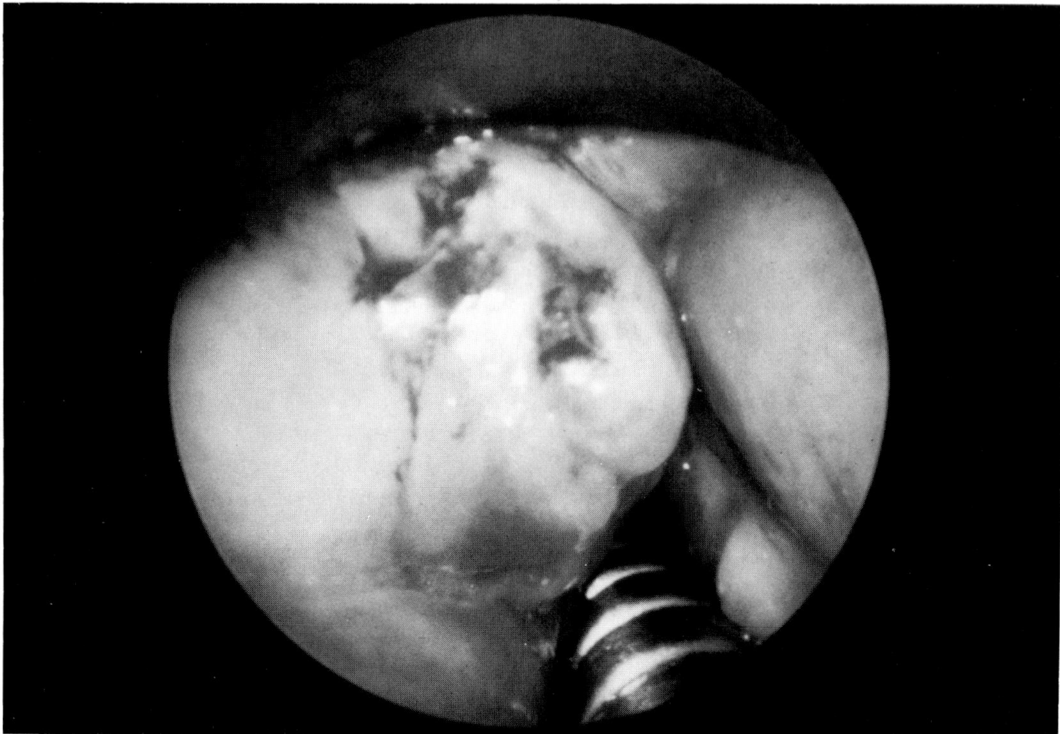

FIGURE 6–38. Areas of erythroplasia are seen in an obstructing left false vocal cord. (Patient of Dr. James Arnold.)

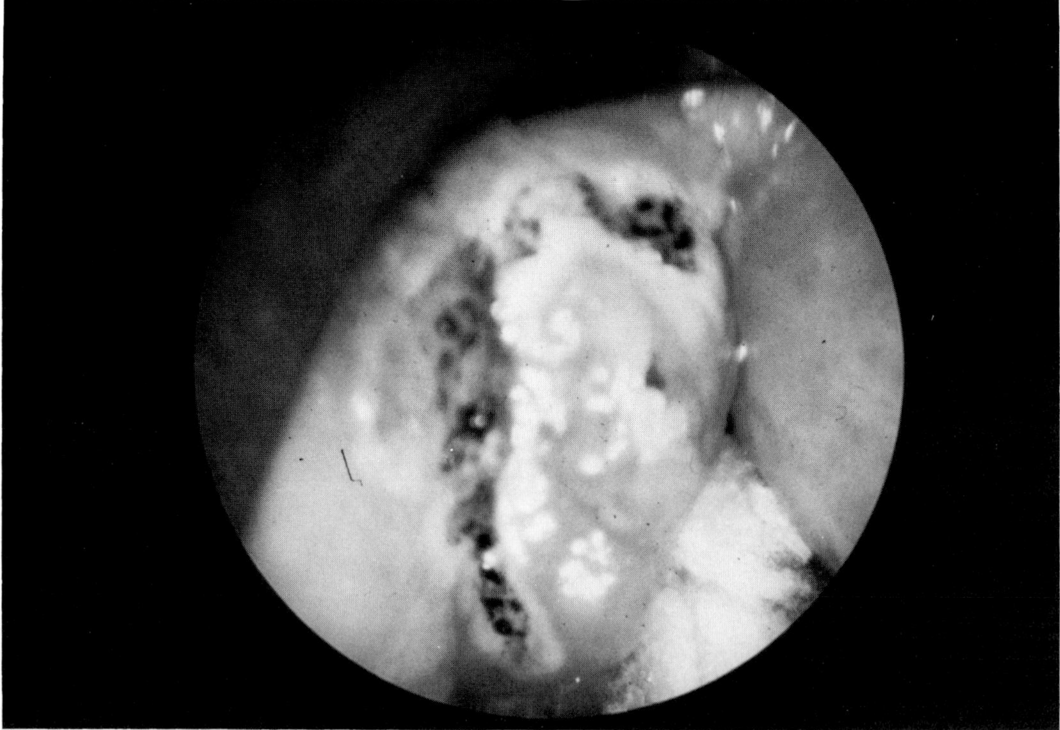

FIGURE 6–39. The false vocal cord lesion in Figure 6–38 has been outlined by the laser.

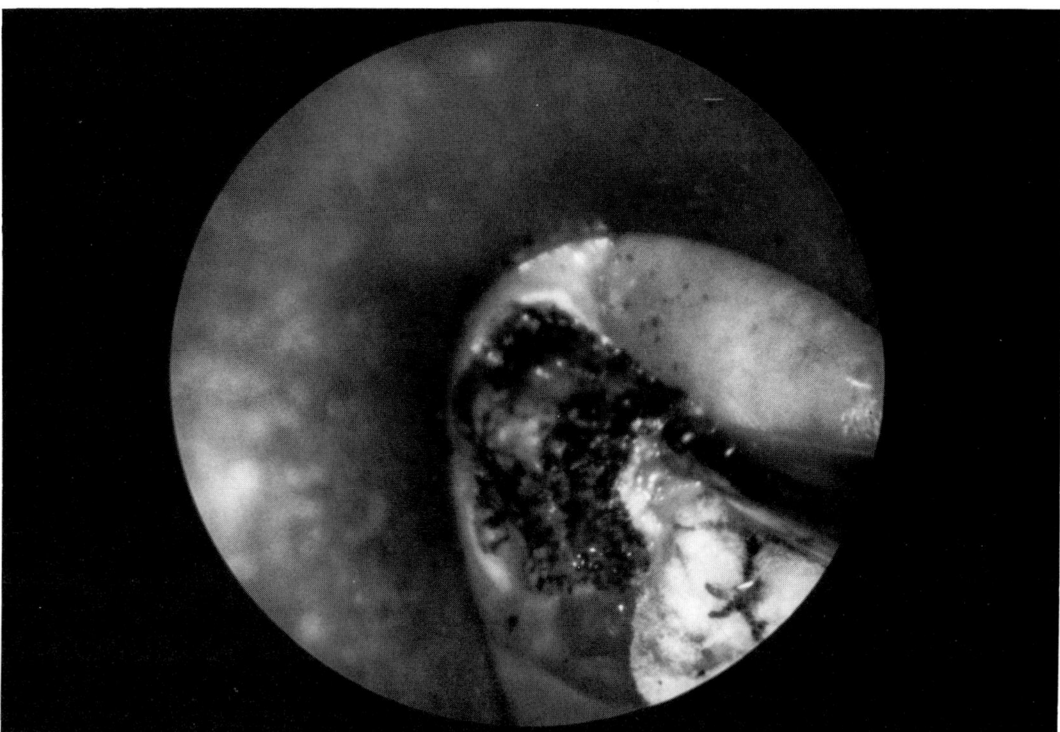

FIGURE 6–40. The lesion (Figs. 6–38 and 6–39) being grasped with a cup forceps. The surgical cottonoid is inferior to the lesion. The specimen is being retracted posteriorly.

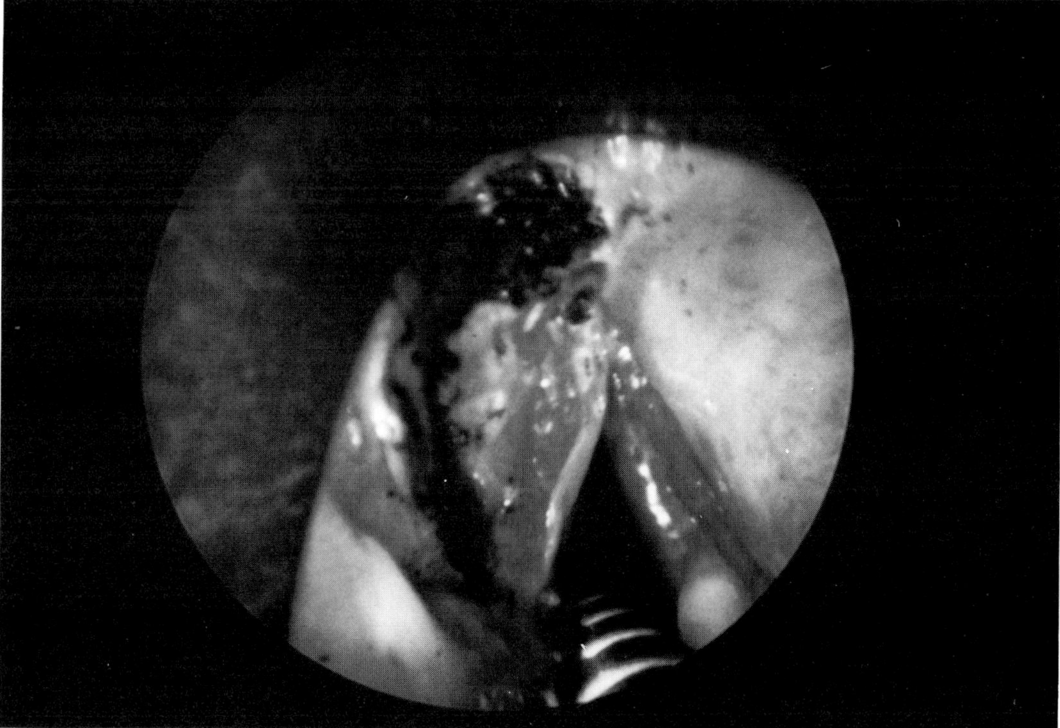

FIGURE 6–41. The false vocal cord lesion (Figs. 6–38 to 6–40) has been excised, revealing the underlying true vocal cord.

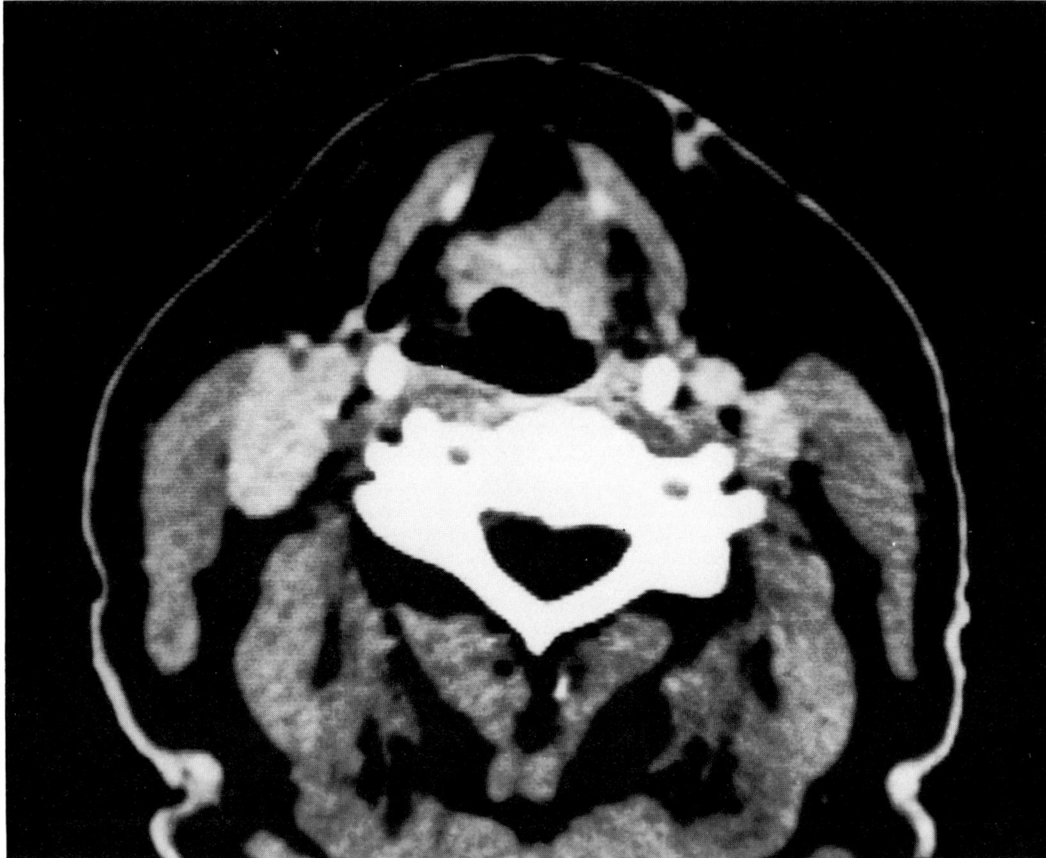

FIGURE 6–42. A CT scan clearly shows preepiglottic space involvement from a supraglottic cancer. Preepiglottic space involvement makes laser excision for cure impossible. However, bulky supraglottic lesions can be debulked, and the patient can subsequently be treated by full course irradiation or surgery as necessary.

lesion with evidence of preepiglottic space involvement. Extension to the preepiglottic space contraindicates laser surgery. As mentioned above, any patient with known vocal cord fixation from aryepiglottic fold or epiglottic cancers does not benefit by laser excision beyond partial cytoreduction for airway maintenance as well.

SPECIAL CIRCUMSTANCES OF LASER THERAPY

Careful observation is required for any patient treated for a laryngeal cancer. In some patients with early cancer of the endolarynx, follow-up visualization is difficult owing to an overlying epiglottis. Usually such problems can be circumvented by using the Hopkins rod system or the flexible nasal pharyngoscope. In exceptional circumstances in which visualization of the vocal cords is difficult with these sophisticated instruments, patients have undergone repeat direct laryngoscopy for follow-up examination. If such a situation exists, an alternative would be a limited epiglottectomy by the method described above to allow adequate visualization. This was successfully done with minimal patient morbidity in the era before development of sophisticated flexible fiberoptic instruments. It may today be of more historical interest than practical need.

Another problem with visualization of the larynx occurs in postirradiation patients. Commonly these patients have significant edema of the epiglottis and, more particularly, of the arytenoid cartilage or aryepiglottic fold area. When edema develops in the postirradiated arytenoid area, and persists for more than 6 months, there should be concern about the potential for residual tumor. In a classic article by Ward and coworkers, the presence of underlying carcinoma was found to be extremely common, mandating biopsy in this situation.[19] The CO_2 laser can be a useful adjuvant to such biopsy. If the presence of tumor has been excluded, and significant arytenoid edema persists, this edema can be easily reduced by laser excision. Such excision should be directed to the soft tissue component of the swelling and should not extend to the underlying arytenoid cartilage.

The principles of epiglottectomy and limited excision of the aryepiglottic fold can be applied to isolated conditions not due to cancer. These are not discussed in this chapter, as the surgical techniques are similar to those already illustrated. The author has had experience with several adult patients with recurrent supraglottitis. Although this can be medically managed, in rare cases supraglottic swelling persists and episodically leads to life-threatening airway obstruction. In these patients the potential airway obstruction can be obviated by a limited epiglottectomy. Epiglottitis due to other entities can also be treated in the same manner. Occasional reports document epiglottitis due to Crohn disease or other inflammatory causes. In such cases, epiglottectomy has allowed extubation in patients who are tracheotomy dependent owing to the severe supraglottic swelling. Obviously such excisions are carefully done in highly selected patients.

OTHER TREATMENT OPTIONS

Use of other medical lasers in cancer of the larynx has been extremely limited. Because of the greater absorption of the argon laser, and especially the neodymium: yttrium-aluminum-garnet (Nd:YAG) laser in tissue, these lasers will unlikely have a significant role in the treatment of early laryngeal cancer. Concern over adjacent tissue damage and subsequent airway edema and obstruction would need to be circumvented to allow clinical use of these lasers. This seems at this time highly unlikely. The use of photodynamic therapy with appropriate photosensitizers also seems unlikely, as the immediate tissue effects of these modalities include edema. Treating carcinoma in situ or tiny T1 glottic cancers by phototherapy is a theoretic possibility, but probably will not confer advantage beyond that already available with the CO_2 laser or other standard techniques.

References

1. Strong MS, Jako GJ: Laser surgery in the larynx. Ann Otol Rhinol Laryngol 81:791, 1972.
2. Jako GJ: Laser surgery of the vocal cords. Laryngoscope 82:2204, 1972.
3. Strong MS: Laser excision of carcinoma of the larynx. Laryngoscope 85:1286, 1985.
4. Schechter GL: Conservation surgery of the larynx. *In* Cummings CW (ed): Otolaryngology–Head and Neck Surgery. St Louis, CV Mosby 1986, p 2095.
5. Miller D: Cryosurgery as a modality in the treatment of carcinoma of the larynx. Laryngoscope 85:1281, 1975.
6. Kaplan MJ, Johns ME, Fitz-Hugh GS, et al.: Stage II glottic carcinoma: Prognostic factors and management. Laryngoscope 93:725, 1983.
7. Lillie JC, DeSanto LW: Transoral surgery of early cordal carcinoma. Trans Am Acad Ophthalmol Otolaryngol 77:92, 1973.
8. Biller HF, Lawson W: Partial laryngectomy for vocal cord cancer with marked limitation or fixation of the vocal cord. Laryngoscope 96:61, 1986.
9. Vaughan CW, Strong MS, Jako GJ: Laryngeal carcinoma: Transoral treatment utilizing the CO_2 laser. Am J Surg 136:490, 1978.
10. Davis RK, Jako GJ, Hyams VJ, Shapshay SM: The anatomical limitations of CO_2 laser cordectomy. Laryngoscope 92:980, 1982.
11. Kirchner JA, Cornog JL, Holmes RE: Transglottic cancer: Its growth and spread within the larynx. Arch Otolaryngol 99:247, 1974.
12. Wang CC: Treatment of glottic carcinoma by mega voltage radiation therapy and results. Am J Roentgenol 120:157, 1974.
13. Abramson AL, Brandsma J, Steinberg B, Winkler B: Verrucous carcinoma of the larynx. Arch Otolaryngol 111:709, 1985.

14. Edstrom S, Johansson SL, Lindstrom J, Sandin I: Verrucous squamous cell carcinoma of the larynx; evidence for increased metastatic potential after irradiation. Otolaryngol Head Neck Surg 97:381, 1987.

15. Blakeslee D, Vaughan CW, Shapshay SM, et. al.: Excisional biopsy in the selective management of T1 glottic cancers: A three-year follow-up study. Laryngoscope 94:488, 1984.

16. Davis RK, Shapshay SM, Strong MS, Hyams VJ: Transoral partial supraglottic resection using the CO_2 laser. Laryngoscope 93:429, 1983.

17. Davis RK, Shapshay SM: Peristomal recurrence: Pathophysiology, prevention, treatment. Otolaryngol Clin North Am 13:449, 1980.

18. Davis RK, Shapshay SM, Vaughan CW, Strong MS: Pretreatment airway management in obstructing carcinoma of the larynx. Otolaryngol Head Neck Surg 89:209, 1981.

19. Ward PH, Calcaterra TC, Kagan AR: The enigma of the postradiation edema and recurrent or residual carcinoma of the larynx. Laryngoscope 85:522, 1975.

CHAPTER 7

LASER BRONCHOSCOPY

Stanley M. Shapshay

Endoscopic diagnosis and therapy of airway disorders have undergone dramatic changes since the development of fiberoptics and laser technology in the past 10 to 15 years. Just as the introduction of the flexible fiberoptic bronchoscope revolutionized diagnostic bronchoscopy and some aspects of therapeutic bronchoscopy, the development of various lasers has extended the capabilities of endoscopic therapy. Combining flexible laser fibers with fiberoptic bronchoscopes has become a reality, particularly with the neodymium:yttrium-aluminum-garnet (Nd:YAG), argon, 532 nm potassium-titanyl-phosphate (KTP-532), and argon dye lasers, but not, unfortunately, with the precise carbon dioxide (CO_2) laser, which cannot be passed through flexible quartz fibers. However, for certain conditions, such as malignant obstruction of the proximal tracheobronchial airway, modified ventilating rigid bronchoscopes of various designs have been extremely useful.

In 1974, Strong and coworkers reported the first laser application in the tracheobronchial tree using a CO_2 laser with a prototypal coupling device.[1] Although this coupling device did not have an aiming and steering mechanism, it was still useful in the treatment of 15 patients (70 bronchoscopic procedures). The CO_2 laser beam was centered down a specially modified rigid bronchoscope, with two thumbscrews controlling the position of the laser beam. Difficulties with beam alignment were found with the smaller pediatric bronchoscopes, and, occasionally, bouncing of the beam within the bronchoscope resulted in dangerous heating of the metallic instrument. Additional limitations associated with the CO_2 coupler system included the lack of a flexible fiberoptic fiber, a dependence on the clumsy articulated arm system intrinsic to the CO_2 laser system, and the limitation of hemostasis to blood vessels of 0.5 mm or less in outer diameter (i.e., capillary blood supply); also, the excellent absorption of the CO_2 in a liquid medium mandated a dry operative field.

Because of the limitations associated with the CO_2 laser in bronchoscopy, an attempt was made to use the argon laser because of its readily available mode of fiberoptic transmission.[2] Unfortunately, unpredictable soft tissue interaction with the argon laser limited its clinical application. Superficial photocoagulation of vascular lesions seemed to be the most appropriate use for the argon laser.

The Nd:YAG laser was introduced in the late 1970s for the treatment of patients with various conditions of the tracheobronchial tree. Initial reports from Toty and associates[3] and Dumon and associates[4] documented the apparent advantages of the Nd:YAG laser, namely excellent hemostasis and an ability to pass readily through available flexible quartz fibers. Since its introduction, this laser has been used extensively by investigators throughout the world both for the palliation of obstructing malignant tumors and for the treatment of benign lesions.[5-7] The major limitations of the Nd:YAG laser, however, soon became apparent: there were unpredictable soft tissue effects and poorly controlled coagulation of deep vessels, especially when compared with those achieved with the more precise CO_2 laser.[8]

Developments in laser bronchoscopy have included contact probes that attach to the Nd:YAG laser fiber and increase the power density for cutting and coagulation[8] (Figs. 7–1, 7–2). Although more precise application of the Nd:YAG laser is possible with these contact probes, which are of different geometric shapes for cutting and coagulation, the endoscopist has greater visibility when using a noncontact mode. It is impossible to visualize directly the degree of tissue damage created by laser impact using the contact probe until the damage is already done.

Another development in laser bronchoscopy has been the use of the KTP-532 laser. The 532 nm KTP wavelength is close to the spectrum of the argon laser; therefore, the same type of tissue interaction is expected. Like the argon laser wavelength, the 532 nm wavelength can be passed through a small quartz fiber (200 microns), which increases power density to permit cutting as well as coagulation. This achieves a compromise between the more precise cutting effects of the CO_2 laser and the superior coagulating properties of the *noncontact* Nd:YAG laser. Both the argon and KTP-532 laser wavelengths are best absorbed by pigment, especially red, which delays their initial absorption by light-colored lesions until desiccation and charring take place.

The application of photodynamic therapy in the tracheobronchial tree continues to be of interest to the bronchologist. Photosensitization of tumors with light-sensitive biologic dyes provides the endoscopist with a highly selective therapy for destroying tumor cells while sparing the normal surrounding tissue. Good tumoricidal effects have been reported by Cortese and Kinsey[9] and others,[10,11] especially with early tumors. Patients with a large bulky obstruction of the airway

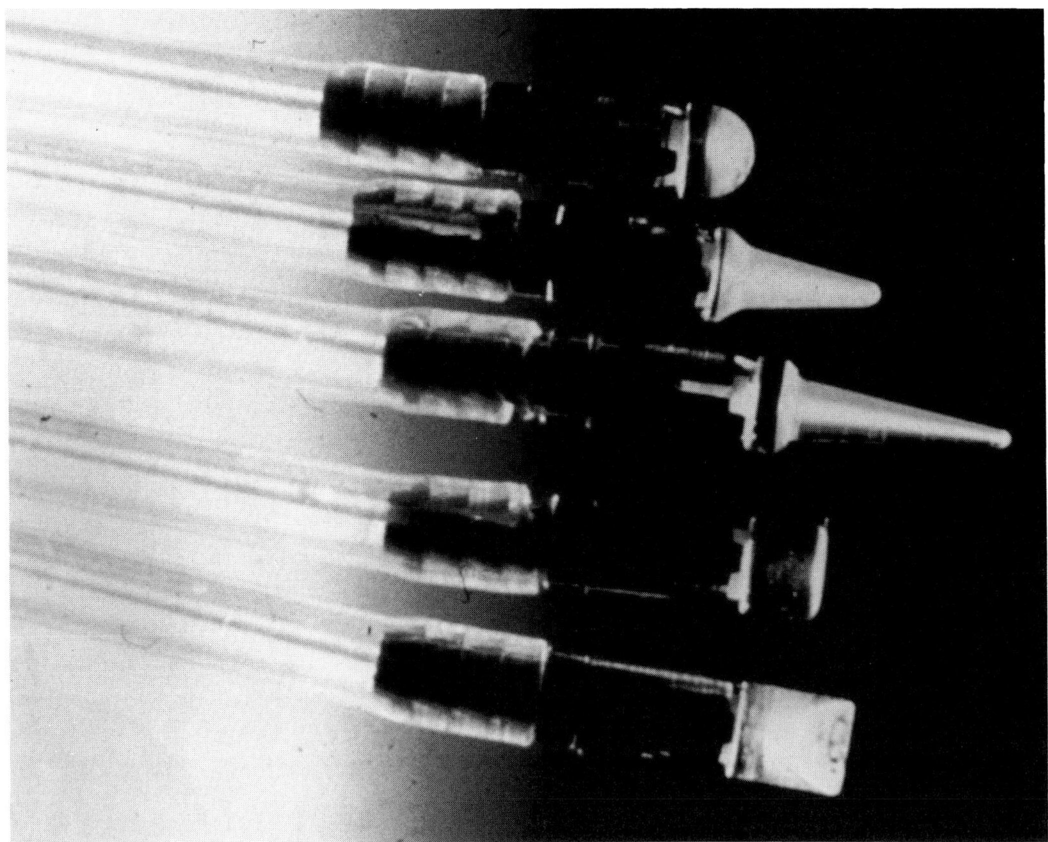

FIGURE 7–1. Artificial sapphire contact tips of different geometric shapes are seen attached to Nd:YAG fibers. The pointed and conical tips are used for cutting, and the flat tips are used for coagulation. (From Shapshay SM: Laser applications in the trachea and bronchi: A comparative study of the soft tissue effects using contact and noncontact delivery systems. Laryngoscope 97[suppl 41]:3, 1987.)

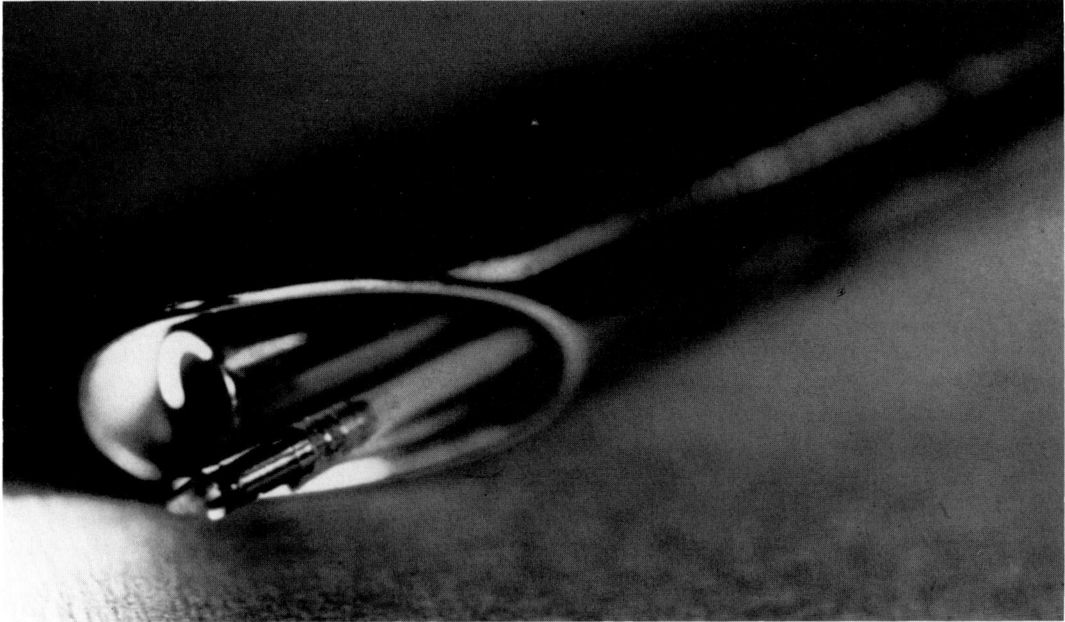

FIGURE 7–2. The distal end of a rigid laser bronchoscopic system. A contact probe is seen with a rigid 0 degree telescope and a semirigid polyethylene suction catheter.

may later require a débriding bronchoscopic procedure for removal of necrotic tumor and debris. Detection of early cancers using a fluorescence technique and subsequent stimulation with a cytotoxic wavelength (630 nm) have been reported to achieve long-term control of early cancers.[9] This effect appears to be the greatest benefit of photodynamic therapy in the tracheobronchial tree. Massive hemorrhage resulting from perforation of the pulmonary artery has occurred after treatment of patients with large bulky tumors involving the paratracheal tissue and the walls of the major blood vessels.

This chapter presents the indications, contraindications, and techniques for using laser technology in the tracheobronchial tree. Major emphasis is placed on the CO_2 and Nd:YAG lasers because their wavelengths are the most commonly used in bronchoscopic applications. In addition, the avoidance of complications and methods of treatment should they occur are considered.

ANATOMIC CONSIDERATIONS

Although the bronchoscopist is expected to know the anatomy of the tracheobronchial tree observed endoscopically, it is also important to have considerable knowledge of the relationships of the large blood vessels of the mediastinum and the airway (Fig. 7–3). Pathologic conditions, such as tracheobronchial cancer, as well as distortions of the anatomy by previous surgery or radiation therapy, complicate therapeutic bronchoscopy.[12]

Trachea. From a vascular point of view, treatment of lesions of the cervical trachea can be accomplished with relative safety. The thoracic trachea, however, descends through the upper third of the thorax, where it has multiple and close relationships with the large blood vessels of the mediastinum.

Arch of Aorta. The arch of the aorta passes on the left anterior aspect of the trachea, making a definite imprint. From the curvature of the arch arises the innominate artery, tightly pressed onto the trachea and passing from left to right toward the base of the neck. The *azygos vein* winds around the right side of the distal trachea before joining the superior vena cava. The *esophagus* lies

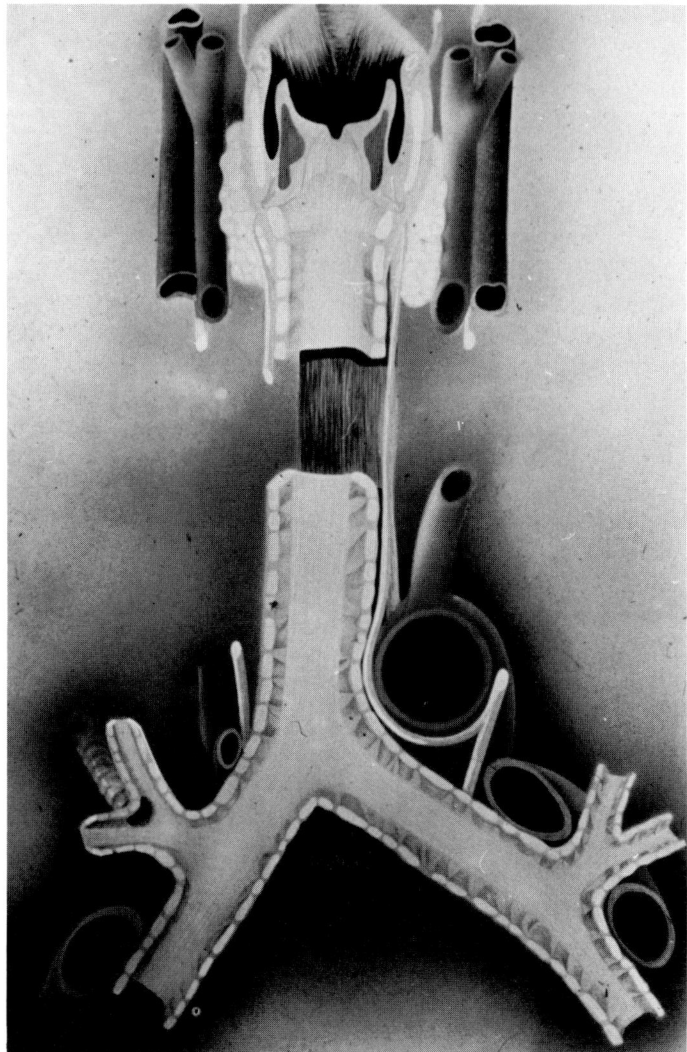

FIGURE 7–3. The vascular relationships in tracheobronchial anatomy. Note the danger areas for the endoscopist: the left distal trachea (innominate artery) and the bronchi of the left upper lobe (pulmonary veins).

in continual close contact with the posterior aspect of the cervical and thoracic tracheal segments. The *left recurrent laryngeal nerve* originates under the arch of the aorta and runs up to the cricoid cartilage in the tracheoesophageal groove. The *right recurrent laryngeal nerve* meets the trachea in the cervical region at the level of the sixth cartilaginous ring.

Carina of Trachea and Mainstem Bronchi. The right main bronchus branches off at a 20 to 30 degree angle from the trachea, and the left main bronchus lies at a 40 to 50 degree angle. Thus, the right main bronchus is more vertical and is easier to intubate with the rigid bronchoscope. Laser applications in the left main bronchus are further hampered because it is longer than the right bronchus (5 cm versus 2.5 cm) and smaller in diameter (11 mm versus 15 mm).

The left main bronchus has more anatomic danger zones than the right main bronchus. The *esophagus* adheres to the first 2 cm of the left bronchus on its posterior aspect; the *arch of the aorta* drapes over it at the front and back; the *bifurcation* of the right and left pulmonary arteries is closely situated to the left main bronchus; and the *pulmonary vein* makes contact at the root of the left upper lobar bronchus. The right main bronchus has the *right pulmonary artery* crossing above it at the level of the right upper lobar bronchus.

Pulmonary Lobes. Treatment of patients with lesions of the left upper pulmonary lobes is risky. Because of its nearly vertical position, the lobe is difficult to intubate with a bronchoscope.

In addition, the pulmonary vein wraps around the back and sides of the left upper lobar bronchus and the pulmonary artery passes over the front.

LASER DELIVERY SYSTEMS

Carbon Dioxide Laser

Until recently, the only option for application of the CO_2 laser was to use a bronchoscopic coupler. The coupling device permitted joining of the articulating arm of the CO_2 laser to a specially modified rigid bronchoscopic system (Fig. 7–4). In 1982, Ossoff and Karlan described their clinical experience using a universal endoscopic coupler for CO_2 laser surgery.[13] This instrument provided direct coaxial vision because the invisible CO_2 laser beam permitted simultaneous transmission of the helium-neon aiming light down the lumen of the bronchoscope, with minimal distortion. Surgeons were able to visualize the precise area of tissue to be vaporized by the invisible wavelength. Included in this set-up was a continuous variable defocusing lens system for laser incision, vaporization, and coagulation. With this system surgeons could vary the spot size of the laser beam as needed. A quick on-off centering screw was designed to facilitate coaxial alignment and disengagement of the bronchoscope from the coupler. Because it weighed only 1 pound, the surgeon was able to grasp the coupler and the attached bronchoscope easily in one hand and perform the bronchoscopic laser procedure in the same fashion as conventional bronchoscopy. A set of custom-designed laser bronchoscopes was used with the universal endoscopic coupler.

Most recently, hollow waveguides able to transmit the CO_2 laser beam have been used on an experimental basis in an attempt to eliminate the bronchoscopic coupling system. Unfortunately, a suitable flexible fiberoptic fiber that is able to transmit the CO_2 laser in flexible fiberoptic bronchoscopes has not yet been developed. Early clinical experience with CO_2 laser waveguides at the Lahey Clinic Medical Center has been encouraging. One advantage of the waveguide transmission

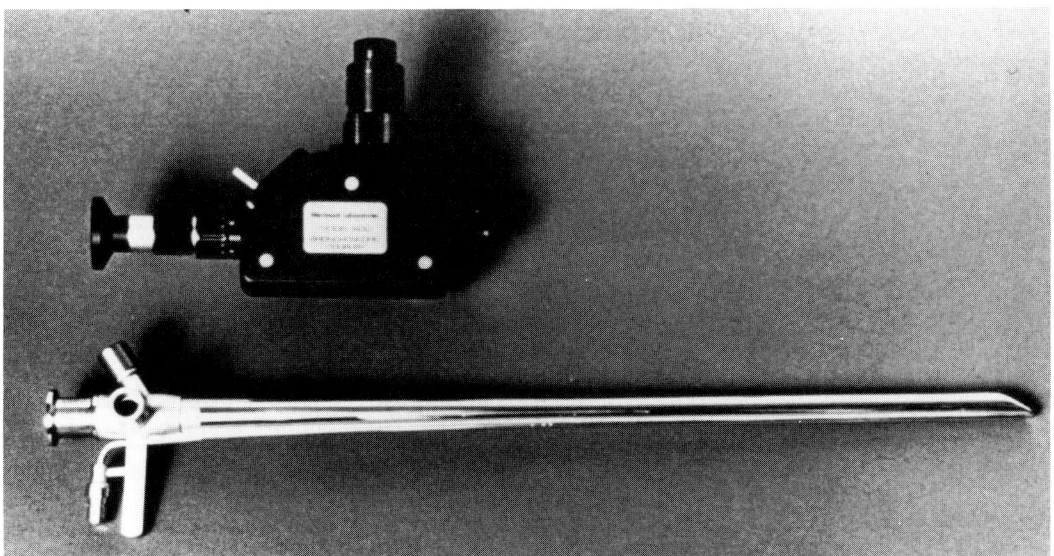

Figure 7–4. The CO_2 laser coupling device *(top)* and a specially prepared ventilating rigid bronchoscope *(bottom)*. The coupling device provides quick on-off attachment to the bronchoscope and also features a convenient aiming device (joystick control) and proximal magnification. (From Shapshay SM: Laser applications in the trachea and bronchi: A comparative study of the soft tissue effects using contact and noncontact delivery systems. Laryngoscope 97(suppl 41):3, 1987).

is the ability to use an open rigid bronchoscopic system rather than a closed coupled system. An open bronchoscopic system gives the bronchoscopist the excellent optics associated with rigid telescopes and permits the simultaneous use of flexible suction catheters to maintain a dry operative field. Unfortunately, the waveguides presently used are rigid, and an appreciable loss of laser power occurs when they are bent. Present waveguides can be as small as 1 mm in outside diameter, but they are still somewhat clumsy to use because of their rigidity and their dependence, again, on an articulated arm system.

Neodymium: Yttrium-Aluminum-Garnet Laser

A flexible quartz fiber approximately 2 mm in diameter can be passed through either a flexible or a rigid bronchoscope. Rigid bronchoscopes of various designs have been specialized for laser fiber application, permitting simultaneous use of flexible suction catheters, laser fibers, and a rigid telescope with either an open or a closed ventilating system (Figs. 7–5, 7–6). The advantages of using a rigid bronchoscope are that it allows secure ventilation, the rapid evacuation of blood clots and secretions through the use of one or two suction catheters, a nonflammable system, palpation of the cartilage-tumor interface, tamponade of bleeding on the tumor surface, the use of a débriding device after photocoagulation, and the use of telescopic optics. The disadvantages of the rigid bronchoscope, compared with flexible fiberoptic bronchoscopes, are limited access to the bronchi of the left main, distal, and upper lobes and the need for general anesthesia.

The advantages of a flexible fiberoptic bronchoscopic system include the ability to perform operations easily with patients under local anesthesia and ready access to upper lobar and distal endobronchial tumors. The disadvantages of the flexible delivery system include a lack of ventilatory control of the compromised airway, minimal suction capability simultaneously with laser use,

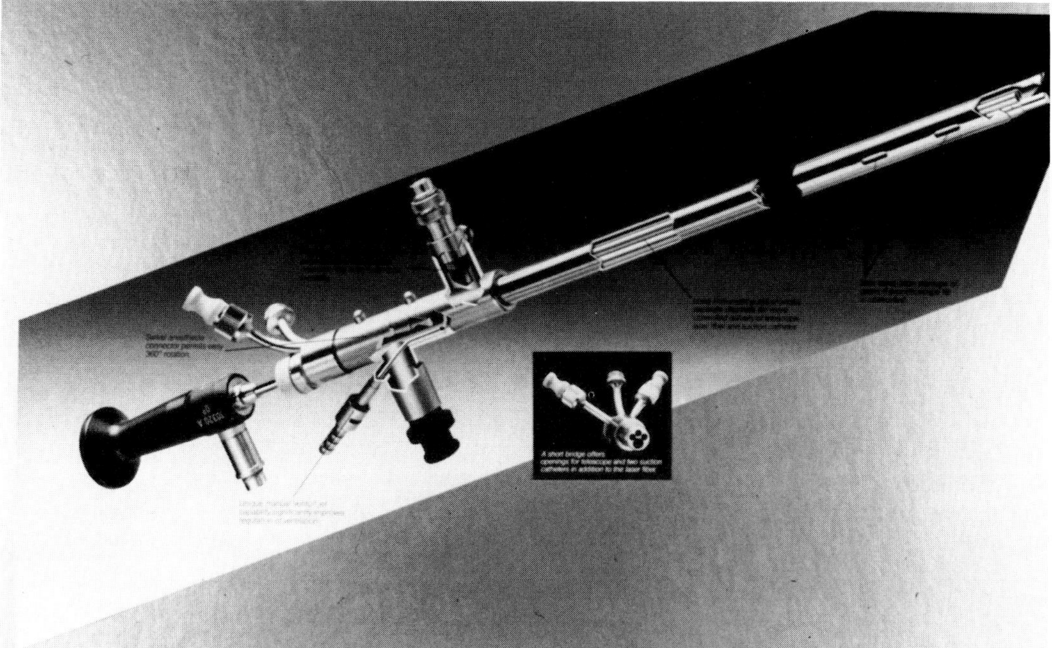

FIGURE 7–5. Universal ventilating bronchoscopic system with a rigid laser fiber. Special features include a retractable prismatic light deflector attached to the bronchoscope, Venturi or side port ventilation attachments, and closed ports for insertion of the laser fiber and suction catheters.

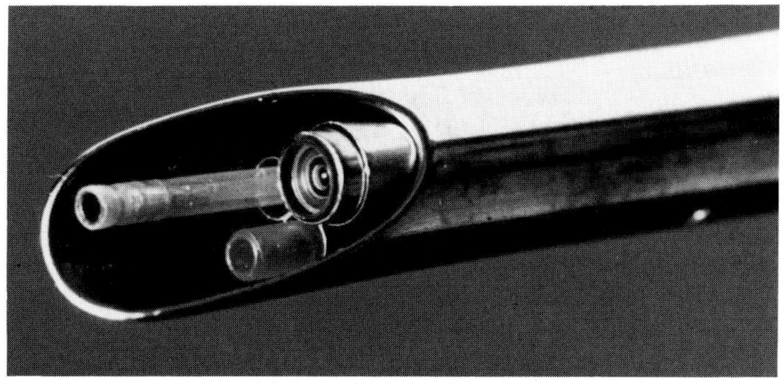

FIGURE 7–6. Distal view of the laser bronchoscope shows the telescope, laser fiber, and suction catheter delivered through an insertion sheath (long bridge). (From Shapshay SM, Beamis JF Jr, MacDonald E: A new rigid bronchoscope for laser fiber application. Otolaryngol Head Neck Surg 96:203, 1987.)

an inability to palpate the tumor at its cartilaginous interface, inefficient evacuation of tumor fragments and debris compared with the open rigid bronchoscopic system, inability to compress the bleeding tumor bed, and risk of igniting the plastic covering of the bronchoscope.[14]

ANESTHESIA AND VENTILATION TECHNIQUES

Often, the use of a rigid bronchoscopic system necessitates the administration of general anesthesics. Although local anesthesia is not contraindicated, the degree of manipulation necessary and the cough reflex, particularly near the carina, usually dictate use of a general rather than a local anesthetic. Before manipulation of the airway, a detailed discussion between the surgeon and the anesthesiologic team is mandatory. The ventilation technique chosen (i.e., spontaneous versus controlled) depends a great deal on the location and degree of the existing lesion. For high grade obstruction from upper tracheal tumors, spontaneous respiration with topical anesthesia is preferred, using 4 per cent lidocaine (Xylocaine) supplemented by intravenous sedation with midazolam (Versed) with titration using fentanyl (Sublimaze) or droperidol (Innovar) as indicated. Patients may require intermittent assisted ventilation if intravenous sedation interferes with spontaneous respiration. For tumors of the distal trachea and main bronchi, a muscle relaxation technique is preferred to ensure cough suppression and controlled ventilation. Atracurium besylate (Tracrium) is currently the muscle relaxant of choice. Venturi jet ventilation (Karl Storz Endoscopy-America, Inc, Culver City, CA) provides an open bronchoscopic system for rapid insertion of instruments and evacuation of tumor fragments and blood clots (Fig. 7–7).

After induction of general anesthesia and adequate relaxation, a specially prepared rigid bronchoscope for laser fiber application (Karl Storz Endoscopy-America) is introduced into the tracheal airway. The Venturi injector is attached to the side arm of the bronchoscope. Adequacy of ventilation is determined by visual inspection of chest excursion and by auscultation. Oxygen (100 per cent at 50 pounds/in^2) powers the Venturi system. The fractional concentration of inspired oxygen (Fi_{O_2}) of the Venturi jet is not lowered during treatment; however, the procedure must be performed with a closed system to prevent fire. Room air drawn in by the Venturi system dilutes the Fi_{O_2} sufficiently to reduce this hazard. With the exception of the laser fiber itself and the heat-resistant semiflexible polyethylene catheters, none of the instruments used in the airway is susceptible to combustion. Oxygenation is monitored constantly with the use of a finger pulse oximeter. With the laser fiber and one or two suction catheters in place and a 0 degree telescope inserted through the proximal open end of the bronchoscope, blood, smoke, and tumor fragments are easily and rapidly removed. Alternatively, rigid laser bronchoscopy can also be performed with side port ventilation as the anesthetic technique; however, a closed system must be used. The most common method of sealing the leak at the level of the vocal cords is to pack the oral pharynx with moist sponges. Using an inflatable rubber cuff around the bronchoscope is potentially dangerous because of its flammability.

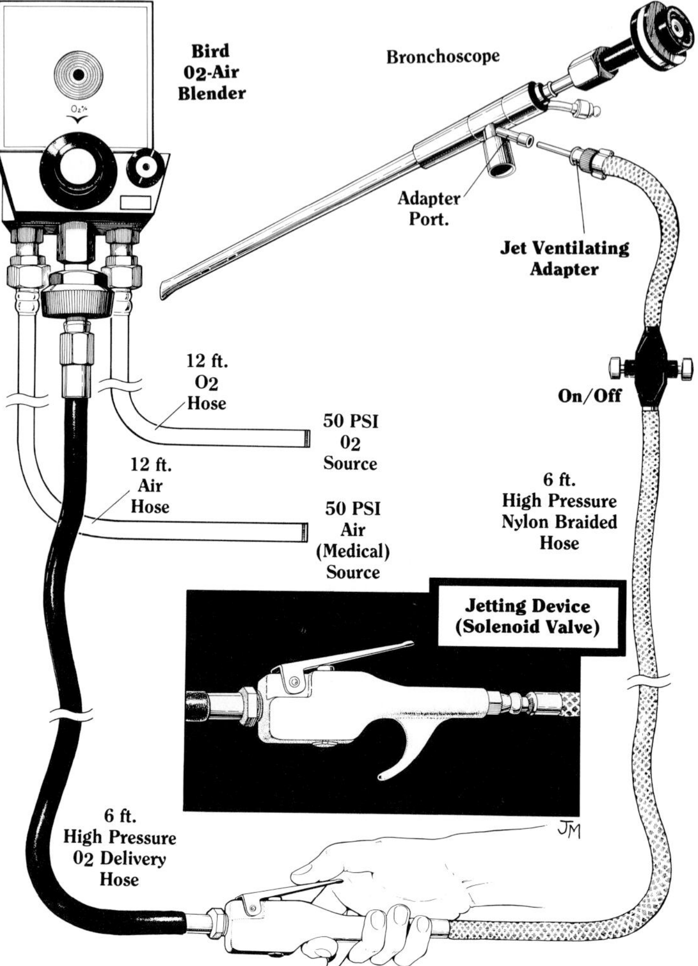

FIGURE 7–7. Venturi jet ventilation system attached to a rigid bronchoscope for laser endoscopy. An oxygen blender reduces the FI_{O_2}, lessening the hazard of fire in the operating environment.

When using the flexible bronchoscope with the Nd:YAG laser fiber, the administration of topical lidocaine and intravenous midazolam hydrochloride is the safest means of inducing anesthesia. A transnasal approach is used, thus avoiding the use of an endotracheal tube and minimizing the chance of fire. Patients breathe spontaneously and receive oxygen by nasal prongs. This technique is usually performed on an outpatient basis with careful cardiac and oxygen saturation monitoring. The procedure is usually reserved for patients who have small lesions with no major airway obstruction.

A video system with a small chip camera on the proximal aspect of the telescope is routinely used and provides excellent documentation. More important, it gives the anesthesiologist and nursing personnel first-hand knowledge of what is happening within the airway, enabling them to coordinate their work with that of the endoscopist.

INDICATIONS, CONTRAINDICATIONS, AND PATHOLOGIC CHANGES

The tracheobronchial condition most frequently encountered is lung cancer, with the most common types being squamous cell carcinoma, adenocarcinoma, and large cell carcinoma. Patients with small cell carcinoma are not usually treated with laser bronchoscopy because alternative means, such as chemotherapy and radiation therapy, are usually effective. A review of the author's experience at the Lahey Clinic Medical Center during 6 years (1982 to 1988) revealed that 222 patients with tracheobronchial tumors underwent 241 laser bronchoscopy treatments. Four patients went on to have open tracheal resection of their tumors. Excluding cases of granulation tissue, Wegener granulomatosis, and sarcoidosis, recurrent respiratory papillomatosis was the benign neoplasm most commonly found (six patients). The most common malignant neoplasm encountered was lung cancer with tracheobronchial obstruction (180 patients). Primary tracheal tumors, such as adenoid cystic carcinoma, squamous cell carcinoma, lymphoma, and carcinoid tumor, were encountered in 16 patients. Twenty-one patients had tracheobronchial metastases from other primary sites, such as the colon, the esophagus, the kidney, the breast, and the thyroid. The most common upper tracheal carcinoma was cancer of the larynx with subglottic extension into the upper trachea (four patients).

The Nd:YAG laser provides the preferred wavelength for malignant neoplasms because these tumors have a greater *propensity* for hemorrhage. The wavelength of the CO_2 laser is preferred for recurrent respiratory papillomatosis of the larynx and the upper trachea, as well as for benign tracheal strictures. It is important to remember that the goal of laser bronchoscopy, particularly for malignant tumors, is palliation of airway obstruction, relief of pneumonitis due to obstruction, and control of tracheobronchial hemorrhage. Palliation is the key focus because patients with early and potentially curable carcinoma of the airway should be treated with open operation or radiation therapy.

Intermediate tumors, such as carcinoid and adenoid cystic carcinoma, are also good indications for endoscopic laser application, especially with the Nd:YAG laser. Carcinoid tumor, when resectable, should be removed by sleeve resection rather than endoscopic laser therapy. Cartilaginous invasion is usually present with carcinoid tumors, necessitating complete resection of the tracheal wall as curative treatment. A so-called iceberg effect occurs in which only the tip of the tumor presents endotracheally, with the rest of the mass in the mediastinum. These tumors are notorious for their high degree of vascularity.

The adenoid cystic carcinoma is less vascular than the carcinoid tumor; however, it is known for submucosal extension. Commonly, long segments of the tracheal wall are affected, frustrating attempts at curative resection. Involvement of margins is not uncommon when these tumors are approached surgically. Fortunately, adenoid cystic carcinoma is a slow-growing mass, and the potential exists for long-term palliation.

LASER APPLICATIONS

Metastases to Trachea

Although bronchoscopy using the Nd:YAG laser can generally be performed for palliative purposes, thyroid and renal carcinomas should be approached with a high degree of caution because of their extremely vascular nature. Both of these tumors—thyroid carcinoma by direct extension and renal carcinoma by metastatic spread—can be extremely dangerous because of the potential for hemorrhage. Defocusing the laser fiber at least 1 to 2 cm from the tumor mass and using the suction catheter to move the tumor about so that thorough photocoagulation can be achieved are necessary before manipulation and subsequent débridement are attempted. Two suction catheters should be available for rapid clearance of blood and secretions.

Esophageal carcinoma with tracheal extension is associated with a poor survival rate. It is the author's policy not to treat such patients because the prognosis is poor and because the nature of the obstruction is submucosal extrinsic compression from the invading esophageal cancer. Treatment is suggested when the invasion of cancer into the trachea is exophytic in nature.

The characteristics of lesions that are most favorable for successful Nd:YAG laser bronchoscopy are endobronchial intraluminal tumor growth, a polypoid growth pattern, a visible distal lumen, a length of obstruction of less than 4 cm, confinement to the tracheal and primary bronchi, and a functioning lung distal to the tumor obstruction. Unfavorable bronchoscopic characteristics include total bronchial obstruction; external airway compression; extensive submucosal disease; a length of obstruction of greater than 4 cm; a lobar or a segmental tumor, especially of the left upper and right upper lobes; and chronic collapse of the lobe or lung. The only absolute contraindication for Nd:YAG laser bronchoscopy is extrinsic compression of the airway, although other unfavorable situations include esophageal carcinoma with extension into the trachea by submucosal invasion and compression, carinal recurrence of tumor after pneumonectomy, tumor-induced tracheobronchial fistula, and, by computed tomography (CT) preoperative assessment, identification of tumor invasion into a major mediastinal blood vessel. The most important evaluations before laser application include conventional linear tomography, which has been helpful in localizing the area of obstruction and demonstrating the characteristics of lesions, and determination of the patency of the distal airway (Fig. 7–8). Routine CT of the chest has not been carried out. Although CT may demonstrate mediastinal anatomy, the airway is not defined well enough in a linear dimension for CT scans to be of value to the bronchoscopist. In general, pumonary function testing, such as with

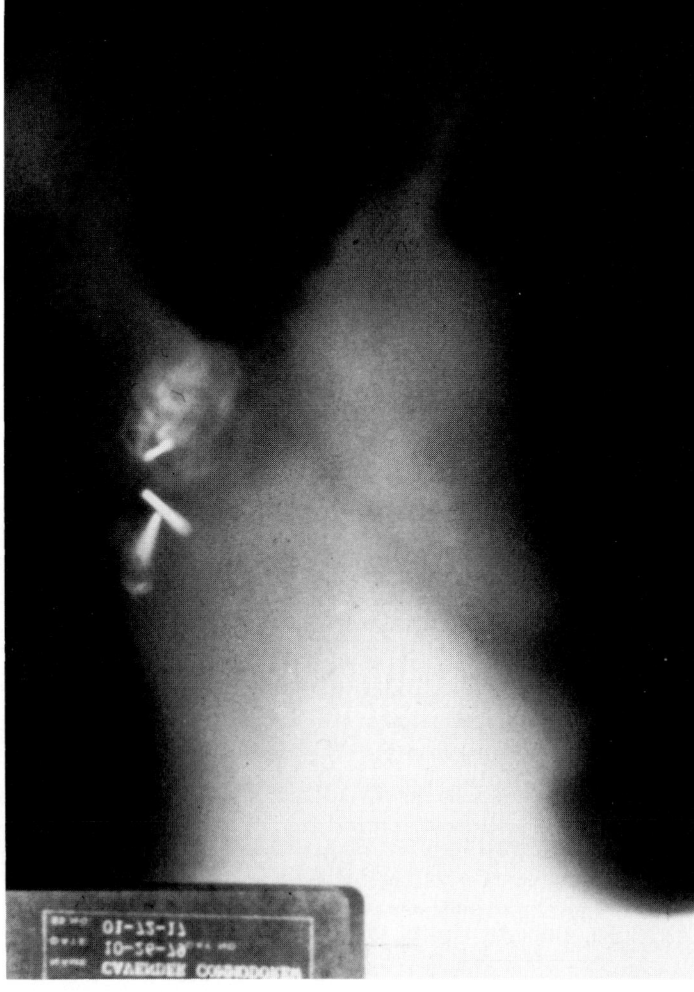

FIGURE 7–8. Tomographic scan of chest reveals extensive compression of both main bronchi by a large mediastinal mass. Radiotherapy failed to control inoperable carcinoma of the lung. This patient was not a candidate for laser palliation.

flow volume loops, has not proved helpful in predicting the need for or outcome of laser therapy. Routine evaluation of baseline arterial blood gas levels is necessary before laser bronchoscopy to assess the need for oxygen therapy before, during, and after the procedure. Routine posteroanterior and lateral radiography of the chest are helpful in evaluating the location and extent of the tumor and the amount of potentially functioning lung distal to the obstruction. The most important assessment is determination of the nature and extent of the obstructing lesion by preoperative fiberoptic bronchoscopy. Often, the distal airway can also be evaluated.

Benign Lesions

Recurrent respiratory papillomatosis is the most frequently encountered benign pathologic condition of the laryngotracheal area (Fig. 7–9). Carbon dioxide laser therapy remains the treatment of choice for patients with this disease (Fig. 7–10), particularly when it occurs in the larynx, where precision is important to preserve laryngeal function. Precise removal of papillomas through the mucosa and submucosa, carefully avoiding injury to the underlying muscles of the vocal cord, is the goal of treatment. The Nd:YAG laser has been useful for more diffuse sessile papillomatosis occurring in the middle to distal trachea beyond the reach of the operating laryngoscope. In fact, the Nd:YAG laser is used to "paint" the sessile lesions with low power defocused laser energy (20 watts) at 0.5 to 1 second exposures. The goal is to photocoagulate the lesion without disturbing the underlying cartilaginous framework. Use of the CO_2 laser may actually be dangerous in cases of tracheal perforation, whereas the Nd:YAG wavelength is preferentially absorbed by the more vascular papilloma rather than the underlying avascular cartilage. Every attempt should be made to avoid tracheotomy in these patients because seeding of the papillomatosis into the tracheobronchial tree commonly occurs.

Lipoma, hamartoma, and chondroma are tumors that are found less commonly on endoscopy. The CO_2 laser using a waveguide-type delivery system with good telescopic optics control is preferable to the Nd:YAG laser for these lesions.

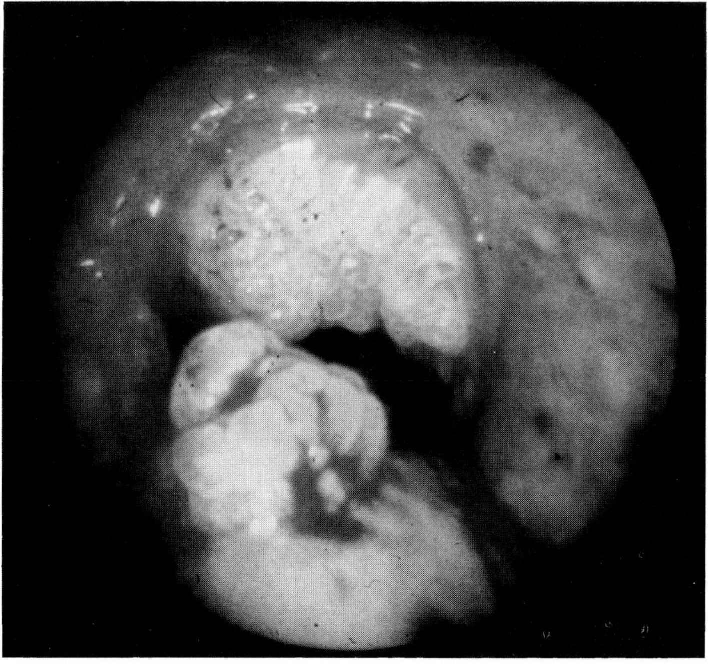

FIGURE 7–9. Endoscopic photograph reveals tracheobronchial papillomatosis of the distal trachea before coagulation and vaporization using the Nd:YAG laser.

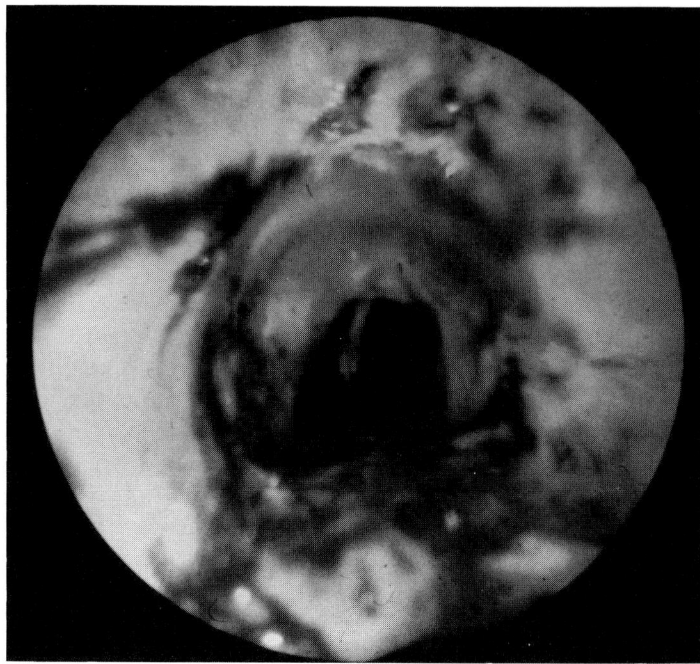

FIGURE 7–10. After removal of tracheobronchial papillomatosis in Figure 7–9. Note satisfactory opening of both main bronchi and good hemostasis. A moderate degree of laser-induced thermal blanching of the distal trachea is seen; however, no subsequent laser-induced stenosis was noted.

Tracheal Stenosis

Tracheal stenosis may occur in three basic situations, namely with concentric webbing, with so-called bottleneck or collapsing cartilage, and with inflammatory-type tissue. Patients with a thin, weblike concentric stenosis can be treated successfully with the CO_2 or the Nd:YAG laser; however, the CO_2 laser is preferred because of its more precise soft tissue interaction. A single radial laser incision is made in each quadrant followed by *gentle* dilation with the bronchoscope (Fig. 7–11). Islands of epithelium that remain between the laser incisions facilitate rapid generation of epithelial cover. Tracheotomy should be avoided if possible because infection from the operative site may complicate healing of the wound. Patients should receive antibiotics for 4 weeks postoperatively; however, steroids should be avoided because a delay in epithelization may occur with their use. More than one treatment using this technique may be necessary to establish a tracheal lumen of near normal dimension.

Unfortunately, only 10 per cent of patients with tracheal stenosis have weblike conditions. The majority of patients have complex stenosis or combinations of intrinsic scarring and malacia of the cartilage, resulting in a bottleneck stenosis that has a high degree of failure with any form of endoscopic treatment. Both the CO_2 and Nd:YAG lasers have been tried with varying success and are best used as temporizing measures before a definitive therapy, such as tracheal resection. Another option for patients with a collapsing tracheal airway is endoscopic resection of the fibrotic tissue with the laser and subsequent insertion of stenting materials to maintain a patent airway. T tube tracheostomy stenting has been used in several patients, who were not candidates for tracheal resection, with good results. It is important to keep the tracheal tube externally plugged so that humidification from the oral cavity and oral pharynx can prevent complications attributable to dry tracheal secretions. The tracheal stent is left in place for 6 months or longer. Alternatively, a tracheotomy may be necessary to palliate the obstructed airway when tracheal resection is not indicated.

Patients with inflammatory or granulation tissue are treated with either the CO_2 or the Nd:YAG laser. When the tissue is pale and granular, the CO_2 laser is preferred because of its better

A

B

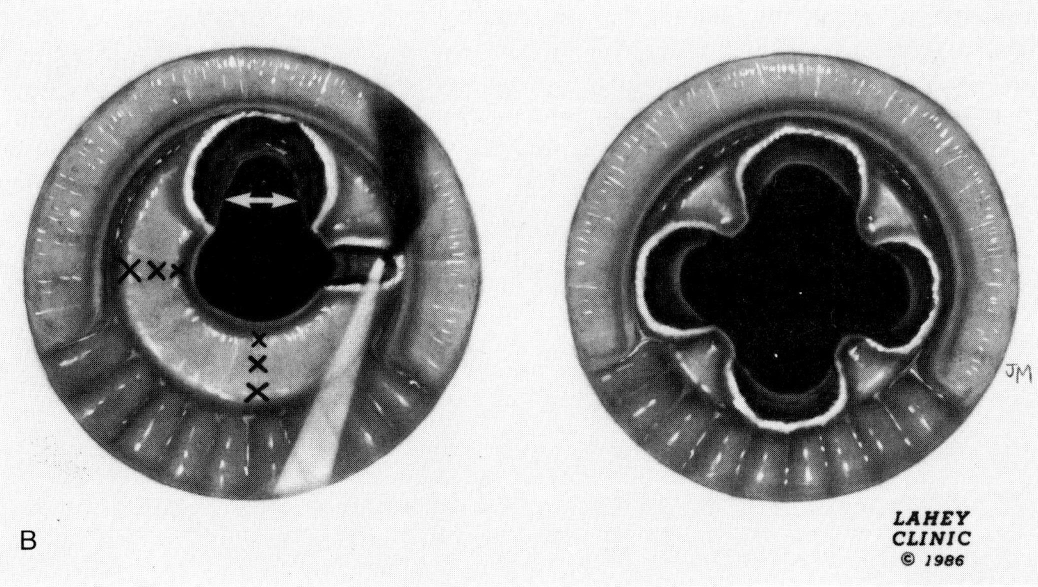

FIGURE 7–11. *See legend on next page.*

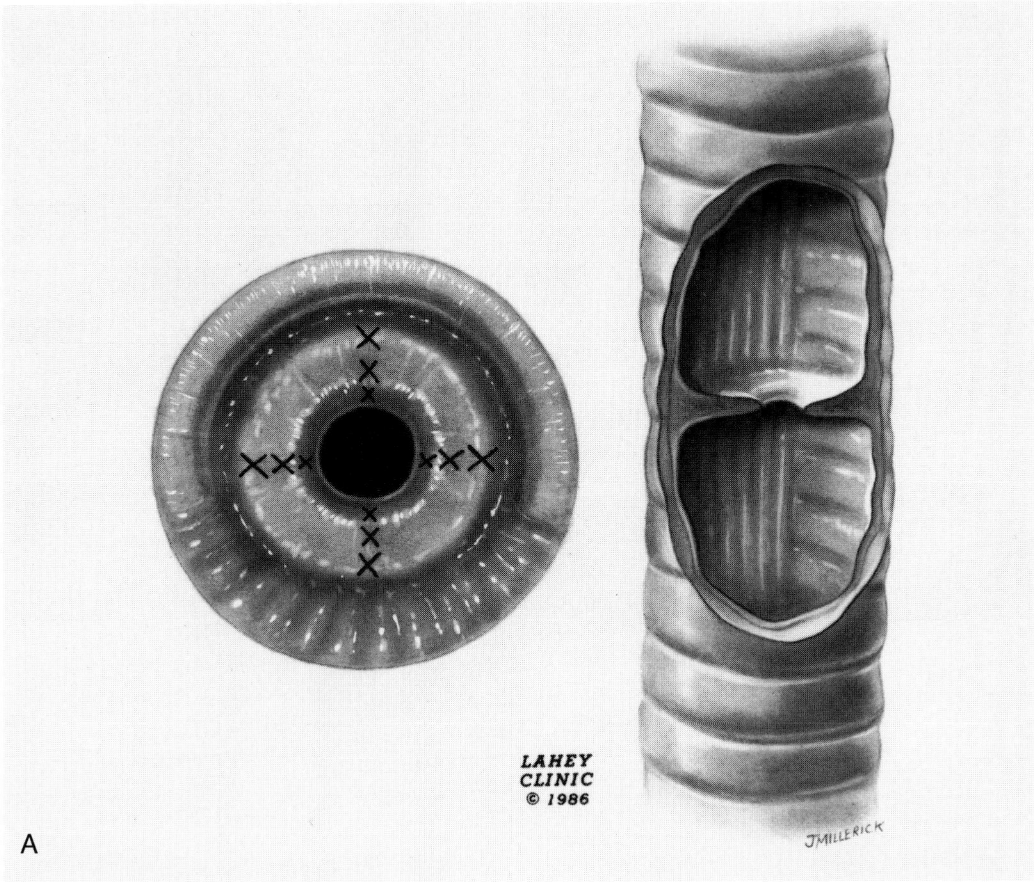

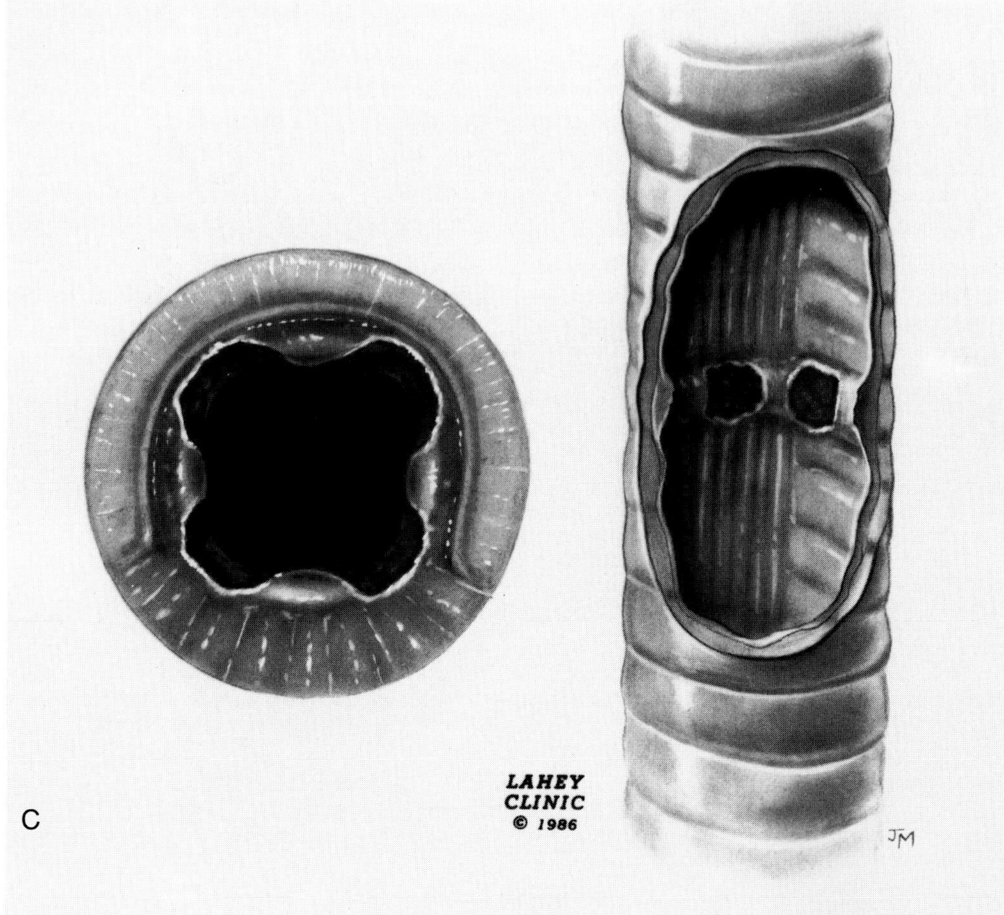

FIGURE 7–11. Laser treatment of a weblike tracheal stenosis. *A,* Radial laser incisions will be made along the Xs. *B,* Radial laser incisions are made (the CO_2 laser is usually used). Note spreading of cicatricial stenosis after the incisions *(arrows).* Recovery is enhanced if islands of epithelium are present between the incisions. *C,* Atraumatic dilation of the stenosis is performed with rigid ventilating bronchoscopes of increasing sizes to achieve a tracheal lumen of normal gauge. (From Shapshay SM, Beamis JF Jr, Hybels RL, Bohigian RK: Endoscopic treatment of subglottic and tracheal stenosis by radial laser incision and dilation. Ann Otol Rhinol Laryngol 96:663, 1987.)

absorption. On the other hand, when an inflammatory vascular component is present, the Nd:YAG laser controls bleeding better than the CO_2 laser. Again, a major advantage of the Nd:YAG laser is ease of application, with telescopic control maintained through the rigid endoscope and flexible suction catheters ensuring a dry operative field.

Obstructing Tumors of Proximal to Middle Trachea

The technique for endoscopic treatment of patients with obstructing tracheobronchial tumors varies with the location of the tumor rather than with the particular histopathologic condition. For tumors obstructing the proximal to middle tracheal region (Fig. 7–12), the rigid laser bronchoscope is inserted and situated above the obstructing tumor. The Nd:YAG laser fiber is passed through the separate bronchoscopic channel, and the laser is activated. Laser power is usually set at 40 to 45

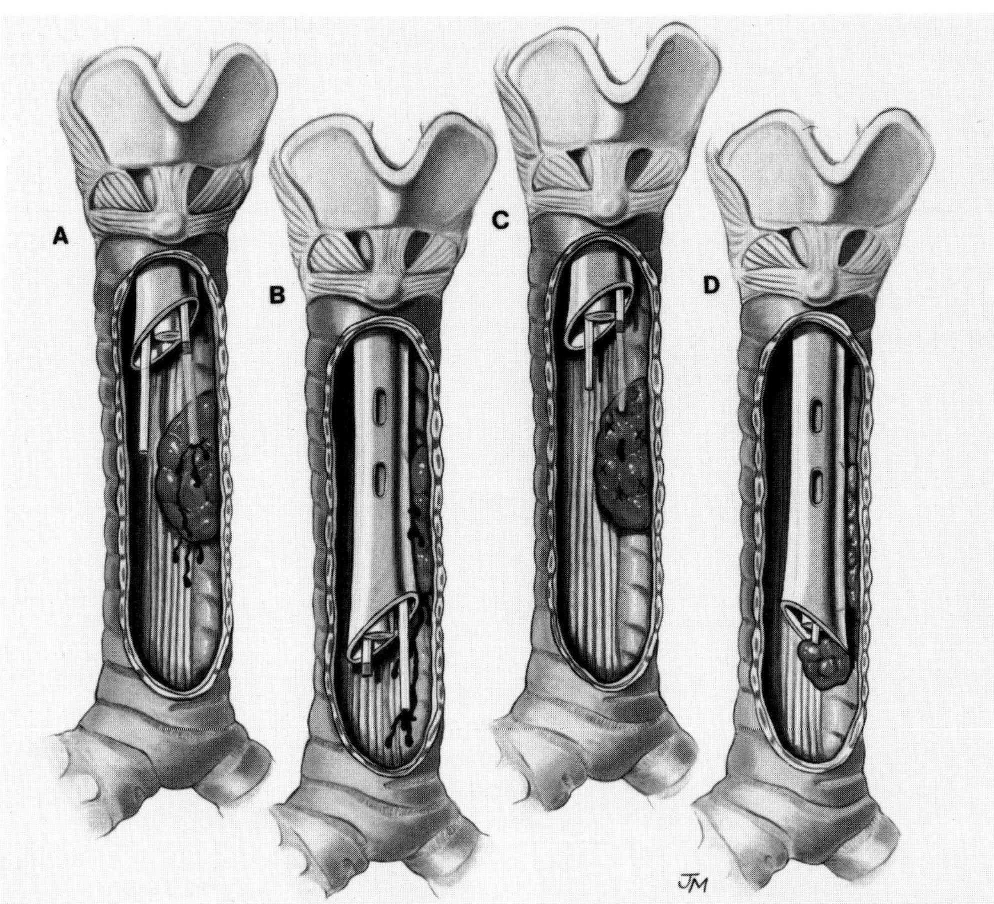

FIGURE 7–12. Procedure for Nd:YAG laser therapy for a proximal tracheal obstruction. *A,* The rigid ventilating bronchoscope is proximal to the tracheal tumor. Good optic control is possible with a 0 degree telescope. The laser fiber is seen coagulating the tumor (40 watts at 1 second exposures with the fiber placed 2 cm from the tumor). A semiflexible heat-resistant polyethylene suction catheter removes debris and secretions. *B,* The bronchoscope is advanced distal to the bleeding tumor for tracheobronchial toilet. The rigid bronchoscope is also used to tamponade the tumor surface for control of hemorrhage. *C,* The bronchoscope is again retracted, and further laser photocoagulation takes place. *D,* The beveled end of the bronchoscope is used to core out photocoagulated tumor. A suction catheter or a foreign body grasping forceps is used to remove these large tumor fragments. (From Shapshay SM: Lasers in diseases of the trachea and bronchi. *In* Fuller TA (ed): Surgical Lasers: A Clinical Guide. New York, Macmillan Publishing Co, 1985, p 54.)

watts with a 0.5 to 1 second pulse duration. Photocoagulation of the tumor is achieved by keeping the tip of the laser fiber approximately 1 to 2 cm from the target surface. A flexible polyethylene suction catheter is kept proximal to the laser fiber, and the 0 degree telescope is used for optic control. Most tumors blanch and seem to shrink during the photocoagulation process. It is important to begin treatment away from the tracheobronchial wall, keeping the laser fiber parallel to the axis of the airway to prevent perforation. Small tumors can be completely vaporized when the power density of laser application is increased by keeping the tip of the fiber 5 mm to 1 cm from the target surface while using 40 to 50 watts of energy. Thorough photocoagulation of large tumors diminishes their blood supply, permitting subsequent mechanical shearing of tumor from the tracheal wall by making a circular screwing motion with the beveled tip of the rigid bronchoscope. This shortens the operative procedure and limits the amount of laser energy applied. Large fragments of tumor can be removed with the flexible suction catheters or, more safely, with optical bronchoscopic foreign body forceps. When most of the tumor is removed, the tumor bed is photocoagulated using 30 to 35 watts of energy at 0.5 to 0.7 second exposures for secure hemostasis. The bronchoscopist should constantly be preoccupied with maintenance of a secure airway with adequate oxygenation. The rigid bronchoscope should be passed distal to the tumor at regular intervals to improve ventilation and provide suctioning of tracheobronchial blood and secretions. Should hypoxemia occur, as indicated by diminished oxygen saturation, laser application should cease, and distal suctioning of the airway should take place.

Obstructing Tumors of Distal Trachea, Carina, and Main Bronchi

Distal tracheal obstruction usually occurs as an urgent problem in the airway. Rapid clearing of the obstruction by intubation of at least one main bronchus (usually the right main bronchus because of its favorable anatomic location) should be performed as soon as possible. The rigid ventilating bronchoscope should be used with the Nd:YAG laser fiber and one or two suction catheters for rapid evacuation of secretions and debris. Rapid photocoagulation of the carinal and right main bronchial tumor is followed by rapid débridement using the rigid bronchoscope as a coring device (Figs. 7–13, 7–14). Bleeding induced by this maneuver is usually controlled by pressure from the bronchoscope and further laser photocoagulation. When the right main bronchus is intubated and the emergency in the airway is resolved, the bronchoscope is withdrawn to the carina and distal trachea and orderly photocoagulation of the remaining tumor is performed. Vaporization of the tumor and periodic débridement of photocoagulated tumor fragments clear the airway, providing a more normal lumen diameter. The Nd:YAG laser is primarily used for photocoagulation, and combining this with mechanical débridement may shorten the operative procedure to less than 45 minutes.

Patients with complete and chronic tumor obstruction of the main bronchi (longer than 3 to 4 weeks) should not undergo laser therapy unless an abscess is present behind the obstructed bronchus. Chronic obstruction of the main bronchus is usually associated with a nonfunctioning distal lung caused by vascular shunting. When the obstruction is a relatively acute condition, photocoag-

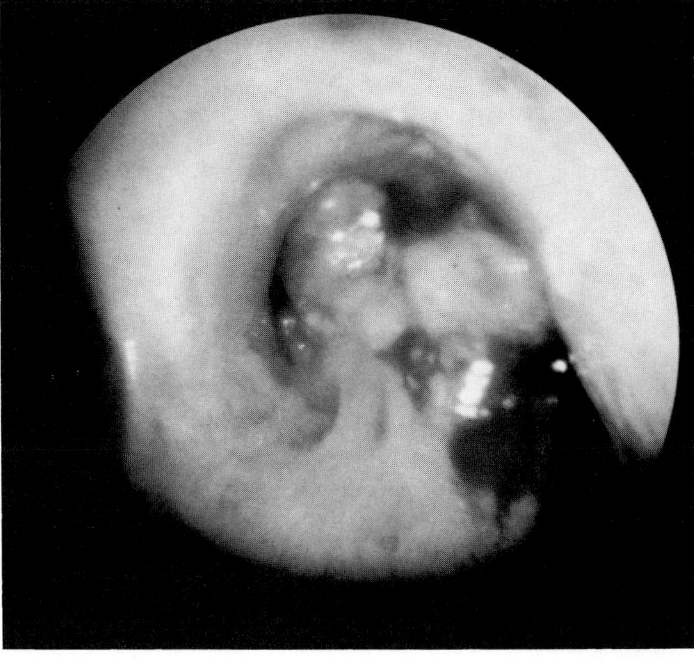

FIGURE 7–13. Endoscopic view of an obstructing metastatic ameloblastoma occluding the right main bronchus.

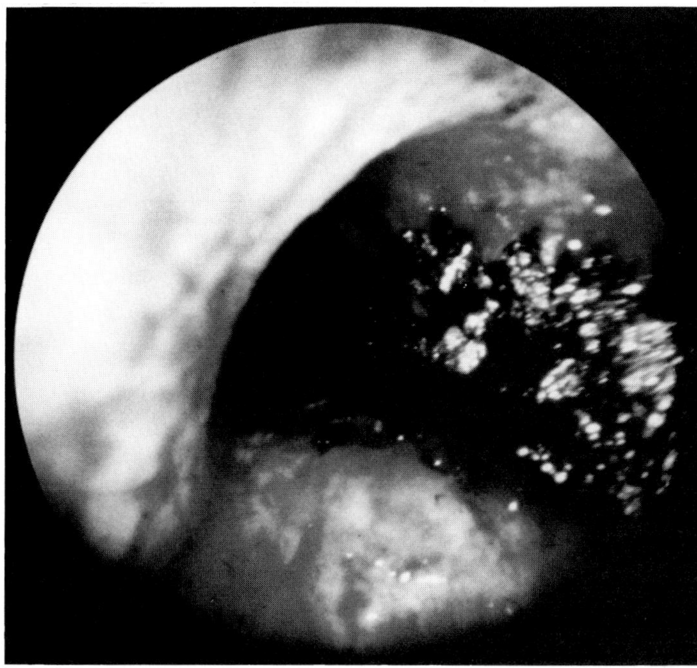

FIGURE 7–14. Immediately after Nd:YAG laser photoablation of the tumor in Figure 7–13. Note the open right main bronchus with a coagulum on the lateral wall. Good hemostasis was achieved with laser use alone.

ulation of the central portion of the tumor mass at a power setting of 40 to 45 watts ultimately vaporizes the central portion of the obstruction. A suction catheter is then used to probe the soft central core of the tumor until it can be passed through the tumor. Distal to the tumor blockage, purulent secretions are often encountered as the obstruction is relieved. The bronchoscope can then be passed safely through the opened area for further débridement of photocoagulated tumor fragments. At this point, it is important to have two suction catheters present because flooding of the airway with purulent secretions may contaminate the more healthy opposite lung. Lateral "safety positioning" of the patient is used with the pathologic lung downward to prevent contamination of the normal lung with purulent secretions. No attempt is made to address distal bronchial seeding of tumor because there is limited access to more distal bronchi, and it is unlikely that these smaller bronchi would remain open regardless of treatment.

Special Considerations with Malignant Tumors

Esophageal Carcinoma with Tracheal Extension

As mentioned above, treatment of patients who have esophageal carcinoma with tracheal extension and obstruction is not usually recommended because these patients have an especially poor survival rate and a high potential for morbidity. The tracheal obstruction is usually submucosal, with extrinsic compression from the invading esophageal carcinoma (Fig. 7–15). Esophagoscopy using the Nd:YAG laser can be performed to relieve the esophageal obstruction and permit better alimentation; however, it is unlikely that a long palliative period could be achieved for the airway, and an iatrogenic tracheoesophageal fistula could result.

Metastatic Tumors of Trachea

Palliation of airway obstruction caused by distal malignant metastasis to the tracheobronchial tree is indicated for selected patients. At times, a slow growth rate occurs in metastases from malignan-

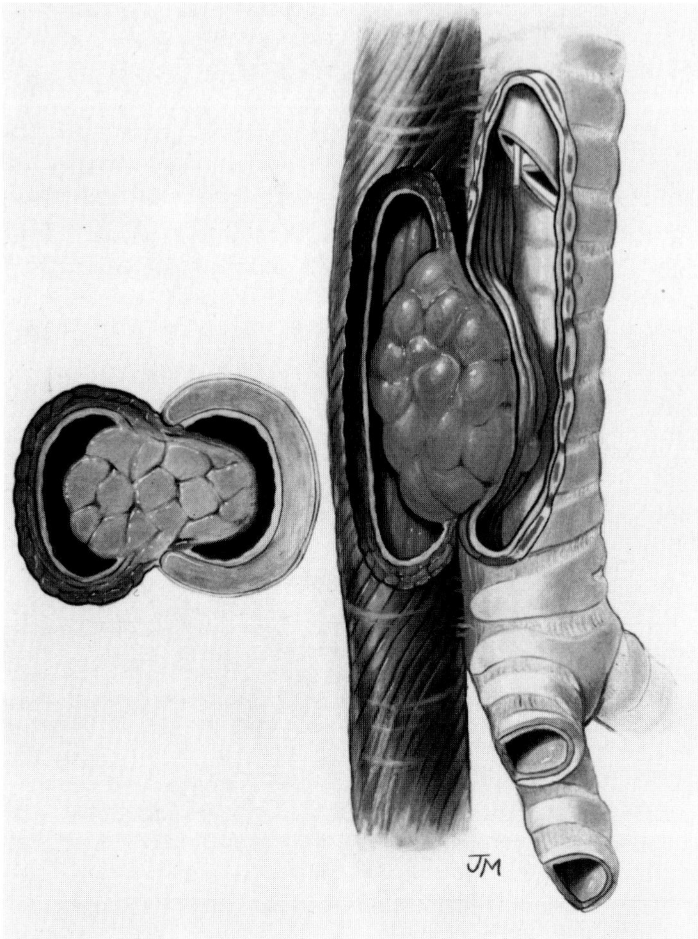

FIGURE 7–15. Esophageal cancer causing tracheal obstruction by submucosal infiltration of the posterior tracheal wall. Neodynium:YAG laser treatment of patients with tracheal obstruction may lead to an esophageal tracheal fistula. Partial palliation of exophytic tumor in the trachea may be achieved. (From Shapshay SM: Lasers in diseases of the trachea and bronchi. *In* Fuller TA (ed): Surgical Lasers: A Clinical Guide. New York, MacMillan Publishing Co, 1987, p 58.)

cies of the colon, the breast, and the uterus. These metastases are often solitary and polypoid in nature. However, tumors with a high degree of vascularity, such as thyroid and renal carcinomas, should be approached with caution. Both of these tumors—thyroid carcinoma by direct extension and renal carcinoma by metastatic spread—can be extremely dangerous because of their high degree of vascularity. Thorough photocoagulation with defocusing of the laser fiber 1 to 2 cm from the tumor is necessary before any manipulation of the tumor takes place. Two suction catheters should be available to provide rapid clearance of blood and secretions should hemorrhage occur.

Intermediate Malignant Neoplasms: Carcinoid and Adenoid Cystic Carcinoma

As mentioned above, carcinoid tumor is notorious for its high degree of vascularity. Fortunately, carcinoid and adenoid cystic tumors respond to Nd:YAG laser photocoagulation, which should take place before any manipulation of the tumor occurs. If possible, however, these tumors should be removed by sleeve resection rather than by endoscopic laser treatment. Adenoid cystic carcinomas are less vascular than carcinoid tumors; however, they are notorious for submucosal extension. Long segments of the tracheal wall may commonly be affected, frustrating attempts at open curative resection. It is not uncommon to encounter involvement of tumor margins when approaching adenoid cystic carcinoma surgically. Fortunately, these tumors grow slowly, and the potential for long-term palliation is good. Laser power of 35 to 40 watts at intermittent 0.7 to 1 second exposures is usually necessary for photocoagulation and débridement of the obstruction.

UNFAVORABLE CONDITIONS FOR LASER BRONCHOSCOPY

Tumor Obstruction in Upper Lobe. Access to the upper lobes, particularly the left upper lobe, is limited, except with use of a flexible fiberoptic bronchoscope. Placement of the laser fiber within the bronchoscope limits flexibility of the instrument, but more important is the difficulty in controlling hemorrhage should it occur in the upper lobes. Generally, patients with these tumors are not treated with laser bronchoscopy. An exception is control of hemorrhage with tumor coagulation as the primary goal.

Carinal Recurrence After Pneumonectomy. Patients undergoing pneumonectomy are especially vulnerable to hypoxemia. Arrhythmia and subsequent cardiovascular collapse may occur, necessitating extremely careful control of bleeding into the remaining lung. Thorough photocoagulation of the carinal recurrence with careful tracheobronchial toilet is important.

Complete Tumor Obstruction After Radiation Therapy. Because of the distortion of the tracheobronchial airway in patients with this condition, it can be difficult to ascertain the direction of the tracheobronchial lumen. Tracheobronchial perforation is certainly a great risk in this situation. If the patient is not symptomatic as a result of chronic obstruction of the airway, treatment is not suggested.

MANAGEMENT OF COMPLICATIONS

Intraoperative Complications

Although the Nd:YAG laser has had a remarkable safety record for more than 10 years, it remains the most powerful and perhaps the most dangerous of available medical lasers. The power density of the Nd:YAG laser is concentrated below the surface of the tissue (as opposed to the surface effect of the CO_2 laser), necessitating intermittent exposure settings of 1 second or less at a power setting of less than 50 watts (usually 40 to 45 watts).

Risk of Combustion with Endotracheal Tubes. In general, the use of endotracheal tubes in bronchoscopic surgery should be avoided because of the risk of combustion, particularly in an oxygen-rich environment. The polyvinylchloride tube should never be used because it is rapidly punctured by both the CO_2 and Nd:YAG laser beams, causing combustion and production of toxic fumes as well as a potential blowtorch effect. External taping of the endotracheal tube does not protect the internal wall from combustion when the Nd:YAG laser is used inside the tube.

Bronchoscopic Fire. Ignition of the sheath of the flexible bronchoscope can cause fire. It is extremely important to be able to see the laser fiber at all times before activating the laser. However, combustion of the flexible bronchoscope most often occurs from ignition of charred tumor fragments or flammable material such as the endotracheal tube. Environmental oxygen should be kept at less that 50 per cent concentration when possible. The immediate response to an endobronchial fire is prompt removal of all flammable materials. When an accident occurs, inspection for tracheobronchial burns and respiratory support should follow. The patient should be treated with antibiotics and steroids to diminish the inflammatory response and decrease the possibility of subsequent scarring. Flammable materials within the rigid bronchoscopic system are the laser fiber itself and the plastic suction materials. The laser fiber should be kept free of debris at all times, and plastic material should be kept proximal to the laser tip if possible.

Perforation of Tracheobronchial Tree. The risk of tracheobronchial perforation with the Nd:YAG laser is much greater than with the CO_2 or the argon laser. The depth of penetration and the extent of scattering are also considerably greater with this wavelength, and its soft tissue interaction is less predictable. Cautious intermittent Nd:YAG laser irradiation using less than 50 watts of power is highly advisable during endoscopy. The Nd:YAG laser fiber should always be used parallel with and never perpendicular to the tracheobronchial wall. The tip of the rigid bronchoscope can be used as a palpating device to help determine the interface of the tumor and the tracheal cartilage. Laser irradiation at continued high power of greater than 40 watts with exposure times of greater than 1 second may cause explosive rupture of the tissues—the so-called popcorn effect. The surgeon may see blanching of the surface of the tissue followed by charring before explosion of tissue.

Hemorrhage. The most common hemorrhagic situation is persistent uncontrolled bleeding of the tracheobronchial tree. Massive hemorrhage is usually caused by perforation of a major pulmonary blood vessel and, fortunately, is a rare complication. However, life-threatening hypoxemia may occur from the accumulation of distal tracheobronchial hemorrhagic secretions. Cessation of tumor resection with immediate tracheobronchial toilet and hemostasis is imperative. Two semi-rigid suction catheters passed through the rigid bronchoscope are used to maintain a dry operative field. The laser is applied at a coagulating power of 30 to 40 watts, with the fiber approximately 2 cm from the target tissue. Coagulation should begin circumferentially around the bleeding site and end at the area itself. Massive bronchial hemorrhage necessitates placing the patient in the safety position with the healthy lung above the affected lung. With the patient in this position, the ventilating bronchoscope is used to evacuate blood and secretions and to achieve patency of the airway. Heroic measures should not be taken when hemorrhage due to perforation of a pulmonary artery occurs. These patients have poor potential for survival and usually do not respond to resuscitative measures.

Hypoxemia. The major cause of death during and after laser resection is hypoxemia. Hypoxemia can arise from distal collection of secretions and debris, as well as from induced respiratory depression caused by anesthetic medications. Uncontrolled hypoxemia leads to cardiovascular complications, such as arrhythmia and bradycardia, as well as myocardial infarction and subsequent cardiac arrest. Constant monitoring of oxygen saturation using a finger pulse oximeter and frequent monitoring of blood gas levels are important with high risk patients. Adequate ventilation and frequent tracheobronchial toilet should be the constant preoccupation of the endoscopist during the laser procedure.

Postoperative Complications

Postoperative septicemia may occur as a result of routine accumulation of secretions and subsequent atelectasis. After laser resection is complete, the flexible bronchoscope is used to clear distal secretions and reexpand the segments of the lung that may have been blocked during the procedure. Postoperative atelectasis is usually a result of insidious accumulation of distal blood clots.

Fortunately, in more than 300 laser bronchoscopies performed between 1982 and 1988 at the Lahey Clinic Medical Center, only one operative death occurred as a result of tension pneumothorax and pericardial tamponade. No major hemorrhage, fire, or postoperative septicemia has occurred. Two patients with severe coronary artery disease died of myocardial infarction in the postoperative period. The risk of complications was analyzed in a large combined series of patients from four medical centers in Europe and the United States that use the same techniques for Nd:YAG laser resection.[15] A total of 1503 laser treatments were performed in 1156 patients. Six deaths occurred in this large series, all of which were attributable to hypoxemia resulting from excessive anesthesia, bleeding, or retained secretions. No perforation, fire, or catastrophic arterial hemorrhage occurred.

References

1. Strong MS, Vaughan CW, Polanyi T, et al.: Bronchoscopic carbon dioxide laser surgery. Ann Otol Rhinol Laryngol 83:769, 1974.
2. Gillis TM, Strong MS, Shapshay SM, et al.: Argon laser and soft tissue interaction. Otolaryngol Head Neck Surg 92:7, 1984.
3. Toty L, Personne C, Colchen A, et al.: Bronchoscopic management of tracheal lesions using the neodymium yttrium aluminum garnet laser. Thorax 36:175, 1981.
4. Dumon J-F, Reboud E, Garbe L, et al.: Treatment of tracheobronchial lesions by laser photoresection. Chest 81:278, 1982.
5. McDougall JC, Cortese DA: Neodymium-YAG laser therapy of malignant airway obstruction: A preliminary report. Mayo Clin Proc 58:35, 1983.
6. Unger M: Bronchoscopic utilization of the Nd:YAG laser for obstructing lesions of the trachea and bronchi. Surg Clin North Am 64:931, 1984.
7. Shapshay SM, Dumon J-F, Beamis JF Jr: Endoscopic treatment of tracheobronchial malignancy: Experience with Nd:YAG and CO_2 lasers in 506 operations. Otolaryngol Head Neck Surg 93:205, 1985.
8. Shapshay SM: Laser applications in the trachea and bronchi: A comparative study of the soft tissue effects using contact and noncontact delivery systems. Laryngoscope 97(suppl 41):1, 1987.
9. Cortese DA, Kinsey JH: Hematoporphyrin-derivative phototherapy for local treatment of cancer of the tracheobronchial tree. Ann Otol Rhinol Laryngol 91:652, 1982.
10. Hayata Y, Kato H, Konaka C, et al.: Hematoporphyrin derivative and laser photoradiation in the treatment of lung cancer. Chest 81:269, 1982.
11. Balchum OJ, Doiron DR: Photoradiation therapy of endobronchial lung cancer: Large obstructing tumors, nonobstructing tumors, and early-stage bronchial cancer lesions. Clin Chest Med 6:255, 1985.
12. Dumon J-F: YAG laser bronchoscopy. New York, Praeger Publishers, 1985, p 9.
13. Ossoff RH, Karlan MS: Universal endoscopic coupler for carbon dioxide laser surgery. Ann Otol Rhinol Laryngol 91:608, 1982.
14. Casey KR, Fairfax WR, Smith SJ, et al.: Intratracheal fire ignited by the Nd:YAG laser during treatment of tracheal stenosis. Chest 84:295, 1983.
15. Dumon JF, Shapshay S, Bourcereau J, et al.: Principles of safety in application of neodymium-YAG laser in bronchology. Chest 86:163, 1984.

ENDOSCOPIC ESOPHAGEAL LASER THERAPY

Kenneth N. Buchi

Jean Marc Brunetaud

HISTORICAL PERSPECTIVE

The development of fiberoptic delivery systems for laser energy in the early 1970s made endoscopic laser treatment possible, clearing the way for a variety of interventional applications in the gastrointestinal tract. Fiberoptic delivery systems are currently available for the argon, neodymium:yttrium-aluminum-garnet (Nd:YAG), and tunable dye lasers. Optical fibers are being developed for the carbon dioxide (CO_2) laser, but are not yet commercially available. Most endoscopic laser therapy in the esophagus and the upper gastrointestinal tract uses the Nd:YAG and argon lasers; tunable lasers are primarily limited to research centers.

When a directed beam of coherent laser energy interacts with tissue, it is absorbed, reflected, or scattered, depending on a number of variables. These include the thermal conductivity of the tissue, the color and surface characteristics of the tissue, the blood circulation in the tissue, the power and duration of the laser pulse, and the wavelength of the laser energy. A few points specifically relating to the gastrointestinal tract are briefly reviewed here.

Much research effort has defined the specific mechanisms of laser-tissue interactions in the gastrointestinal tract, including the depth of penetration, coagulation times, and perforation times in the stomach,the intestine, and colon.[1-5] Excellent summaries of these investigations are available for those interested in pursuing this information in greater detail.[6,7] There have been no animal studies specifically looking at the tissue interactions in the esophagus, but most of the principles are similar throughout the gastrointestinal tract. It is important to remember that the wall of the esophagus is thinner than the gastric wall, which increases the risk of full thickness coagulation. In addition, the esophagus does not have a serosal surface, which makes a free perforation more likely if full thickness coagulation does occur.

This experimental information is conceptually helpful and important to understand. However, findings from the controlled laboratory situation are not directly applicable to clinical endoscopic laser use. In the laboratory, the variables of power, duration, and distance from the target are precisely controlled. When actually working in the esophagus, the target tissue is often moving owing to peristalsis, respiratory excursions, or cardiac motion. The distance from the fiber to the target is never constant, so the laser spot size and the resultant energy density is continually changing. This energy density, or power density, determines how much energy is converted to heat at the point the laser beam strikes the tissue. As contractions occur or as the esophagus is distended by air or gas insufflation, the thickness of the esophageal wall is also constantly changing, which varies potential perforation times. Overlying blood or secretions may obscure the target and diffuse, absorb, or reflect the laser energy.

The endoscopist must thus use not only the known information about ideal laser-tissue interaction, but also clinical judgment and visual cues to help assess the effect of laser energy on the specific lesion being treated. As the laser energy is absorbed by the target tissue and converted to heat, increasing tissue temperatures lead progressively to cell death, protein coagulation, vascular constriction, and finally water and tissue vaporization. These changes are visible endoscopically and help predict the ultimate outcome of the laser-tissue interaction (Table 8–1). Although spanning a continuum of effects, ultimate tissue results can be divided into two major categories: Below 100°C, varying degrees of tissue coagulation occur. Above 100°C, vaporization or ablation of tissue occurs. Coagulation is useful for treating bulky esophageal malignancies, benign or premalignant mucosal lesions, arteriovenous (AV) malformations, and other bleeding lesions in the esophagus. Coagulation can typically be achieved with power settings of 2 to 10 watts with the argon laser, and 20 to 70 watts with the Nd:YAG laser. The ablative effect destroys obstructing neoplastic tissue or cuts through tissue to treat anatomic lesions, such as strictures or cysts. Higher power settings are required to ablate or cut tissue, typically 60 to 100 watts with the Nd:YAG laser.

The initial applications of laser energy through endoscopes were directed toward coagulation of actively bleeding lesions, or lesions that had recently bled and were at risk for rebleeding. Dwyer and colleagues[8] and Fruhmorgen and colleagues[9] first used the argon laser to control bleeding in the stomach in 1974. Kiefhaber and associates used the higher power of the Nd:YAG laser for the same purpose.[10] During the subsequent 10 years, a number of uncontrolled[11–15] and controlled studies[16–25] confirmed the feasibility, and in selected instances the desirability, of using endoscopic lasers to treat gastrointestinal bleeding. Interestingly, however, a number of new instruments and approaches to the therapy of bleeding have been developed in the 1980s,[26,27] and the use of lasers for this problem has declined significantly. A few specific indications for laser application for bleeding lesions remain, and they are discussed below.

Table 8–1. THERMAL EFFECTS OF LASER–TISSUE
INTERACTIONS

Tissue Temperature	Physiologic Event	Endoscopic Tissue Appearance	Ultimate Outcome
45°C	Cell death, edema, vasodilation	Erythema, edema	Cell death, inflammation
60°C to 80°C	Protein coagulation, contraction of collagen and blood vessels	Tissue turns gray or white; blood turns black	Cell death, slough and ulceration, followed by repair
100°C	Tissue water vaporizes	Hole or ulcer in tissue; brown base	Tissue ablated
210°C	Dehydrated tissue burns	Black tissue glows and disappears; sparks may form	Tissue ablated

In the early 1980s, the use of endoscopic laser therapy began to expand beyond therapy for bleeding lesions. Dixon and colleagues first established that small gastrointestinal mucosal lesions could be ablated with a minimal risk of perforation.[28,29] Simultaneously, Fleischer and coworkers described the use of the Nd:YAG laser's ability to coagulate tissue for the palliative treatment of obstructing esophageal malignancies.[30] These innovative applications allowed a broader array of endoscopic laser treatments in the digestive tract and led to the use of lasers throughout the world for palliative tumor therapy, mucosal lesion ablation, and other applications such as stricture treatment and cyst drainage.

LASER APPLICATIONS

Neoplasia

The palliation of gastrointestinal malignancies is one of the more appealing applications of endoscopic laser surgery and the most frequently used in the 1980s. All areas of the gastrointestinal system that are accessible to fiberoptic endoscopes can potentially be treated, but the greatest experience is with neoplasms of the esophagus, the colon, and the rectum.

Malignancies in hollow organs frequently do not become symptomatic until they are large enough to cause bleeding or obstruction. At this stage, most are incurable by surgical resection, yet surgery is often necessary for palliation. Radiation therapy plays a role in these patients as well, but has undesirable systemic side effects, and its use is limited by potential damage to the adjacent normal tissue.[31]

Other palliative therapies available for esophageal malignancies include simple dilation with or without stent placement, radiation therapy, chemotherapy, and bipolar electrocoagulation. Dilation is relatively easy to perform, but rarely achieves any symptomatic benefit for longer than a few days. It is thus primarily used to improve access to the tumor for the delivery of other treatment modalities. Radiation therapy and chemotherapy are often employed as adjuvant methods to prolong the symptom-free period following endoscopic recanalization. Laser treatment is the most widely used endoscopic therapy to establish lumen patency. Bipolar electrocoagulation is a newer modality; experience with its use is only beginning to accumulate, but it has potential advantages in selected patients.

The management of obstructing or bleeding tumors with these endoscopic treatment modalities does not necessarily improve survival rates in patients when compared with those achieved with surgery or radiation therapy. It does offer several important advantages: It requires only intravenous sedation, avoiding the risks of general anesthesia and major surgery. It can usually be performed on an outpatient basis, thus reducing medical costs and avoiding prolonged hospital stays. It can be applied on a repetitive schedule, because there is no limiting cumulative dose for laser or bipolar electrical energy. Finally, systemic side effects are uncommon, thus increasing patient acceptance of the therapy.

Indications and Results of Laser Surgery

The major indications for laser therapy of esophageal tumors are the relief of obstruction and the control of bleeding. Although small tumors can theoretically be ablated for potential cure, such tumors should ideally be surgically resected for cure if they are found. Laser treatment is not effective in relieving pain and thus is not indicated solely for pain control.

The earliest esophageal tumor work in the United States was that of Fleischer and colleagues, who reported the successful relief of dysphagia in five patients with obstructing squamous cell carcinomas of the esophagus.[30] Subsequently, Fleischer and Sivak reported their experience with 40 patients who were not candidates for surgical or radiation therapy.[32] Most of these patients had dysphagia with 90 per cent or greater occlusion of the esophageal lumen. Thirty-seven of the 40 patients improved symptomatically following laser treatments, with endoscopically determined luminal diameters increasing from a mean of 2.8 mm to 11.5 mm. Clinical improvement lasted for 3 to 6 months, and some patients were successfully retreated. Five patients (12 per cent) developed a tracheoesophageal fistula or perforation. Two of those were clearly laser related, but the other three occurred as long as 6 months following laser treatment and may have been related to the underlying tumor.

Mellow and Pinkas reported similar early results in 11 patients and also noted a significantly increased median survival time of 36 weeks compared with a 17 week survival for matched historical controls.[33] They suggested that the improved survival time was due to the patients' ability to maintain better nutrition after laser canalization. This explanation is attractive, but has not been verified.

In Europe, much of the early work with laser treatment of esophageal tumors was performed at the University of Lille. Since 1979, 115 patients have been treated there, with nearly two thirds of the patients undergoing laser therapy as their first means of palliation. One third were treated with laser therapy after radiation or surgical therapy failed or symptoms recurred.[34]

Ninety-nine of these patients had significant dysphagia and extensive tumor. Laser therapy successfully restored swallowing capability and improved nutrition in 76 of these patients (83 per cent), with an average of two treatment sessions. The average duration of improvement was 4 months (130 days). Four major complications (4 per cent) occurred, including two tracheoesophageal fistulas, one acute gastric dilation requiring a gastrostomy placement, and one fatal posttreatment hemorrhage.

The experience at the University of Utah Laser Institute includes 35 patients; 32 (91 per cent) achieved successful relief of dysphagia with an average of 2.3 treatment sessions. Two thirds of the patients had inoperable or recurrent squamous cell carcinomas, whereas the remainder had adenocarcinomas arising at the gastroesophageal junction or in underlying columnar esophageal mucosa. Three tracheoesophageal fistulas (9 per cent) developed in this group, all in patients who were treated without prior dilation via the prograde method. No perforations have occurred since the procedure was changed to include routine prelaser dilation.

At both centers, factors associated with unsuccessful relief of dysphagia, even if the lumen can be recanalized, have been identified. Patients with tumors involving the proximal esophagus often can swallow little or nothing even after opening of the lumen to as much as 14 to 15 mm, a problem also reported at other centers.[35,36] Tumors involving the gastroesophageal junction do not respond well if the junction makes a horizontal angulation before entering the stomach, again a problem seen by others.[35] Patients who present after the failure of prior therapies have not responded as well at Lille as those who underwent laser as primary therapy,[34] although this has not made a difference in other's series.[35] A prospective series from the Mayo Clinic[36] reported that patients with adenocarcinomas had more improvement in swallowing than those with squamous cell carcinomas (93 per cent improved versus 56 per cent), but this has not been a factor elsewhere.

The reported worldwide experience with laser palliation for esophageal malignancy now totals nearly 2000 patients,[30,32–43] and it is likely that many more than that number have been treated but not reported. This combined experience confirms the feasibility of palliative laser therapy, with results consistently similar to those outlined above in experienced hands: Improvement in swallowing can be achieved in 80 to 90 per cent of patients, but is less likely to occur if the tumor involves the upper one third of the esophagus, makes a horizontal angle at the gastroesophageal junction, or has an extensive extrinsic component.[33–37,43] Major complications, including perforation, tracheoesophageal fistulas, and delayed hemorrhage, occur in 5 to 10 per cent of patients.[33–37,40,42,43] The duration of improvement in the ability to swallow ranges from 4 to 20 weeks, with the average approximately 8 weeks.

The risk of major complications and the relatively short duration of symptomatic improvement have continued to stimulate interest in the development of adjuvant or different means of achieving similar palliative effects. Several centers now combine laser therapy to reestablish lumen patency and allow improved nutrition with subsequent radiotherapy, chemotherapy, or intraluminal radiation,[44–46] in an effort to extend the symptom-free duration after treatment. As yet, no large series of patients has been evaluated to assess results.

New and Future Therapies

The other newer methods of palliative therapy are being actively evaluated currently. The BICAP tumor probe (Circon ACMI, Stamford, Ct) is a bipolar electrocoagulation device incorporated into a flexible shaft with an olive-shaped distal segment (Figure 8–1). It delivers circumferential electrical energy to coagulate tissue to a depth of 1 to 2 mm. The probes are available in sizes from 6 to 15 mm in diameter and are powered by a 50 watt generator. The 12 mm or 15 mm size is most commonly used, usually after prior dilation of the tumor stenosis over a guide wire. A 15 mm hemicircumferential probe is available, ostensibly for treating noncircumferential tumors. It is difficult to position correctly, however, and is not recommended for use.

Preliminary reports confirmed the efficacy of the BICAP tumor probe, but major complications, including fistula formation, perforation, and delayed bleeding, occurred in 20 per cent of cases.[47] As experience has accumulated, however, the complication rate has decreased. The largest published series comparing BICAP with Nd:YAG laser therapy is that of Jensen and colleagues, who treated 14 patients with each modality.[48] Both treatments achieved functional success by improving ability to swallow in 86 per cent of patients, and there was no significant difference between the groups in number of treatment sessions, weight change, improvement of tumor performance score, or survival time.

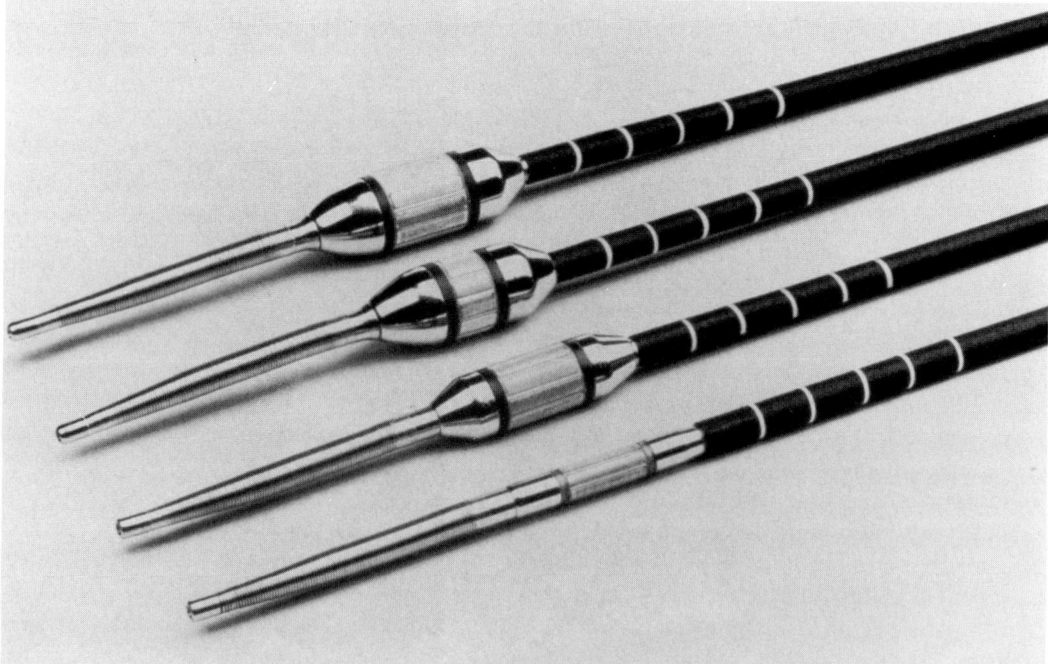

Figure 8–1. BICAP tumor probes, which range in size from 6 mm in diameter *(bottom)* to 15 mm in diameter *(top)*. (Courtesy of Circon ACMI, Stamford, CT.)

One patient treated with the BICAP probe developed a tracheoesophageal fistula. None of the laser-treated patients developed fistulas or perforations, although three did develop posttreatment strictures, which required dilation. Minor complications included chest pain, in three laser-treated and one BICAP-treated patient, and post treatment edema, in four laser-treated and two BICAP-treated patients.

These investigators believe that BICAP therapy and Nd:YAG laser therapy are complementary palliative options. With the BICAP tumor probe the treatment of submucosal, long, or proximal esophageal tumors is faster and easier, but only if the tumor is circumferential. The Nd:YAG laser is preferred for noncircumferential tumors, short strictured areas, and tumors that are exophytic or located in the distal esophagus.

Similar results have been reported by other investigators with fewer numbers of patients.[49,50] It appears likely that the BICAP tumor probe will have an established role in the palliative treatment of esophageal tumors, particularly because it has the advantages of portability and lower cost.

Clinical experience is also accumulating in the use of tissue-sensitizing agents, which allow more precise photoradiation therapy to be applied to tumor tissue with less risk of damage to surrounding normal tissue. Currently the most commonly used sensitizing agent is a derivative of porphyrin called hematoporphyrin derivative, or dihematoporphyrin ether (DHE). This agent is injected intravenously and is retained with greater affinity by malignant than by normal tissue. Subsequent exposure to light in the 625 to 635 nm wavelength stimulates a photochemical reaction in the DHE, producing tumor cell death or damage by a mechanism thought to involve the production of singlet oxygen.[51]

McCaughan and associates reported the successful use of this phototherapy in 16 patients with obstructing esophageal cancers.[52,53] Twelve patients were able to eat standard diets following treatment, with a 1 to 19 month follow-up. The mean survival was 6.5 months, although three patients died in the first month from complications of their disease. Treatment-related complications were minimal, with three patients developing posttreatment edema or stricture that required dilation.

Other reports have shown similar results in small numbers of patients.[54,55] Many details of this therapy have yet to be delineated, such as the ideal doses of DHE and light and the ideal timing of light therapy after injection of DHE.

The use of endoscopic ultrasonography for more accurate localization and staging of esophageal malignancy is also being evaluated in a few centers.[56] This has the potential, along with videoendoscopy and computer image enhancement, to allow much more precision in identifying and delivering treatment modalities to abnormal tissue, while sparing adjacent normal tissue.[57] Such advances offer much promise for future use, and it is likely that laser applications in various forms will continue to expand for the palliative and, perhaps eventually, for the curative treatment of esophageal and other gastrointestinal malignancies.

Laser Methods

Laser photoablation of esophageal malignancies can be accomplished in two ways: coagulation of the tumor, which then is allowed to slough over the 48 to 72 hours following treatment, or vaporization of the tumor with immediate tissue destruction. Laser energy can be delivered to the tumor in a prograde fashion, beginning at the proximal tumor margin as described by Fleischer and colleagues,[30,32] or in a retrograde fashion, starting at the distal tumor margin and treating proximally as the endoscope is withdrawn (Fig. 8–2).

Before treatment, intravenous access is obtained. Sedation is achieved using a combination of meperidine and either diazepam or midazolam, titrating the dose slowly to achieve a drowsy state. The endoscope is then advanced to the tumor and, if possible, through the tumor into the stomach. If the endoscope cannot pass, a guide wire is introduced through the residual esophageal lumen,

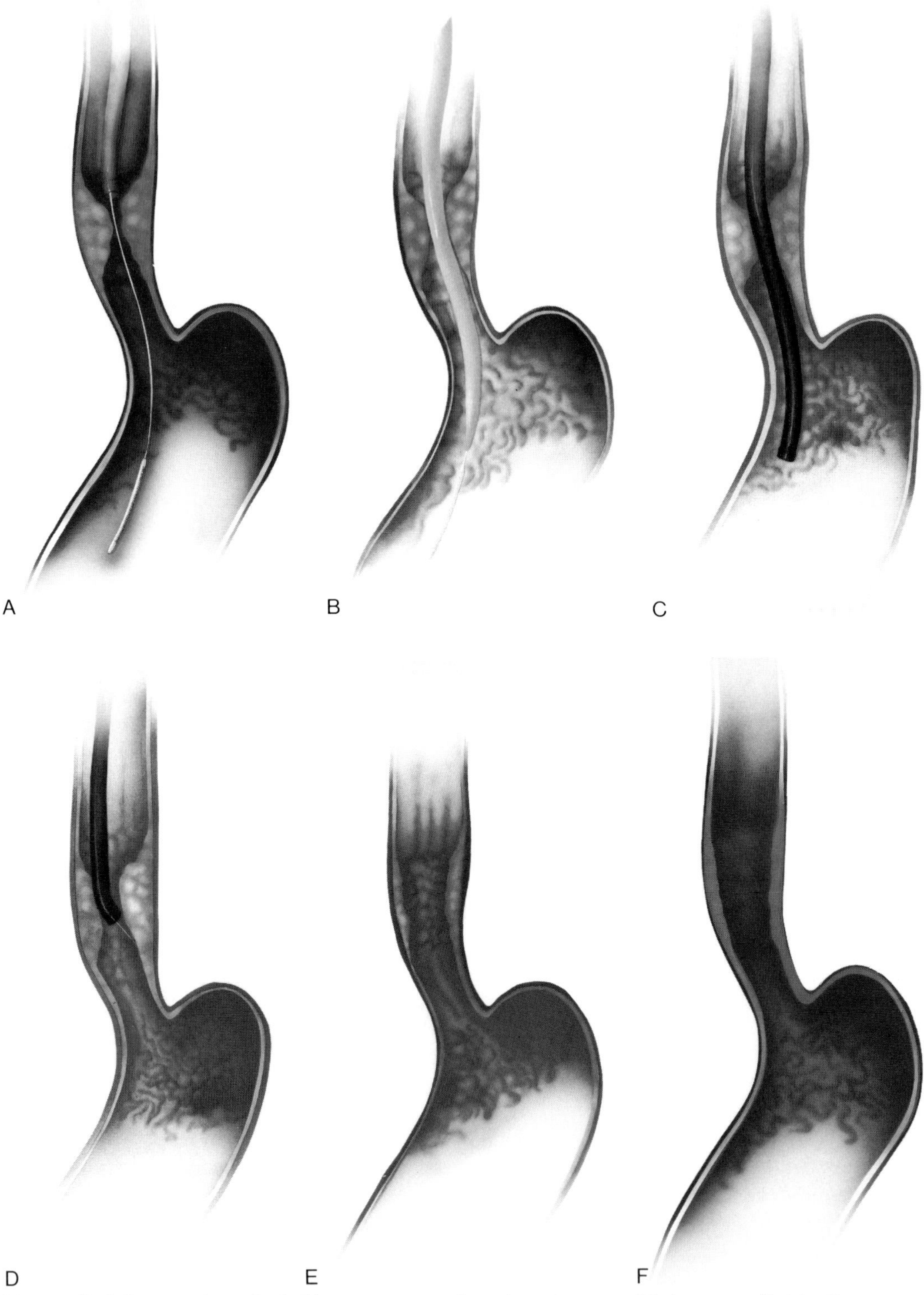

FIGURE 8–2. Retrograde method of laser treatment of esophageal cancer, dilating tumor first to allow access for laser therapy. *A*, Endoscopic placement of guide wire through the tumor. *B*, Dilation over the guide wire with polyvinyl dilators. *C*, Endoscope advanced through the tumor, ready to begin laser treatment. *D*, Laser energy directed circumferentially at the tumor, moving from the distal margin to the proximal margin. *E*, After treatment, the surface of the tumor has been coagulated to a depth of 1 to 3 mm. *F*, Two to 4 days later, the coagulated tumor tissue has sloughed away, leaving an enlarged lumen through the tumor.

confirming appropriate placement, when necessary, with fluoroscopy (Fig. 8–2A). The tumor is then progressively dilated using polyvinyl dilators (Savary-Guillard) passed over the guide wire (Fig. 8–2B). When beginning with a narrow lumen (2 to 3 mm), the tumor is dilated to 9 to 11 mm to minimize the risk of perforation and to allow the subsequent passage of a pediatric endoscope through the tumor. If the initial lumen diameter is at least 5 to 6 mm, it can usually be safely dilated to 14 to 15 mm, allowing a standard upper endoscope to pass for delivery of the laser energy.

Following dilation, the endoscope is again advanced through the tumor to the distal margin, either during the same treatment session over the guide wire, which is still in place, or under direct vision a day or two after dilation. A 600 micron sheathed quartz fiber is placed through the endoscope channel, and the coaxial air or nitrogen flow is set at 5 to 10 cc/second to avoid overdistention of the esophagus and the abdomen. Laser energy is then directed at the visible areas of the tumor in a circumferential manner, treating proximally as the endoscope is withdrawn (Fig. 8–2C, D). Power settings are chosen to achieve coagulation of the tumor as indicated by a color change to whitish or gray brown, but avoiding vaporization. Powers of 40 to 65 watts with the Nd:YAG laser and pulse durations of 0.5 to 1.0 second are usually adequate.

Treatment continues until all visible areas of tumor have been coagulated (Fig. 8–2E). It is helpful to advance the endoscope into the stomach frequently during treatment to aspirate air, smoke, and secretions.

The treated tumor tissue sloughs away 2 to 4 days postoperatively (Fig. 8–2F), at which time the patient can be retreated if clinically necessary. Initial treatments are performed once or twice a week until dysphagia is relieved, and subsequent treatments are performed as symptoms recur, usually at about 6 to 8 week intervals.

The prograde method of treatment, as initially described by Fleischer and associates,[30,32] does not use dilation when the endoscope cannot pass through the tumor. Instead, visible areas of tumor at the proximal margin are coagulated as described above, beginning at the luminal surface and working circumferentially toward the esophageal wall. Two to three days later, the necrotic tumor is débrided either with a large bore evacuator tube or through the endoscope. Treatment is then directed at the newly exposed tumor tissue farther down the esophageal lumen. This process continues until the tumor is progressively cored through to the distal margin, treating about 1.5 to 2 cm at a session. The prograde method is time consuming, requires more initial treatment sessions on average, and is difficult to perform safely if the residual lumen is eccentric or irregular. This method has thus largely been replaced by the retrograde method.

Some centers prefer to use higher powers (80 to 100 watts) to vaporize the tumor and enlarge the esophageal lumen at the time of the initial treatment session, rather than allowing coagulated tissue to slough away. There are no direct comparative studies to show that one method is safer or more effective than the other. Vaporization does have some procedural drawbacks. It generates large amounts of smoke and debris, which must be evacuated and which accumulate on the endoscope tip, obscuring vision. It also requires general, rather than intravenous, anesthesia, which eliminates one of the major benefits of palliative laser therapy outlined above.

Following the laser treatment, patients are typically observed in the outpatient recovery area for 2 to 4 hours until their anesthesia has worn off and they are taking liquids orally. Patients are maintained on a liquid diet for the initial 24 hours after treatment and are encouraged to advance their intake to soft and then solid foods over the 2 to 4 days during which tissue sloughing occurs. The decision to repeat laser treatment depends on the patient's ability to swallow after 4 days.

BICAP Tumor Probe Methods

The coagulation effect of the tumor probe on tissue is not visible during treatment. The probes are thus tested before use by connecting to the generator and placing a drop of saline on each metallic stripe of the probe. The generator is set at a power of 2 watts on the dial, with a 1 second pulse duration, and the foot pedal is activated. Visible bubbling of the saline drops should occur at these settings; if not, the probe should not be used.

The probe chosen should be the same size as the largest polyvinyl dilator used for stricture dilation. A probe that is too large cannot pass through the strictured area, whereas one that is too small does not have the firm tissue contact necessary to conduct the electrical current.

Initial treatment requires a 3 day hospitalization. Dilation to 12 to 15 mm is done on day 1, using the Savary-Guillard dilators over a guide wire as described for laser treatment (Fig. 8–3A, B). On day 2, a guide wire is passed endoscopically through the dilated tumor, and the proximal and distal extents of the tumor are measured. The endoscope is then removed, and the tumor probe is passed over the guide wire (Fig. 8–3C). The probe is advanced the measured distance to engage the distal extent of the tumor. When possible, a pediatric endoscope is passed to observe the proximal extent of the tumor.

The generator is set at a power of 8 to 10 watts, with a 2 second pulse duration. Five pulses of 2 seconds each are delivered, and the probe is withdrawn to the next segment as determined by probe length (Fig. 8–2D). Each segment is coagulated five times until the proximal end of the tumor is reached. The tumor probe is then removed, and the malignant stricture is reexamined endoscopically to confirm that all segments have been coagulated (Fig. 8–3E).

Following treatment, the patient is observed overnight for potential complications and is discharged on postoperative day 3. Follow-up endoscopy and retreatment is determined by symptoms, as with Nd:YAG laser therapy.

Bleeding

Although an extensive body of experience exists for the treatment of gastrointestinal bleeding with endoscopic lasers,[6–25] little of it pertains directly to bleeding lesions in the esophagus. The two most frequent sources of bleeding in the esophagus are esophageal varices and Mallory-Weiss tears. Together they make up about 25 to 30 per cent of all upper gastrointestinal bleeding sources.[58,59]

Many patients with bleeding esophageal varices were included in the early uncontrolled trials of laser therapy for gastrointestinal bleeding. Although initial hemostasis was usually achieved in these trials, the rate of recurrent bleeding (30 per cent) was much higher than that for other bleeding lesions.[10,11,14,60] Similar problems with recurrent bleeding were experienced during controlled trials that included lesions other than bleeding peptic ulcers.[19,20]

The only study that deals exclusively with bleeding from esophageal varices is that of Fleischer.[24] Initial hemostasis was achieved in 70 per cent of his patients using the Nd:YAG laser. Recurrent bleeding was common, however, and only 30 per cent of the patients had lasting hemostasis. Most endoscopists believe that endoscopic injection sclerosis is a more appropriate method to manage variceal bleeding,[61,62] although Keifhaber continues to use the Nd:YAG laser for initial control of bleeding, followed by injection sclerosis to maintain hemostasis.[63]

Several controlled and uncontrolled series also include a few patients with Mallory-Weiss tears.[10,14,15,19,21,60] None of these reports specifically addresses the efficacy of laser treatment for the tears, but the patients who re-bled or in whom complications of laser treatment were seen were not those with Mallory-Weiss tears. The laser appears to be effective in that situation, and this inference is supported by experience at the Universities of Utah and Lille.

Other lesions that may bleed in the esophagus include ulcers, esophagitis, vascular malformations, and malignancies. The first three of these are uncommon bleeding sources, but all have been treated with endoscopic lasers. Laser treatment is effective, but these lesions can also be treated effectively with other thermal modalities.

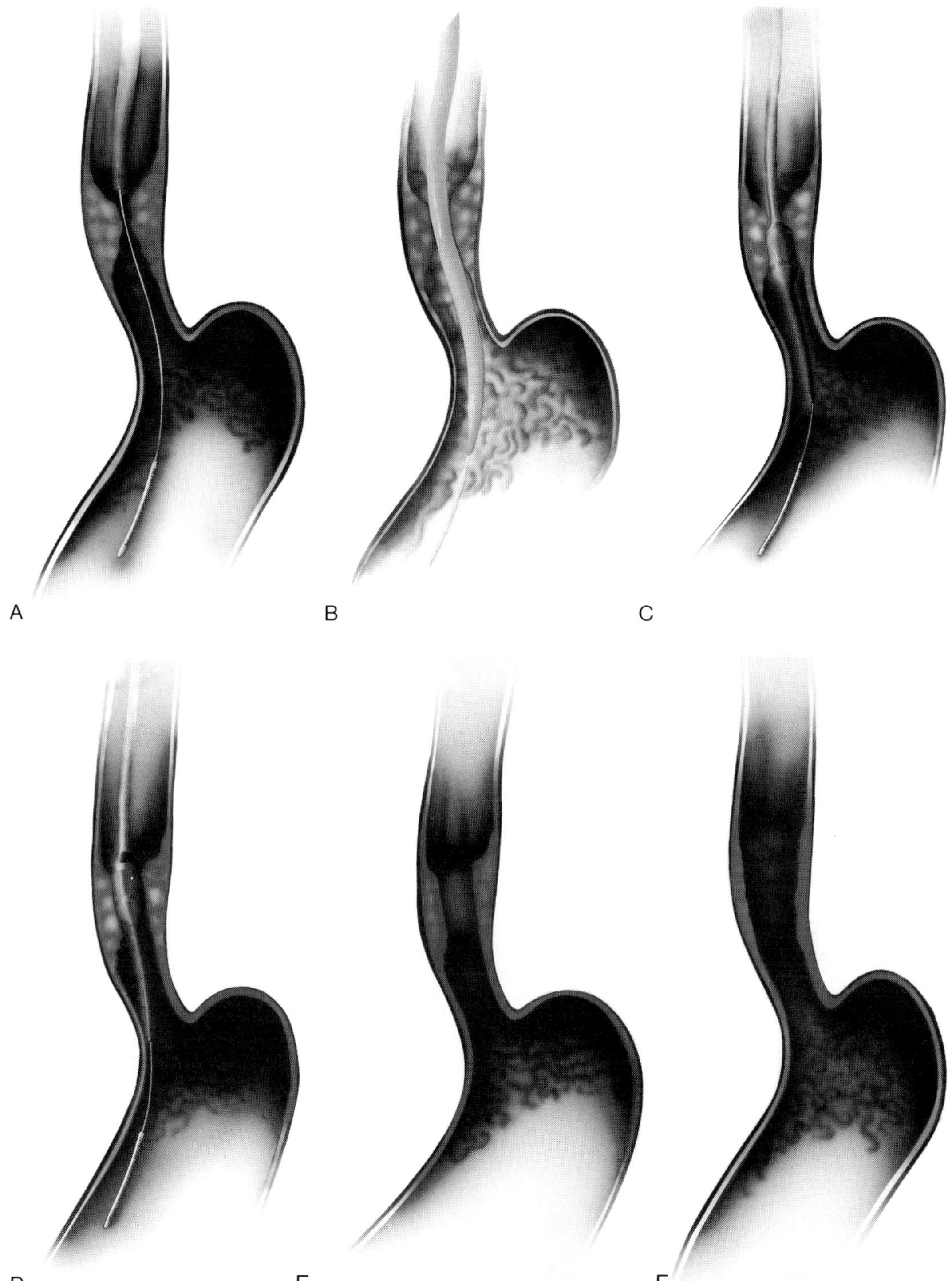

FIGURE 8–3. Treatment of an esophageal cancer with the BICAP tumor probe. *A, B,* The tumor is dilated, when necessary, over an endoscopically placed guide wire, in a manner similar to that in laser treatment (Fig. 8–2). *C,* The tumor probe is passed over the guide wire and advanced a measured distance to engage the distal segment of the tumor. *D,* Five 2-second treatment pulses are delivered at each tumor segment. The BICAP probe is then withdrawn the length of the cautery segment, and treatment is applied again. This sequence is repeated until the entire length of tumor has been coagulated. *E,* After treatment, the surface of the tumor has been coagulated to a depth of 1 to 3 mm. *F,* Two to 4 days later, the coagulated tumor tissue has sloughed away, leaving an enlarged lumen through the tumor.

Although not systematically addressed in these studies, the complication rates with the use of endoscopic laser to treat gastrointestinal bleeding are less than those observed with palliative tumor therapy. Perforation occurs in about 1 per cent of patients treated, whereas increased hemorrhage during laser treatment occurs in about 5 per cent of patients.[64]

Methods

The goal of laser photocoagulation of bleeding lesions is to create a cuff of edema around the bleeding point, which cuts off the inflow of blood to the source. The Nd:YAG laser requires adequate power to achieve tissue coagulation, usually 50 to 80 watts with 0.3 to 1.0 second applications. The energy is directed circumferentially around the active bleeding point and about 0.5 cm away. As the laser contacts the tissue, thermal shrinking of the mucosa occurs immediately. After a few minutes, this treatment produces a cuff of edema around the bleeding point, which usually reduces blood flow from the central lesion,[65] and often complete cessation of bleeding follows. If bleeding continues after the edema cuff forms, the laser energy may be directed centrally at the bleeding source to effect coagulation. Such direct laser energy, however, can induce further, massive bleeding and must be used with great caution if it is used at all. Short applications of higher powers with the Nd:YAG laser are more efficacious than longer applications at lower power,[66] but again the visible tissue reaction is often the best guide of effective energy delivery in the clinical setting (Fig. 8–4).

The argon laser is effective for the treatment of vascular malformations that may occur in the esophagus.[67–69] Vascular malformations may be hereditary, as in hereditary hemorrhagic telangiectasis (HHT), and can be responsible for blood loss beginning at an early age. Most are acquired, however, often in association with aortic valvular disease, portal hypertension, or renal disease.

Vascular malformations are particularly amenable to laser therapy. They are mucosal; they are rarely more than 1 to 2 mm deep; and, owing to their vascularity, they absorb light energy well in

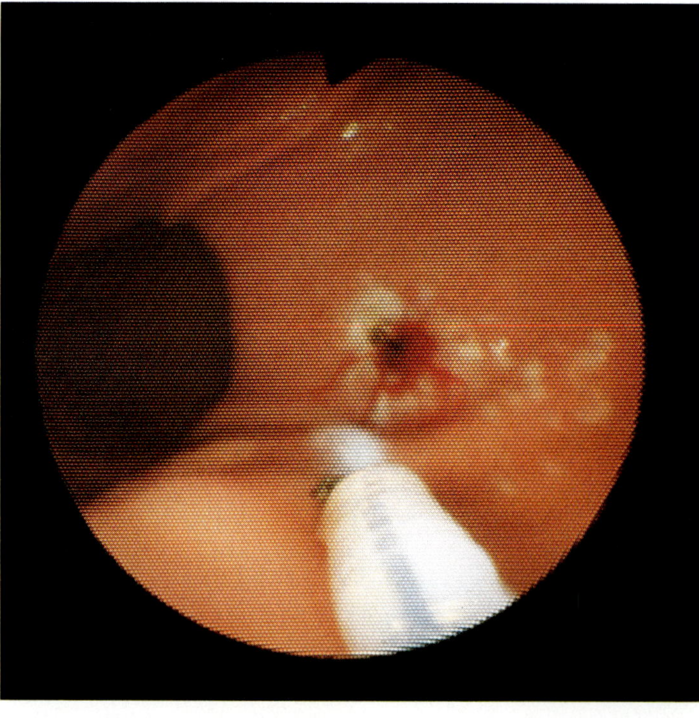

FIGURE 8–4. Laser treatment of a bleeding gastric arteriovenous malformation. The laser energy is directed circumferentially around the bleeding point to achieve a ring of whitish coagulation. The edema and coagulation then slow or stop the active bleeding, and the central lesion can be coagulated.

the argon laser wavelength. When these lesions are less than 2 mm in diameter, they are coagulated with a direct laser pulse. If larger, they are typically treated in a circumferential manner, as for an actively bleeding lesion, moving from the periphery to the center of the lesion. The argon laser is set at power outputs of 3 to 5 watts, with a spot size of 2 mm and applications of 1 to 5 seconds in duration. The resulting energy densities of 200 to 300 joules/cm^2 effectively coagulate most vascular lesions.

Benign Stenosis

The ability of the Nd:YAG laser to vaporize and ablate tissue can be used for incisional therapy of nonmalignant esophageal lesions. Successful incisional enlargement of congenital rings and webs of the esophagus has been described.[15] The Nd:YAG laser is set at 70 to 80 watts, and 0.5 second pulses are delivered to three or four quadrants of the ring (Fig. 8–5). Passage of the endoscope or a bougie through the ring then ruptures it at the treated points.

Several reports describe the use of lasers to enlarge postoperative strictures or anastomoses.[15,70–72] The technique is similar to that described for webs, although the total number of pulses required is usually greater, the incision is made on only one or two quadrants of the stricture, and subsequent dilation is usually not required.

The Nd:YAG laser has also been used to enlarge inflammatory strictures, most reflux induced, with a few due to caustic ingestions.[63,73,74] The reported results in more than 20 patients are good, but most of these patients also had daily postlaser dilation to maintain improvement. In the authors' experience, strictures longer than 1 or 2 cm do not respond well to laser treatment. The coagulation and inflammation caused by the laser energy often results in restenosis as the treated area heals. The beneficial results reported in the literature are probably attributable as much to the frequent dilation as to the laser treatment.

Benign Mucosal Lesions

The uniform, shallow depth of coagulation from the argon laser suggested that it might be appropriate for the ablation of benign gastrointestinal mucosal lesions. Dixon and colleagues reported animal and human studies verifying that colonic mucosa and mucosal polyps could be ablated with a minimal risk of perforation.[28]

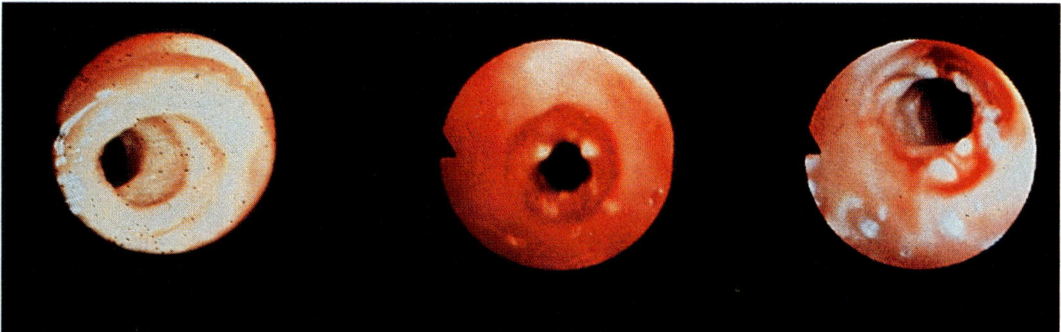

Figure 8–5. *Left,* Endoscopic view. Distal esophageal mucosal ring. *Center,* The Nd:YAG laser was used to coagulate a 2 mm spot on each of the four quadrants of the ring. *Right,* After coagulation, the endoscope was passed easily through the ring, rupturing it at the coagulated spots. A small amount of bleeding was seen, which quickly stopped.

Subsequently, the argon laser has been used to ablate multiple polyps on a recurrent basis in patients with hereditary polyposis syndromes.[62] It is also used for sporadic small, sessile adenomas in the colon and the stomach when standard resection cannot be performed.[15,29] Although such lesions are not seen in the esophagus, the argon laser could certainly be used for small mucosal lesions in the esophagus.

One innovative application of the argon laser was to ablate residual columnar mucosa in a patient who had undergone esophagectomy with a colonic interposition for dysplasia in a Barrett esophagus.[15] After ablation, the treated area reepithelized with squamous mucosa, suggesting that this might be a potential primary therapy in the future for eliminating columnar metaplasia in the esophagus.

References

1. Fruhmorgen P, Reidenbach HD, Bodem F, et al.: Experimental examinations on laser endoscopy. Endoscopy 6:116, 1974.
2. Silverstein FE, Protell RL, Gilbert DA et al.: Argon versus neodymium YAG laser photocoagulation of experimental canine gastric ulcers. Gastroenterology 77:491, 1979.
3. Dixon JA, Berenson MM, McCloskey DW: Neodymium-YAG laser treatment of experimental canine gastric bleeding: Acute and chronic studies of photocoagulation, penetration, and perforation. Gastroenterology 77:647, 1979.
4. Rutgeerts P, Van Trappen G, Geboes K, et al.: Safety and efficacy of neodymium-YAG laser photocoagulation: An experimental study in dogs. Gut 22:38, 1981.
5. Hunter JG, Burt RW, Becker JM, et al.: Colonic mucosal lesions: Evaluation of monopolar electrocautery, argon laser, and neodymium:YAG laser. Curr Surg 41:373, 1984.
6. Swain CP: Endoscopic Nd:YAG laser control of gastrointestinal bleeding. *In* Joffe SN (ed): Neodymium-YAG Laser in Medicine and Surgery. New York, Elsevier Science Publishing Co, 1983, p. 15.
7. Silverstein FE, Gilbert DA, Feld AD, et al.: Laser photocoagulation: Experimental and clinical studies. *In* Papp JP (ed): Endoscopic Control of Gastrointestinal Hemorrhage. Boca Raton, FL, CRC Press, 1981, p 87.
8. Dwyer RM, Yellin AE, Craig J, et al.: Gastric hemostasis by laser phototherapy in man. JAMA 236:1383, 1976.
9. Fruhmorgen P, Bodem F, Reidenbach HD, et al.: Endoscopic laser coagulation of bleeding gastrointestinal lesions with report of the first therapeutic application in man. Gastrointest Endosc 23:73, 1976.
10. Kiefhaber P, Nath G, Moritz K: Endoscopic control of massive gastrointestinal hemorrhage by irradiation with a high power neodymium YAG laser. Prog Surg 15:140, 1977.
11. Kiefhaber P: Survey data. *In* Papp JP (ed): Endoscopic Control of Gastrointestinal Bleeding. Boca Raton, FL, CRC Press, 1981, p 103.
12. Fleischer D: Lasers and gastroenterology. Am J Gastroenterol 79:406, 1984.
13. Dixon JA: General surgical and endoscopic applications of lasers. *In* Dixon JA (ed): Surgical Application of Lasers. Chicago, Year Book Medical Publishers, 1983, p 72.
14. Kiefhaber P: Laser endoscopic experience. Brussels, 5th International Symposium on Digestive Endoscopy, 1982.
15. Hunter JG, Bowers JH, Burt RW, et al.: Lasers in endoscopic gastrointestinal surgery. Am J Surg 148:736, 1984.
16. Swain CP, Bown SG, Storey DW, et al.: Controlled trial of argon laser photocoagulation in bleeding peptic ulcers. Lancet 2:1313, 1981.
17. Vallon AG, Cotton PB, Laurence BH, et al.: Randomised trial of endoscopic argon laser photocoagulation in bleeding peptic ulcers. Gut 22:228, 1981.
18. Jensen DM, Machicado GA, Tapia JI, et al.: Endoscopic argon laser photocoagulation of patients with severe upper gastrointestinal bleeding. Gastorintest Endosc 28:151, 1982.
19. Ihre T, Johansson C, Seligson U, et al.: Endoscopic YAG-laser treatment in massive upper gastrointestinal bleeding. Scand J Gastroenterol 16:633, 1981.
20. Escourrou J: Survey data. *In* Papp JP (ed): Endoscopic Control of Gastrointestinal Hemorrhage. Boca Raton, FL, CRC Press, 1981, p 103.
21. Rutgeerts P, Van Trappen G, Broeckaert L, et al.: Controlled trial of YAG laser treatment of upper digestive hemorrhage. Gastroenterology 83:410, 1982.
22. Swain CP, Bown SG, Salmon PR, et al.: Controlled trial of Nd:YAG laser photocoagulation in bleeding peptic ulcers. Gastroenterology 84:1327, 1983.
23. MacLeod IA, Mills PR, MacKenzie JF, et al.: Neodymium yttrium aluminum garnet laser photocoagulation for major haemorrhage from peptic ulcers and single vessels: A single blind controlled study. Br Med J 286:345, 1983.
24. Fleischer D: Endoscopic Nd:YAG laser therapy for active esophageal variceal bleeding. Gastrointest Endosc 31:4, 1985.
25. Krejs GJ, Little KH, Westergaard H, et al.: Laser photocoagulation for the treatment of acute peptic ulcer bleeding. N Engl J Med 316:1618, 1987.
26. Fleischer D: Endoscopic therapy of upper gastrointestinal bleeding in humans. Gastroenterology 90:217, 1986.
27. Johnston JH: Endoscopic thermal treatment of upper gastrointestinal bleeding. Endosc Rev 2:12, 1985.

28. Dixon JA, Burt RW, Rotering RH, et al.: Endoscopic argon laser photocoagulation of small sessile colonic polyps. Gastrointest Endosc 28:162, 1982.
29. Richey GD, Dixon JA: Ablation of atypical gastric mucosa and recurrent polyps by endoscopic application of laser. Gastrointest Endosc 27:224, 1981.
30. Fleischer D, Kessler F, Haye O: Endoscopic Nd:YAG laser therapy for carcinoma of the esophagus: A new palliative approach. Am J Surg 143:280, 1982.
31. Bloomer WD, Hellman S: Normal tissue responses to radiation therapy. N Engl J Med 293:80, 1975.
32. Fleischer DE, Sivak MV: Endoscopic Nd:YAG laser palliation for obstructing esophagogastric carcinoma. Lasers Surg Med 3:172, 1983.
33. Mellow MH, Pinkas H: Endoscopic therapy for esophageal carcinoma with Nd:YAG laser: Prospective evaluation of efficacy, complications, and survival. Gastrointest Endosc 30:334, 1984.
34. Brunetaud JM, Maunoury V, Cochelard D, et al.: Palliative treatment for esophagogastric cancer by laser photoablation. Laser Surg Med (in press).
35. Fleischer D, Sivak MV: Endoscopic Nd:YAG laser therapy as palliation for esophagogastric cancer. Gastroenterology 89:827, 1985.
36. Ahlquist DA, Gostout CJ, Viggiano TR, et al.: Endoscopic laser palliation of malignant dysphagia: A prospective study. Mayo Clin Proc 62:867, 1987.
37. Fleischer D, Sivak MV: Endoscopic Nd:YAG laser therapy as palliative treatment for advanced adenocarcinoma of the gastric cardia. Gastroenterology 87:815, 1984.
38. Groisser VW: YAG laser therapy of gastrointestinal tumors. Gastrointest Endosc 30:311, 1984.
39. Imaoka W, Okuda J, Ida K, et al.: Treatment of digestive tract tumor with laser endoscopy: Experimental and clinical studies. In Atsumi K, Nimsakul N (eds): Laser Tokyo '81. Tokyo, Inter Group Corp, 1981, p 5–7.
40. Cello JP, Gerstenberger PD, Wright T, et al.: Endoscopic neodymium-YAG laser palliation of nonresectable esophageal malignancy. Ann Intern Med 102:610, 1985.
41. Naveau S, Zourabichvili O, Poitrine A, et al.: Traitement palliatif des cancers de l'oesophage et du cardia par le laser YAG neodyme. Gastroenterol Clin Biol 11:364, 1987.
42. Peitrafitta JJ, Cartsens MH, Dwyer RM: Endoscopic laser therapy for the treatment of malignant esophageal obstruction. Lasers Surg Med 7:487, 1987.
43. Ell C, Demling L: Laser therapy of tumor stenoses in the upper gastrointestinal tract: An international inquiry. Lasers Surg Med 7:491, 1987.
44. Fleischer D: The laser in gastroenterology with emphasis on upper gastrointestinal malignancies. Symposium held at World Congress of Gastroenterology, Sao Paolo, Brazil, September 12, 1986. Gastrointest Endosc 33:119, 1987.
45. Fleischer D: Esophageal cancer and therapeutic cloggology. Gastrointest Endosc 34:147, 1988.
46. Jung M, Diezler P, Colemont L, Manegold BC: Treatment of inoperable obstructing cervical esophageal carcinoma. Gastrointest Endosc 34:178, 1988.
47. Johnston JH, Fleischer D, Petrini J, Nord HJ: Palliative bipolar electrocoagulation of obstructing esophageal cancer. Gastrointest Endosc 33:349, 1987.
48. Jensen DM, Machicado G, Randall G, et al.: Comparison of low-power YAG laser and BICAP tumor probe for palliation of esophageal cancer strictures. Gastroenterology 94:1263, 1988.
49. Rutgeerts P, Van Trappen G, Broechaert L, et al.: BICAP tumor probe treatment of esophageal and colorectal carcinoma: comparison with YAG laser therapy. Gastrointest Endosc 33:177, 1987.
50. Fleischer D: A comparison of endoscopic laser therapy and BICAP tumor probe therapy for esophageal cancer. Am J Gastroenterol 82:608, 1987.
51. Weishaupt KR, Gomer CJ, Dougherty TJ: Identification of singlet oxygen as the cytotoxic agent in photo-inactivation of a murine tumor. Cancer Res 36:2326, 1976.
52. McCaughan JS, Hicks W, Laufman L, et al.: Palliation of esophageal malignancy with photoradiation therapy. Cancer 54:2905, 1984.
53. McCaughan JS, Williams TE, Bethel BH: Palliation of esophageal malignancy with photodynamic therapy. Ann Thorac Surg 40:113, 1985.
54. Thomas RJ, Abott M, Bhathal PS et al.: High-dose photoirradiation of esophageal cancer. Ann Surg 206:193, 1987.
55. Hayata Y, Kato H, Okitsu H, et al.: Photodynamic therapy with hematoporphyrin derivative in cancer of the upper gastrointestinal tract. Semin Surg Oncol 1:1, 1985.
56. Murata Y, Yoshida M, Akimoto S, et al.: Evaluation of endoscopic ultrasonography for the diagnosis of submucosal tumors of the esophagus. Surg Endosc 2:51, 1988.
57. Fleischer DE: Endoscopic therapy for gastrointestinal neoplasma: From science fiction to science (editorial). Mayo Clin Proc 62:954, 1987.
58. Peterson WL, Barnett CC, Smith HJ et al.: Routine early endoscopy in upper-gastrointestinal-tract bleeding. N Engl J Med 304:925, 1981.
59. Gilbert DA, Silverstein FE, Tedesco FJ, et al.: The national ASGE survey on upper gastrointestinal bleeding. III. Endoscopy in upper gastrointestinal bleeding. Gastorintest Endosc 27:94, 1981.
60. Brunetaud JM, Mosquet L, Sabben G, et al.: Photocoagulation laser des hémorragies digestives graves du tractus digestif supérieur. Acta Gastroenterol Belg 45:47, 1982.
61. Sivak MV: Esophageal varices. In Sivak MV (ed): Gastroenterologic Endoscopy. Philadelphia, WB Saunders Co, 1987, p 342.
62. Buchi KN, Brunetaud JM: Endoscopic gastrointestinal laser therapy. In Dixon JA (ed): Surgical Application of Lasers, 2nd ed. Chicago, Year Book Medical Publishers, 1987, p 95.
63. Kiefhaber P: Indications for endoscopic neodymium-YAG laser treatment in the gastrointestinal tract. Twelve years' experience. Scand J Gastroenterol 22(suppl 139):53, 1987.

64. Johnston JH: Complications following endoscopic laser therapy. Gastrointest Endosc 28:135, 1982.
65. Dwyer RM: The technique of gastrointestinal laser endoscopy. *In* Goldman L (ed): The Biomedical Laser. New York, Springer-Verlag, 1981, p 20.
66. Johnston JH, Jensen DM, Mantner W, et al.: Nd:YAG Laser treatment of experimental bleeding canine gastric ulcers. Gastroenterology 79:1252, 1980.
67. Waitman AM, Grant DZ, Chateau F: Argon laser photocoagulation treatment of patients with acute and chronic bleeding secondary to telangiectasia. Gastrointest Endosc 28:153, 1982.
68. Jensen D, Machicado G, Tapia J, et al.: Endoscopic treatment of hemangiomata with argon laser in patients with gastrointestinal bleeding. Scand J Gastroenterol 17(suppl 78):182, 1982.
69. Bowers JH, Dixon JA: Argon laser photocoagulation of vascular malformations in the GI tract: Short term results. Gastrointest Endosc 28:126, 1982.
70. Sasako M, Iwasaki M, Konishi T, et al.: Clinical application of the Nd:YAG laser endoscopy. Lasers Surg Med 2:137, 1982.
71. Chen P, Wu C, Chang-Chien C, Liaw Y: YAG laser endoscopic treatment of an esophageal and sigmoid stricture after end-to-end anastomosis stapling. Gastrointest Endosc 30:258, 1984.
72. Sander R, Poesl H: Nd:YAG laser treatment of non-neoplastic GI stenoses. Gastrointest Endosc 32:170, 1986.
73. Sander R, Poesl H, Spuhler A: Management of non-neoplastic stenoses of the GI tract—a further indication for Nd:YAG laser application. Endoscopy 16:149, 1984.
74. Sander R, Poesl H: Treatment of non-neoplastic stenoses with the neodymium-YAG laser: Indications and limitations. Endoscopy 18(suppl 1):53, 1986.

CHAPTER 9

Laser Surgery for Benign Conditions in the Oral Cavity and Oropharynx

Michael H. Stevens

R. Kim Davis

The use of the laser in this anatomic location may be confusing to the neophyte and experienced operator alike. The reasons for this are several: One is that various wavelengths are applicable because of their unique suitability for specific lesions in the oral cavity and the oropharynx. Another is that there are a wide variety of diagnostic entities in the oral cavity and the oropharynx for which lasers have been used. A third reason is that, because of the theoretic advantages of lasers, they have been used successfully in clinical settings in which their actual advantages over traditional techniques unfortunately have not been documented. This chapter therefore attempts to help the reader understand when use of the laser really represents a clear advantage and when it does not. A methodical approach utilizing known safety factors is emphasized. Possible applications of each kind of laser are enumerated. Even though many surgeons may have access to only one laser, one should be aware of the unique capabilities of other lasers. Thus the individual patient can be referred to another surgeon with access to a laser that is better suited to the problem. The authors' experience with specific diagnostic entities is utilized to try to eliminate some of the confusion about laser treatment.

INDICATIONS

Many benign lesions involving the oral cavity and oropharynx are particularly well suited for the use of the laser. This is because of the advantages that apply to the use of lasers in other anatomic locations in the head and neck as well as those that are specific for the oral cavity and the oropharynx. These advantages include increased precision, better hemostasis, and decreased postoperative edema and pain, as well as less postoperative scarring and better wound healing,[1] than with conventional techniques. Fewer postoperative complications and less morbidity with less chance of airway compromise or dehydration produce shorter hospitalization time and a shorter operating time. Because of the laser's ability to control bleeding, treatment of vascular lesions, lingual tonsillectomy, tongue resections, and treatment of extensive leukoplakia or multicentric lesions are particularly well managed by lasers.

Limitations of the laser, however, include conditions in which resection of bone or osteotomies are required. Because of the high power density that is required of the laser under these circumstances, any cutting of bone is best not done with the laser.[2] In addition, deep extension of the lesions into buccal fat or lip muscle is also best not treated by the laser.

LASER CONSIDERATIONS

Although the ruby laser was the first to be used medically,[3] the carbon dioxide (CO_2) laser has probably been used more often than any other and for a wider variety of reasons. This is true in the oral cavity and the oropharynx. This is because the carbon dioxide wavelength is absorbed by water and all biologic tissues. It can be used as a scalpel to excise tissue for biopsy and can also vaporize tissues rapidly with negligible damage to the surrounding tissue. One can vary the spot size, the exposure time, and the power with most commercial CO_2 lasers.

The neodymium:yttrium-aluminum-garnet (Nd:YAG) laser is particularly suitable for darkly pigmented tissues, such as vascular lesions. However, because of its long extinction time and larger beam diameter, this laser causes more damage to surrounding tissue and has an energy distribution over a larger volume. It, therefore, is uniquely advantageous for deep vascular lesions, such as cavernous hemangiomas, because it can provide hemostasis of vessels several millimeters in diameter.

The argon laser is also absorbed by blood and pigmented tissues. Its beam is located in the visible light spectrum so focusing is rather easy. Because of absorption by vascular tissues, it provides hemostasis that is superior to that achieved with the CO_2 laser and can control vessels 1 to 2 mm in size. It has been used extensively for superficial lesions because it lacks the deep penetration of the Nd:YAG laser. It has an advantage in that it can be transmitted by flexible fibers that can be hand held, allowing better facility in aiming the beam. Lesions such as port wine stains, capillary hemangiomas, telangiectasias, and tattoos are particularly well suited for treatment with this laser. The disadvantage of this laser is that the operator has to wear orange or red glasses to protect her or his eyes. This causes more difficulty in accurately controlling any bleeding that does occur when treating vascular lesions.

Another laser that has been used in the oral cavity and the oropharynx is the potassium-titanyl-phosphate (KTP) laser. It is similar to the argon laser, but its beam frequency (532 mm) is closer to the wavelength of hemoglobin; therefore, it is thought to be better absorbed by vascular lesions. The other advantages are similar to those of the argon laser; however, it is more expensive. Both the KTP and argon lasers produce wavelengths in the visible range, eliminating the necessity for an aiming beam, which is needed for the CO_2 and Nd:YAG lasers. When a small spot size and precise aiming are required, there may be some difficulty with the CO_2 and Nd:YAG lasers that require a separate aiming beam. In the oral cavity, however, this is not an important consideration.[4]

SAFETY FACTORS

Although lasers are precise, they are potentially dangerous; therefore, there are important precautions that must be strictly adhered to. This applies to their use in the oral cavity or the oropharynx as well as in any other head and neck location. Because the anesthesiologist is competing with the surgeon for airway space, one of the chief hazards of the use of the laser is ignition of the endotracheal tube. This can be prevented by the use of either a metal tube or a rubber Rusch tube wrapped with aluminum foil. When working in the anterior oral cavity, the use of nasotracheal intubation can help reduce the chance of hitting the tube with the laser beam. When working in the oropharynx, covering the nasotracheal tube with saline-saturated cottonoids is essential; if the procedure is a prolonged one, repeated saturation is necessary. Decreasing the concentration of oxygen below 40 per cent and avoiding the use of nitrous oxide are adjunctive safety measures.

The next most important safety consideration is protection of the eyes. This includes not only the eyes of the patient and the operator but also those of ancillary personnel in the operating room. Warning signs should be placed on the doors at the entrance to the operating room. Saline-soaked eye pads are placed on the patient, and safety lenses are then positioned over these and taped in place for use of the argon, Nd:YAG, and KTP lasers. The color of the safety lenses depends on the type of laser that is used. For example, green lenses are appropriate for the Nd:YAG laser and orange to red for the KTP and argon lasers. The eyes are protected only by saline-soaked gauze sponges for the CO_2 laser, and operating room personnel wear clear lens glasses. It is important that the safety glasses worn by the surgeon and other personnel have side guards in addition to the lenses in front. The CO_2 laser primarily causes injuries to the cornea, whereas the others injure the retina because of their absorption properties.[6]

Special attention needs to be given to the skin of the face. The authors place a towel over the patient's face and secure this in place. Cloth rather than paper drapes should be used. It is important in working in the oral cavity that the lips and nose also be protected. The teeth are also covered with saline-soaked sponges or a tooth guard to avoid enamel burns.

Before proceeding, particularly with the CO_2 and Nd:YAG lasers, it is important to focus the beam to make certain that it is accurate at the start of each case. Use of a noncontinuous mode is an additional safety factor, because it limits exposure time. General anesthesia is preferred, although small lesions in the anterior portion of the mouth in a cooperative patient can easily be removed with local anesthesia. When general anesthesia is used, the patient should be paralyzed to avoid any motion. Often assistants are employed to provide retraction to gain exposure in the oral cavity, and there is a chance of injuring them with either reflection of the beam or direct impact of the beam on their hands in a microscope-mounted delivery system. Therefore caution must be exercised.

One of the difficulties with the use of the laser in the oral cavity and the oropharynx is that of poor exposure. This may be accentuated by prominent incisor teeth, trismus, or obscure location of the lesion. This may limit exposure so much that the use of the laser may be contraindicated.[7]

LASER APPLICATIONS

Vascular Lesions in Oral Cavity and Oropharynx

Most hemangiomas and all arteriovenous (AV) malformations of the tongue and the floor of the mouth represent discomforting and potentially serious clinical problems. Although the exact figure for overall incidence is not available from the literature, approximately 50 percent of all hemangiomas and 70 per cent of all lymphangiomas occur in the head and neck. Although many vascular malformations occurring in this area are isolated, these lesions may occur as a component of a number of systemic conditions such as Osler-Weber-Rendu, blue rubber bleb nevus, and Maffucci syndromes.

Patients with lingual AV malformations typically have complaints of recurrent bleeding, usually resulting from tongue biting. Other common presenting symptoms include pain, from either engorgement or trauma, and symptoms related to the volume of the lesion, namely difficulty in breathing, chewing, swallowing, or speaking. Most nonlaser treatment modalities employed for these problems have unsatisfactory results. Aggressive excision procedures, including CO_2 laser excision, often lead to recurrence or unacceptable functional disability owing to the removal of large amounts of lingual or intraoral tissue. Although these lesions are progressive, they are not truly neoplastic, and therefore a treatment centered on control of symptoms rather than wide excision of the lesion with its attendant functional disability is appropriate. The argon, KTP, or Nd:YAG laser can be used to photocoagulate these lesions with good success rates.[8]

The argon laser is best used to photocoagulate superficial vessels and to vaporize superficial blood vessels or lymph-containing vesicles. Treatment is usually carried out at power settings of 2 to 4 watts, in a continuous mode, utilizing a 600 micron fiber at a 1 cm distance and developing a 2 mm spot size. This represents approximately 75 watts/cm^2 with a total delivered energy level of 1000 to 4000 joules. As the argon laser output is at the 488 to 514 nm range, this wavelength is strongly absorbed by hemoglobin and penetrates to a depth of only 1 mm. Energy is applied with the argon laser in a "targeted spot" fashion to control specific sites of bleeding. A continuous ("painting") technique is useful in more confluent lesions.

In a situation such as hereditary hemorrhagic telangiectasia, the lips are also commonly involved and a much better cosmetic result can be obtained by using the argon laser than by trying any excision modality. Local anesthesia can easily be used in a cooperative patient, and laser treatment can be done in an outpatient setting. Large, superficial confluent areas of capillary hemangioma or port wine stains are often approached using a spot technique rather than treating the whole lesion at one setting. This allows the surgeon to treat again at a later time and avoids the potential necrosis or slough of the entire area with resultant scarring and poor healing.

Figure 9–1 shows a capillary-cavernous hemangioma of the tongue of a young child. This lesion was symptomatic as a result of bleeding during feeding. The lesion was initially controlled using the argon laser in a painting fashion. The child had resolution of bleeding for 3 months until bleeding recurred during bottle feedings. Therefore, the lesion was treated with the Nd:YAG laser in a targeted spot fashion (Fig. 9–2). This led to complete resolution of bleeding through a follow-up period of 1 year.

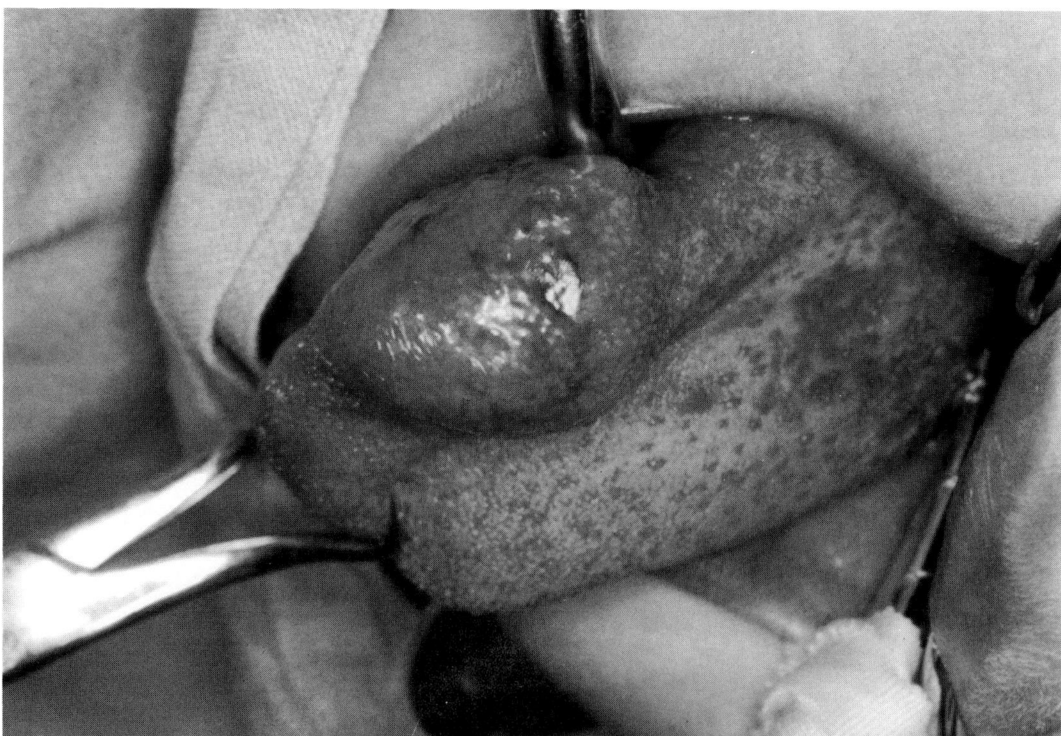

FIGURE 9–1. Capillary-cavernous hemangioma of the tongue of a young child.

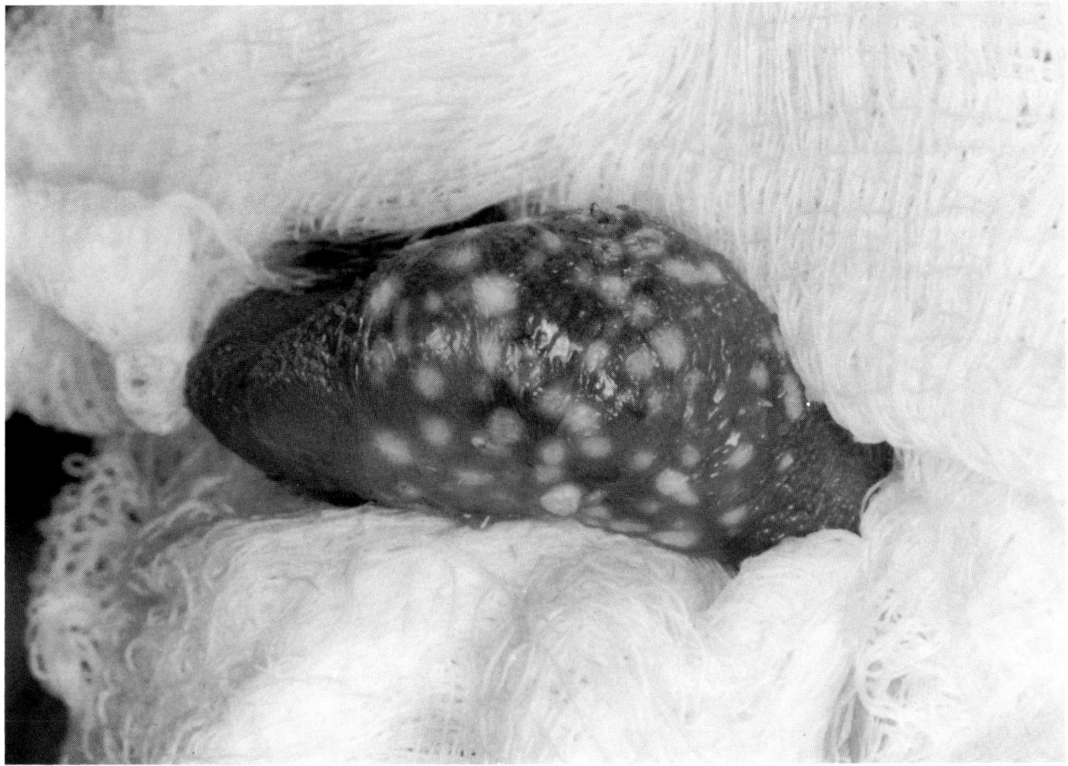

FIGURE 9–2. Lesion in Figure 9–1 after treatment with the Nd:YAG laser using spot technique.

The Nd:YAG laser can be cautiously used in the treatment of cavernous hemangiomas and AV malformations.[9–11] This is accomplished at a power setting of 30 to 50 watts with a 600 micron fiber at a 1 cm distance, using a 2 mm spot size for 0.2 to 0.5 second pulse duration. This represents 1000 to 3000 watts/cm^2 with a total delivered energy amount of 400 to 6000 joules. As the Nd:YAG laser output is at 1060 nm, this wavelength penetrates to a depth of 3 to 4 mm.

The Nd:YAG laser energy must be delivered in a spot fashion. The margins for each 2 mm application must be placed at least 2 mm apart to avoid overlap resulting from scattering of laser energy and subsequent necrosis. It must be remembered that large vessels that are more than 4 mm in diameter are not controlled well by the Nd:YAG laser, and additional methods of hemostasis, such as suture ligature or electrocautery, may need to be used in these instances.

Figure 9–3 shows a hemangiolymphangioma in the floor of the mouth, which frequently bled with trauma. Excision of the lesion would have produced unacceptable morbidity to the patient. This area was treated in a targeted spot fashion with the laser with good resolution of symptoms (Fig. 9–4).

Figures 9–5 and 9–6 show the pre- and post-operative views of an extensive hemangiolymphangioma of the tongue treated by Nd:YAG laser photocoagulation. The vascularity of the patient's lesion is greatly decreased, and the actual size of the tongue itself was not decreased (Fig. 9–6). The patient, however, experienced significantly less swelling of her tongue after laser therapy. Prior to therapy, on arising each morning the patient would often have to spend up to 45 minutes decreasing the size of her tongue to allow it to come back in the mouth. Following treatment with the Nd:YAG laser, this symptom completely resolved. Some experimental evidence suggests that excision to debulk lymphangiomatous lesions with the CO_2 laser coupled with Nd:YAG laser photocoagulation may confer the best long-term prognosis for these lesions. This needs to be studied more extensively.[12]

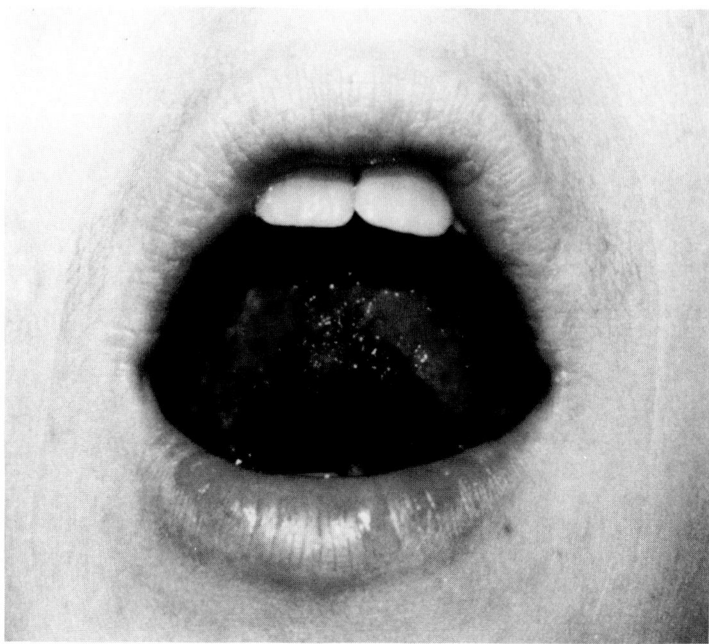

FIGURE 9–3. Hemangiolymphoma of the floor of the mouth. This was easily traumatized, leading to recurrent bleeding.

When large cavernous hemangiomas are approached with the Nd:YAG laser, caution must be used to photocoagulate the vessels without rupture and significant hemorrhage. This can be done by holding the laser fiber 3 to 4 cm from the area to be treated, thereby developing a greater thermal effect without the vaporization potential seen at closer application ranges. If an extensive amount of surgery is necessary and a large volume of tissue is photocoagulated, notable postoperative swelling and airway obstruction can develop. In cases of extensive treatment, patients must be intubated with a nasal tracheal tube for 1 to 2 days after therapy. Excision of limited areas is often done with the patient under local anesthesia on an outpatient basis.

Superficial tongue lesions can be effectively treated using the argon laser. This often can be done under local anesthesia and offered on an outpatient basis. Deeper lesions or lesions producing

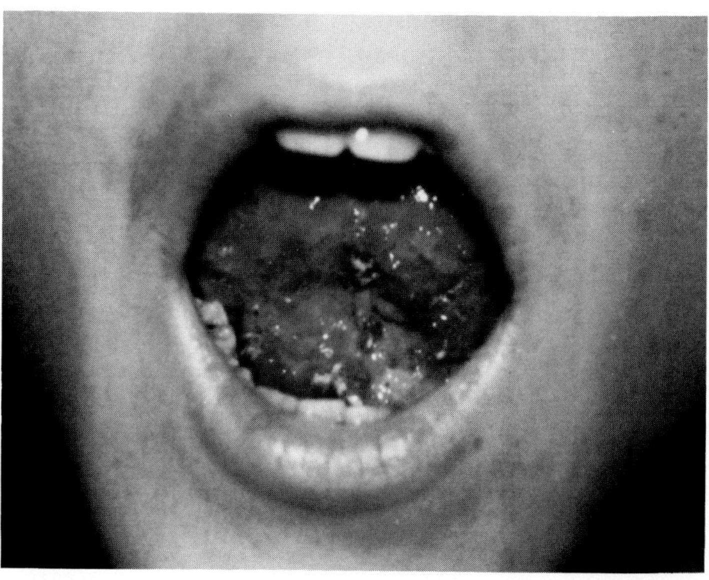

FIGURE 9–4. Postoperative appearance of the lesion in Figure 9–3 after laser treatment using the spot technique. The vascular lesion has been obliterated with preservation of most normal tissue.

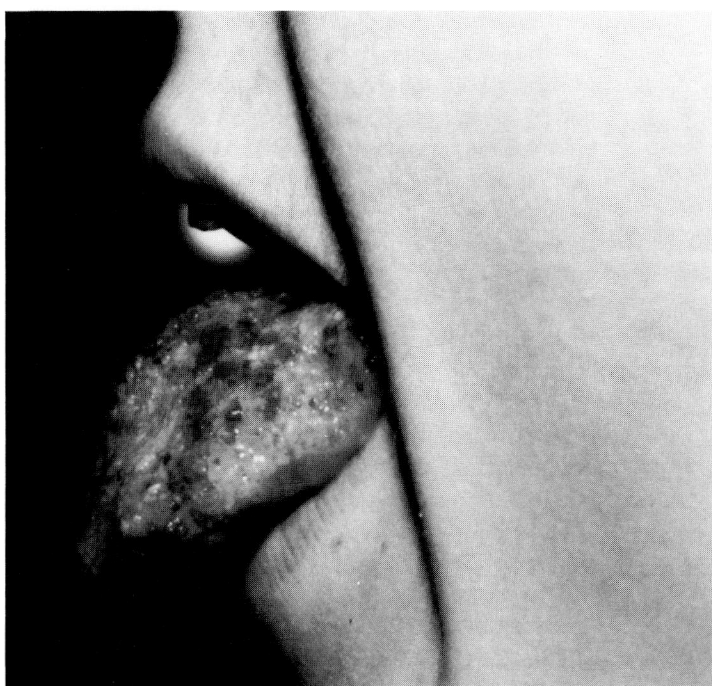

FIGURE 9–5. This extensive hemangiolymphoma of the tongue would swell extensively at night, forcing the tongue out of the mouth in the morning.

symptoms attributable to volume effect are more effectively treated with the Nd:YAG laser or with the argon and Nd:YAG lasers in combination. The Nd:YAG laser is the instrument of choice for debulking of lesions. These patients are hospitalized with careful airway management to include nasotracheal intubation for 24 to 48 hours if necessary.

Lymphangiomas can also be treated by laser photocoagulation or by laser excision. Carbon dioxide laser excision is effective in bulky lymphangiomas in which loss of some normal tongue or intraoral tissue does not lead to undue postoperative morbidity.[13] Such CO_2 laser excision has

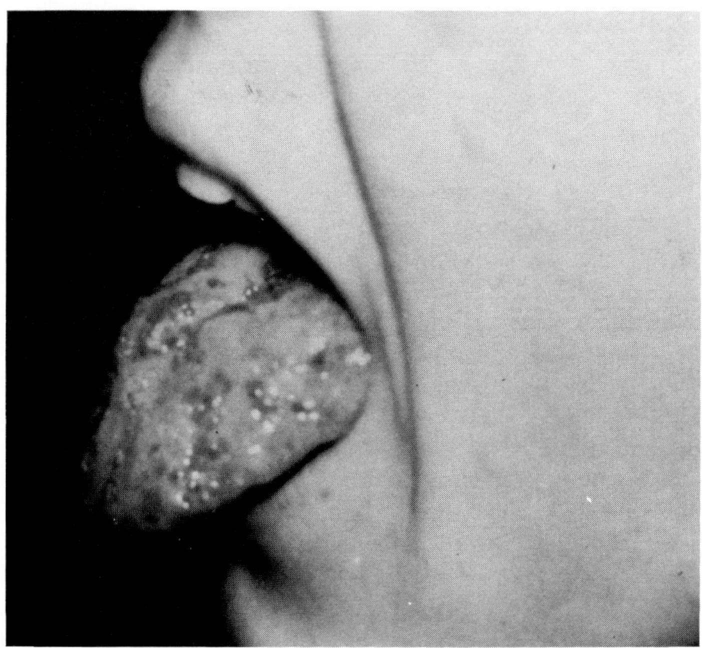

FIGURE 9–6. The postoperative appearance after Nd:YAG laser photocoagulation of the lesion in Figure 9–5 shows a decrease in vascularity. The most important difference was functional, with the degree of night-time swelling markedly decreased.

proved particularly helpful in the palliation of lymphangiomas that involve the entire tongue and the lateral oropharynx. These lesions become symptomatic when growth causes impingement of the lesion on the supraglottic larynx. Simple vaporization of these lesions after biopsy can yield long-term symptom-free intervals.

An alternative to laser excision is to debulk these lesions using the Nd:YAG laser. Lesions are treated in a targeted spot fashion, which causes some regression of the lesion. In this way, normal tissue is not excised, in the hope of decreasing morbidity. It is expected that extensive Nd:YAG laser treatment of these lesions leads to scarring in the treatment bed, which itself may become symptomatic. Whether Nd:YAG photocoagulation is a better method of palliation than simple excision must yet be studied.

In summary, the CO_2 laser is effective in debulking lymphangiomatous lesions and in treating capillary hemangiomas if loss of tissue does not result in functional disability. Superficial vascular lesions, such as the troublesome bleeding areas from hemangiolymphangiomas, can effectively be treated with the argon laser. Deep lesions, such as cavernous hemagiomas, are clearly best treated with the Nd:YAG laser. Caution must be exercised in use of the Nd:YAG laser not to overtreat by using confluent painting techniques. Such use will almost invariably lead to significant loss of tissue. The role of the KTP laser in vascular lesions of the oral cavity and the oropharynx is yet to be evaluated fully. It is likely that KTP laser effects most closely parallel those of the argon laser.

Lingual Tonsillectomy

Although lingual tonsillectomy is not commonly performed, there are patients who have recurrent lingual tonsillitis that is accompanied by significant dysphagia and occasionally even inspiratory stridor because of marked hypertrophy of the lingual tonsils.[14] The laser offers distinct advantages in this procedure. Previous excision attempts have generally included the use of electrocautery. Electrocautery techniques have significant disadvantages, which include poor exposure because of the difficulty of surgical access, bleeding, and postoperative swelling. Surgical difficulty is further compounded because there is no capsule around the lingual tonsil, and so excision is of necessity subtotal and incomplete.

The authors have used the CO_2 laser to great advantage in these cases: After draping the patient, the best access is obtained by using a Jako laryngoscope. A mouth guard is inserted to protect the teeth and the gums from excessive pressure. The laryngoscope must be moved from side to side, as each side is usually done separately, particularly if there is extensive hypertrophy present. An initial biopsy is taken, which is important in some cases to rule out lymphoma. This can be done with a regular forceps or with the laser. Following this, the CO_2 laser is used, usually with a continuous mode of about 8 to 10 watts and a spot size of 1.0 to 1.5 mm. Lower power settings can be used, but the procedures become excessively time consuming. At 8 to 10 watt settings, excellent hemostasis has been seen during the vaporization of the lingual tonsil. Although the patient has postoperative pain, it is probably less than that with traditional electrocautery techniques because of the reduced intraoperative manipulation. Should it be necessary, retreatment can also be accomplished with minimal morbidity. Care must be taken to protect the endotracheal tube with saline-soaked sponges. Because the lingual tonsil can extend down toward the larynx, the authors recommend the use of methylene blue–colored saline in the cuff of the endotracheal tube, as well as protection of the posterior pharyngeal wall with saline-soaked cottonoids. The authors have not experienced significant bleeding during the procedure or in the postoperative period in any patients they have treated.

This experience suggests that patients undergoing lingual tonsillectomy have less postoperative pain and more rapid recovery periods. There are, however, no studies in the literature regarding the amount of pain that is experienced by patients following lingual tonsillectomy with the laser versus that resulting from traditional techniques.

Palatine Tonsillectomy

Although several investigators have used the laser for removal of tonsils, it is the authors' opinion that definitive studies have not been done to document the advantages of the laser. Removal of the tonsils can be accomplished either by a hand-held applicator or by the use of the operating microscope. Although the adenoid can be removed by the laser at the same time by reflection of the beam off mirrors, the authors have not done adenoidectomy with the laser. Safety precautions as mentioned above are again applicable in this situation, particularly with regard to protection of the endotracheal tube. One of the authors (MHS) prefers the hand-held fiber to the microscope mount, because of ease of exposure. The CO_2 laser has been used, as well as the argon and KTP lasers, for tonsillectomy.

The technique of argon laser tonsillectomy is described: For speed of dissection, 10 to 12 watts is a good power setting. Generally either a 600 mm fiber or a 300 mm fiber can be used with the hand-held device. The end of the fiber is placed 1 cm or less from the tissue to obtain a spot size of about 1 mm. This allows fairly rapid cutting. The tonsil is grasped and pulled toward the midline; then the mucosal incisions are made, following which the laser is used to identify the capsule and the tonsil is removed from its bed. An assistant is employed to suction away the smoke. Any small pieces of tonsillar tissue that are left can be vaporized. In the experience of one of the authors (MHS) the argon laser has resulted in a virtually bloodless field. Usually only 1 to 2 ml of blood on each side has been lost because small bleeders can be well controlled with the laser.

Investigators have reported successful tonsillectomy using the CO_2 laser[15] and the KTP laser. Although some reports have described shortened operative time, the author (MHS) has not found this to be the case. Other researchers also suggested that laser surgery causes less postoperative pain, but at the present time there is no study in the literature other than antecdotal statements to substantiate this claim. In many cases the placebo effect may be playing a significant role, wherein the physician tells the patient beforehand that because she or he is using the laser, the patient will have less pain. Studies evaluating the degree of pain after tonsillectomy with the laser are necessary.

The author (MHS) is currently involved in a single blind study wherein the argon laser is used to remove one tonsil and electrocautery is used to remove the other tonsil. The patient does not know which tonsil is removed with the laser. At the time of this writing, 30 cases have been done. Findings so far indicate that there is little bleeding with either technique. There is slightly more bleeding with the electrocautery technique. The amount of blood loss has usually ranged from 5 to 10 ml versus 1 to 2 ml with the laser. Although the laser does a better job of hemostasis intraoperatively, the difference when one considers the minimal amount of blood loss involved is not important. There has not been a significant decrease in operative time. If there were a time savings because of fewer bleeding vessels to coagulate, this would represent an advantage. Both the argon and KTP lasers, however, necessitate the use of colored glasses by the operating team, which make detection of bleeding that does occur more difficult.

So far there has been no significant difference in the amount of pain experienced postoperatively by the patient between the two sides in this study. Some patients have reported more pain on the laser side, whereas others have reported more pain on the electrocautery side. Therefore, in view of the substantial expense of laser use, laser tonsillectomy does not appear to be cost effective at this time. To offset the cost of the laser, one would have to significantly reduce operative time or postoperative pain or other complications, such as bleeding, and reduce the necessity for rehospitalization to make this technique one that should be endorsed. As this study progresses, further information will be obtained regarding what advantages the laser might have in tonsillectomy.

Uvulopalatoplasty

Uvulopalatoplasty is commonly performed by otolaryngologists, and the laser would seem to have some theoretic advantages in doing this procedure. One advantage should be the ability to achieve hemostasis, and others would be decreased postoperative pain and improved healing. The author (MHS) has therefore undertaken to perform the uvulopalatoplasty on one side with electrocautery and on the other side with the laser. Experience so far has shown no significant difference in healing, postoperative pain, or bleeding. There is slightly more bleeding near the midline with electrocautery in the area of the musculus avulae, but again this difference is insignificant. Principally because of the cost to the patient, the authors, therefore, cannot recommend the routine use of the laser in uvulopalatoplasty. That the laser can be used for a given procedure does not necessarily mean that it should be used simply because it is easier or more enjoyable for the surgeon. The benefit to the patient must be kept foremost in mind and must be paramount when considering the use of any new techniques.

Tongue Resection

Potential advantages of the laser in this instance seem to be self-evident and principally involve the control of bleeding. Although tongue resection can be accomplished with electrocautery, significantly more tissue injury is anticipated; potentially better healing can be accomplished with less pain with laser resection. Although a large study reported decreased pain in 100 procedures wherein the tongue was resected with the use of the CO_2 laser,[16] again one wonders what the placebo effect might be. This was an uncontrolled study, therefore, the additional cost to the patient may not be justified. Again, this is a procedure in which the laser can be used, but the question is, should it be used? Possible indications for laser application include benign or malignant tongue lesions, glossoptosis, and sleep apnea. Potential advantages include decreased bleeding, decreased swelling, and improved healing. Several lasers potentially can be used for this, including the CO_2 argon, and KTP lasers. If the argon laser is used, a unit in which a higher power is obtainable would be recommended for purposes of increasing the speed of the resection. Handheld or microscope-mounted delivery systems can be used, depending on the surgeon's preference. Large posterior lesions would probably be best handled with a consideration of performing a tracheotomy at the same time for airway control.

Diffuse Leukoplakia Treatment

An ideal use of the laser is for excising large areas of leukoplakia with minimal morbidity and bleeding.[17] Small areas of involvement could be vaporized. The advantages previously reported have been increased speed of removal, better hemostasis, reduced recurrence rate, and excellent wound healing. After excision the area is left open for healing by second intention. Biopsy should always be done on areas of ulceration or erythematous change that may be suggestive of cancer.

Therapy for Floor of Mouth Lesions

There are some unique lesions in the floor of the mouth that the laser can treat with some advantage. The CO_2, argon, or KTP laser could be used in treating ranulas by excising and/or vaporizing the roof of the cyst. Using the laser to seal the edge of the excised tissue may allow the marsupialized area to stay open without the need for sutures at the edge of the excision. Anticipated advantages would be less pain because of decreased manipulation and lack of necessity to use sutures.

This use has not been reported in the literature, and the authors do not have experience with it. One of the reasons for considering the use of the laser in this instance is the potential decrease in stenosis of Wharton duct. In the past this was thought to represent an important advantage, particularly in dealing with lesions such as floor of the mouth tumors. A recent study, however, suggests that the lasers do not have a distinct advantage over electrocautery or the knife in this particular instance.[18] Patients had just as many postoperative symptoms referable to obstruction of the submandibular gland with or without the laser.

Other Uses of the Laser in the Oral Cavity and Oropharynx

Removal of a lingual thyroid by laser surgery has the potential advantages cited for laser tongue resection.[19] Papillomas involving the soft palate or other areas can be easily removed with the laser, as can benign pleomorphic adenomas, pyogenic granulomas, or denture-induced hyperplasia.[20] Other benign lesions such as fibromas, chronic candidiasis, erosive lichen planus, benign cysts, amyloid tumors, granular cell myoblastoma, myxoma, or neurilemomas could be excised with the laser.[20] In all of these applications, the surgeon should consider whether using the laser represents a cost effective advantage to the patient.

References

1. Andrews AH, Polyani TG, Grybauskas VT: General techniques and clinical considerations in laryngologic laser surgery. Otolaryngol Clin North Am 16:800, 1983.
2. McDonald GA, Simpson GT: Transoral resection with carbon dioxide laser. Otolaryngol Clin North Am 16:843, 1983.
3. Simpson GT, Polyani TG: History of the CO_2 laser in otolaryngologic surgery. Otolaryngol Clin North Am 16:739, 1983.
4. Polyani TG: Laser physics. Otolaryngol Clin North Am 16:759, 1983.
5. Hayes DM, Gaba DM, Goode RL: Incendiary characteristics of a new laser-resistant endotracheal tube. Otolaryngol Head Neck Surg 95:37, 1986.
6. Ossoff RH, Duncavage JA: The CO_2 laser in otolaryngology–head and neck surgery: Advantages, precautions, administrative considerations, and complications. In Johnson JT, Blitzer A, Ossoff RH, Thomas JR (eds): Instructional Courses, Vol I. St Louis, CV Mosby Co, 1988, p. 67.
7. McDonald GA, Simpson GT: Transoral resection with carbon dioxide laser. Otolaryngol Clin North Am 16:840, 1983.
8. Apfelberg DB, Bailin P, Rosenberg H: Preliminary investigation of KTP/532 laser light in the treatment of hemangiomas and tattoos. Lasers Surg Med 6:38, 1986.
9. Dixon JA, Davis RK, Gilbertson JJ: Laser photocoagulation of vascular malformations of the tongue. Laryngoscope 96:537, 1986.
10. Shapshay SM, David LM, Zeitels S: Neodymium-YAG laser photocoagulation of hemangiomas of the head and neck. Laryngoscope 97:323, 1987.
11. Rosenfeld H, Sherman R: Treatment of cutaneous and deep vascular lesions with the Nd:YAG laser. Lasers Surg Med 6:20, 1986.
12. Primrose WJ, McDonald GA, O'Brien MJ, et al.: Synergistic effects of sequential carbon dioxide and neodymium: yttrium aluminum garnet laser injuries. Experimental observations and measurements. Ann Otol Rhinol Laryngol 96:47, 1987.
13. White B, Adkins WY: The use of the carbon dioxide laser in head and neck lymphangioma. Lasers Surg Med 6:293, 1986.
14. Joseph J, Reardon E, Goodman M: Lingual tonsillectomy: A treatment for inflammatory lesions of the lingual tonsil. Laryngoscopy 94:179, 1984.
15. Martinez SA, Atkin DP: Laser tonsillectomy and adenoidectomy. Otolaryngol Clin North Am 20:271, 1987.
16. Carruth JAS: Resection of the tongue with the carbon dioxide laser: 100 cases. J Laryngol Otol 99:887, 1985.
17. Chu FW: CO_2 laser treatment of oral leukoplakia. Laryngoscope 98:125, 1988.
18. Mihail R, Zajtchuk JT, Davis RK: Incidence of Wharton's duct stenosis in floor of the mouth cancers excised with scalpel or cautery vs CO_2 laser. Head Neck Surg 4:241, 1987.
19. Crockett DM, McGill RJI, Healy GV, Friedman EM: Benign lesions of the nose, oral cavity and oropharynx in children: Excision by carbon dioxide laser. Ann Otol Rhinol Laryngol 94:489, 1985.
20. Frame JW: Removal of oral soft tissue pathology with the CO_2 laser. J Oral Maxillofac Surg 43:850, 1985.
21. Evans PHR, Frame JW, Brandrick J: A review of carbon dioxide laser surgery in the oral cavity and pharynx. Laryngol Otol 100:67, 1986.

CHAPTER 10

LASER SURGERY for Oral Cavity and Oropharyngeal Cancer

R. Kim Davis

Soon after the introduction of microsurgery with the carbon dioxide (CO_2) laser in the larynx, attention was directed to other soft tissue applications of this therapeutic modality. One of the first procedures investigated was treatment of premalignant lesions of the oral cavity.[1] Leukoplakia, a white lesion that in a small percentage of cases can overlie a superficially invasive malignancy, was one of the first lesions treated. This lesion can involve a small aspect of intraoral mucosa or can extend through the buccal mucosa and the gingivobuccal areas in the floor of the mouth. When leukoplakia has appeared as an isolated small lesion, it typically has been removed by limited excision followed by primary closure. It also has been treated by electrocautery excision, electrofulguration, and cryosurgery. All of these modalities have been successful in limited lesions, but led to problems with the more extensive areas of leukoplakia occasionally seen. In light of this, it was only natural that the CO_2 laser was investigated to determine if it represented a better therapeutic modality.

Leukoplakia has been treated two ways historically with the laser: (1) by excision using the laser as a cutting instrument after outlining the lesion or (2) by laser vaporization. When lesions are vaporized, a laser is used simply to paint over the surface of the lesion, thereby destroying it. Generally vaporization is used for extensive lesions. The problem with this technique is that it is not possible to examine a surgical specimen to determine if cancer exists in any area on the underface of this lesion.

Laser surgery was also used for erythroplasia, a red-appearing lesion, that much more frequently is precancerous. The best treatments with the laser involved excisional biopsy of erythroplastic areas. The step from treatment of erythroplasia to that of T1 squamous cell carcinomas of the oral cavity was not a large one, as the surgical techniques involved in excision of small cancers are similar to those best used in erythroplasia.[2]

Initial use of the laser in the oral cavity was accomplished in one of two ways: (1) using microsurgical technique with the CO_2 laser delivered to the tissues using a micromanipulator or (2) delivering laser energy using handpieces (the handpiece served in essence as a scalpel without microscopic attachment). The microsurgical technique offered microscopic precision and excellent visualization. Both techniques were successfully used for leukoplakia, erythroplasia, and early cancer.

Use of the CO_2 laser to remove erythroplasia and leukoplakia, especially as excisional biopsy procedures, represented an application of the laser technique in place of other commonly used methods of biopsy. The advantage of laser use was the better hemostasis obtained and, especially with microscopic guidance, the better visualization obtained. This use of the laser was much in concert with standard oncologic principles of performing biopsy before making decisions concerning therapy. When the laser was used for excision of early cancer, the question of the oncologial soundness of this approach became an issue. With small T1 cancers, the laser effectively could be used to resect the lesions with a wide margin of normal tissue in the same manner as any other surgical technique. In this sense laser surgery is indeed oncologically sound and confers the advantages cited above over other methods of excision. The questions concerning laser application with T1 oral cavity cancer are the same questions that pertain to any surgical technique relating to early stage cancer in the oral cavity or the oropharynx.

In contrast to lesions in the glottic larynx, stage I cancer in the oral cavity can have a great propensity for spread to distant sites.[3–7] A critical review of the United States and European literature concerning survival rates is presented in Table 10–1. Distressingly, survival rates with either surgery or irradiation alone for early oral cavity cancer are much lower than expected. Although it can be argued that such reports reflect cancers inadequately treated by either modality, it is nonetheless the case that early oral cavity cancers are cured in much lower percentage than early cancer in the laryngeal area.

It is generally considered that surgery alone in early oral cavity cancer can effectively treat the primary site, but if neck dissection is not added to the primary cancer resection, treatment failure can occur in the neck owing to occult metastatic spread at the time of initial presentation. With irradiation therapy, the occult spread to the neck is generally effectively treated, whereas the primary lesion may not be most satisfactorily treated. If interstitial implantation is added to external beam irradiation therapy, the rates of local control in the oral cavity itself become much higher, but at the expense of significant morbidity from radiation ulceration and radionecrosis when lesions lie adjacent to the mandible. The obviously important question then becomes, which of these modalities is best? and second, when should standard combined therapy be used? Although these issues again do not pertain to laser surgery directly, they have relevance for laser use when laser application is the surgical modality selected.

Table 10–1. SURVIVAL RATES WITH EARLY ORAL CAVITY CANCER

Stage	3 Year NED Status, European	
	Number of Patients	*All Modalities (%)*
I	161	68
II	241	52
III	231	39
IV	169	17

Stage	3 Year NED Status, United States		
	Surgery (%)	*Irradiation (%)*	*Both (%)*
I	48	52	82
II	33	52	74
III & IV	31	15	46

NED, No evidence of disease.

One of the most helpful methods of determining the magnitude and type of therapy to be used in oral cavity malignancy involves using the laser as an excisional biopsy tool. It is possible to excise small floor of the mouth or tongue carcinomas (T1 lesions) with minimal morbidity. Such excision is done with the standard wide margins, which would allow this surgery to have the same results as a standard surgical approach. The advantages of better hemostasis and excellent visualization, when the laser is attached to an operating microscope, make laser use in this manner a reasonable choice. After the biopsy specimen has been removed and oriented in a standard manner, routine histopathologic examination is undertaken.

In an interesting paper from Japan,[8] the investigators not only used routine histologic examination, but also used Jakobsson's criteria, which are listed in Table 10–2. These histologic criteria have been well studied in Scandinavia. Although they are somewhat difficult to determine, these criteria have been reliable in identifying which cancers have a more threatening prognosis. The most important single factor listed is cancer mode of invasion. When the cancer deeply infiltrates adjacent tissue as single cell or cordlike extensions, the propensity for local treatment failure and neck metastases becomes markedly greater. Using this criterion as a guide, it is possible to determine which patients need more extensive surgery at the primary site as well as neck dissection versus those requiring postoperative irradiation after the initial laser excision procedure.

When the initial lesion is size T2 (between 2 and 4 cm in largest diameter) or larger, combined therapy almost always is necessary. The role of the laser can be that of the excision modality when surgery is opted for, or laser surgery can be used for limited excisional or incisional biopsy prior to definitive therapy. Laser use for purely incisional biopsy confers no advantage over other standard techniques and is probably best not used.

Use of laser surgery in advanced cancer of the oral cavity has little role except in certain experimental situations in stage IV cancer (see below).

CANCER DETECTION WHEN PATIENTS HAVE DIFFUSE LEUKOPLAKIA AND/OR ERYTHROPLASIA

When patients have areas of leukoplakia or erythroplasia, the total extent of tumor is often difficult to detect visually. It is true that areas of erythroplasia (as mentioned above) much more often are sites of microinvasive cancer. Erythroplasia must be excised, and the specimen should be carefully studied histologically. The more problematic situation involves leukoplakia. Cancer presence is more difficult to determine. The concept of field cancerization is an additional factor that leads to difficulty in determining the true extent of aerodigestive tract cancer. This was originally proposed by Slaughter and is based on the premise that carcinogens in the aerodigestive tract work diffusely throughout the entire tract.[9] Whereas obvious cancer may develop at one site, severe dysplasia may be present in another location but not be clinically evident. One of the methods to deal with this problem involves the use of the supravital stain toluidine blue.[10]

Toluidine blue is a nuclear stain that specifically stains DNA. As dysplastic and cancerous cells normally have higher concentrations of DNA, these areas stain more intensely when toluidine

Table 10–2. JAKOBSSON'S CRITERIA (Tumor–Host Relations)

1. Cellular response
2. Vascular invasion
3. Stage of invasion
4. Mode of invasion
   a. Well-defined border
   b. Cords, less marked borderline
   c. Groups of cells, no distinct borderline

blue is applied. Figure 10–1 shows an area of leukoplakia in the oral cavity. When the dye is added, several areas stain intensely, which did not have a clinically different appearance (Fig. 10–2). Biopsy directed to these spots has the greatest chance of proving the presence of malignancy.

Cancer detection has been facilitated by the introduction of photodynamic cancer identification.[11] This technique involves the administration of a photoactive compound, such as the dye hematoporphyrin or dihematoporphyrin ether (DHE). DHE is a purified hematoporphyrin derivative that is taken up in the perivascular stroma around tumor cells. Approximately 24 to 48 hours after intravenous injection of DHE, the concentration near tumor cells is significantly greater than the concentration surrounding other normal oral cavity cells. When the oral cavity is exposed to a Wood lamp, a fluorescence is seen in the areas of greatest DHE uptake. Figure 10–3 shows a T1 squamous cell cancer before DHE administration. Figure 10–4 shows the area of fluorescence when the floor of the mouth is exposed to a Wood lamp. Biopsy can be directed to these areas.

LASER APPLICATIONS

Severe Dysplasia and Carcinoma in Situ

Carcinoma in situ as well as severe dysplasia is best treated by excision techniques. As mentioned above, the most specific technique involves use of the CO_2 laser coupled to the operating microscope. Exposure to the anterior floor of the mouth is obtained by placing a Jennings mouth gag or a bite block and placing a suture through the tongue and retracting this to the side. The microscope is then positioned, and the area is outlined as shown in Figure 10–5. After the circumferential laser incision is made, the mucosa around the lesion retracts greatly. Silk traction sutures are placed, and

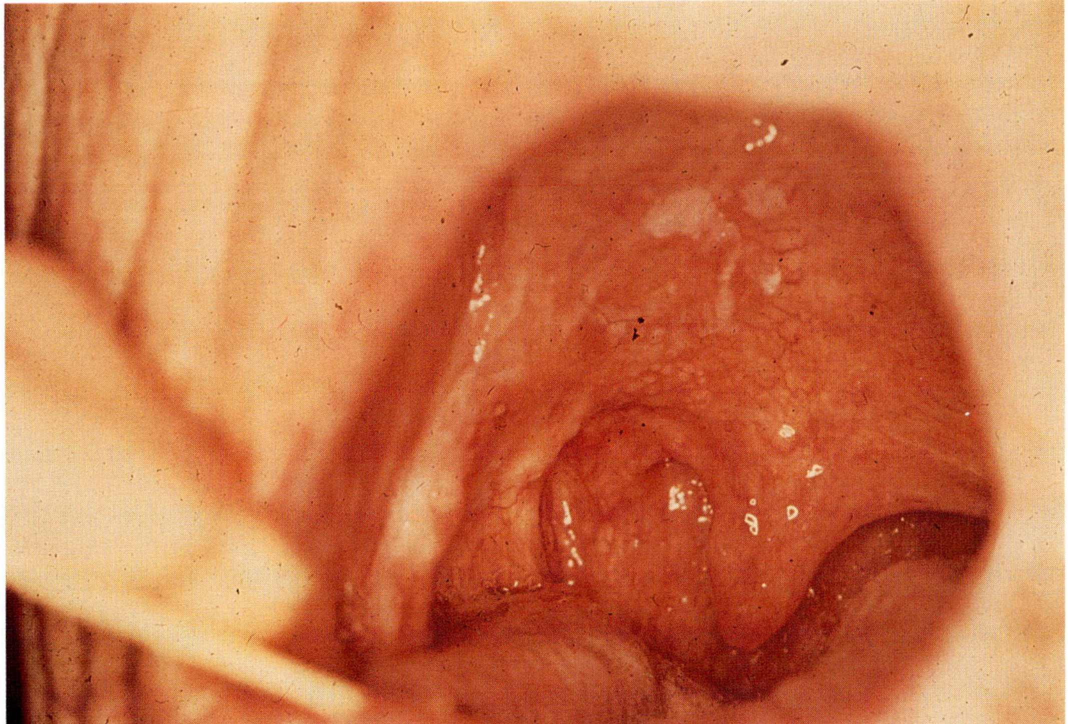

FIGURE 10–1. Areas of leukoplakia on the palate of a patient.

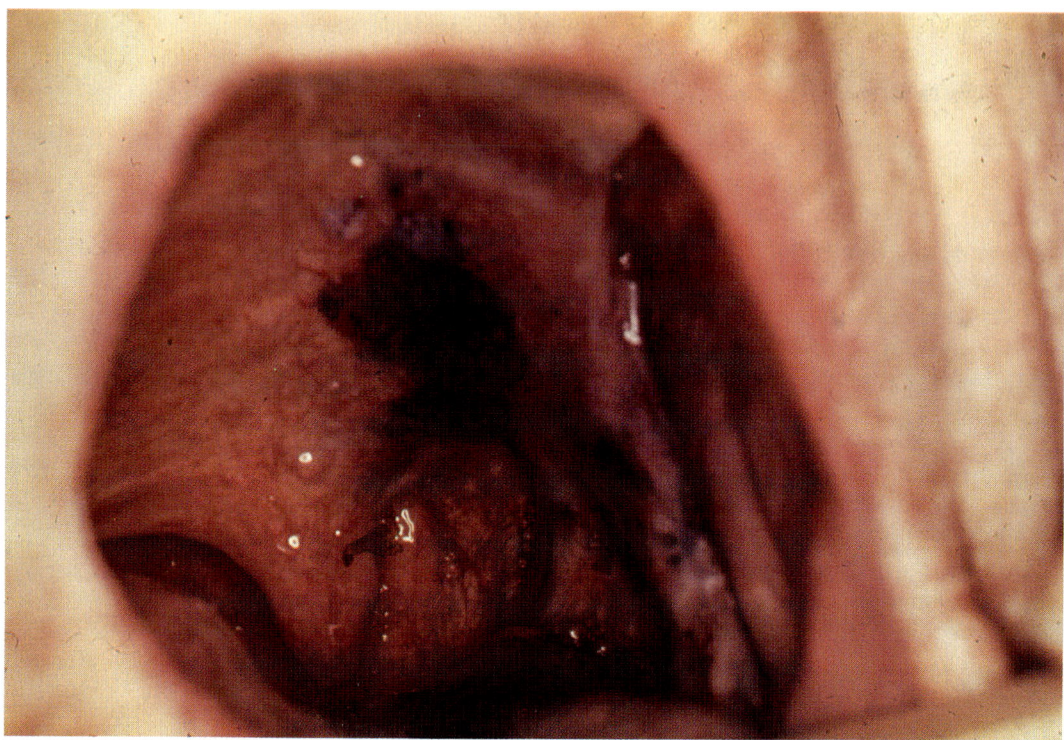

FIGURE 10–2. The supervital stain toluidine blue was applied to the palate. Note the areas of intense staining, which indicate areas most likely to be cancerous. Also note that the areas of leukoplakia well seen in Figure 10–1 do not intensely stain and probably do not reflect cancer presence.

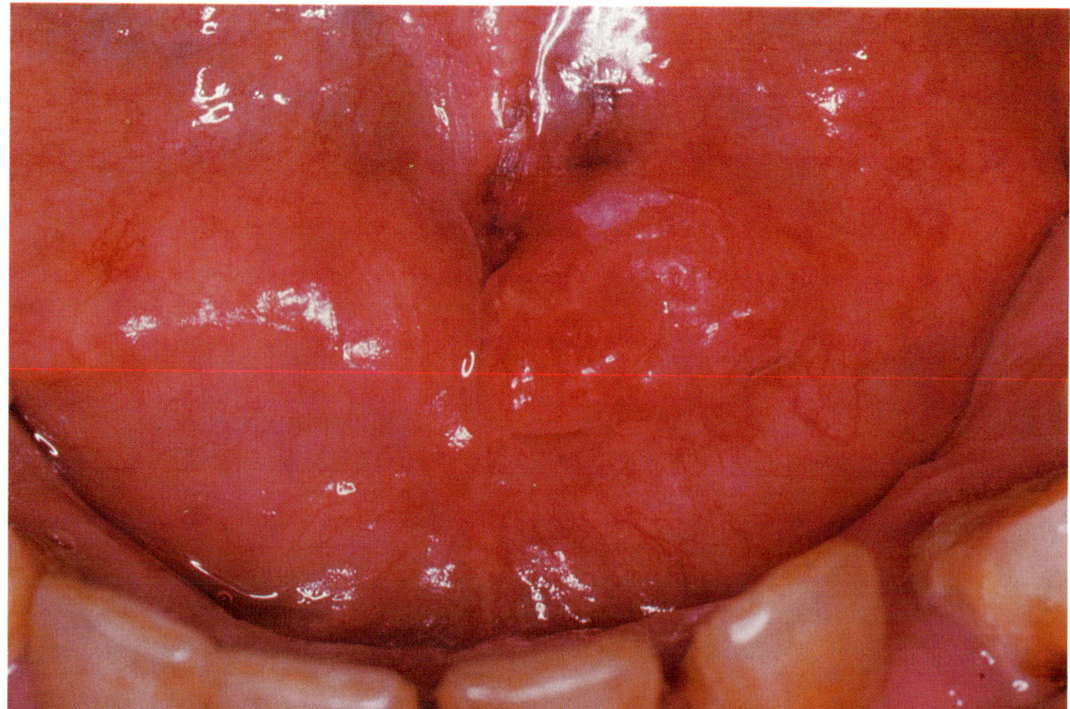

FIGURE 10–3. A stage I squamous cell carcinoma of the anterior floor of the mouth. (Courtesy of James Hill, M.D., deceased.)

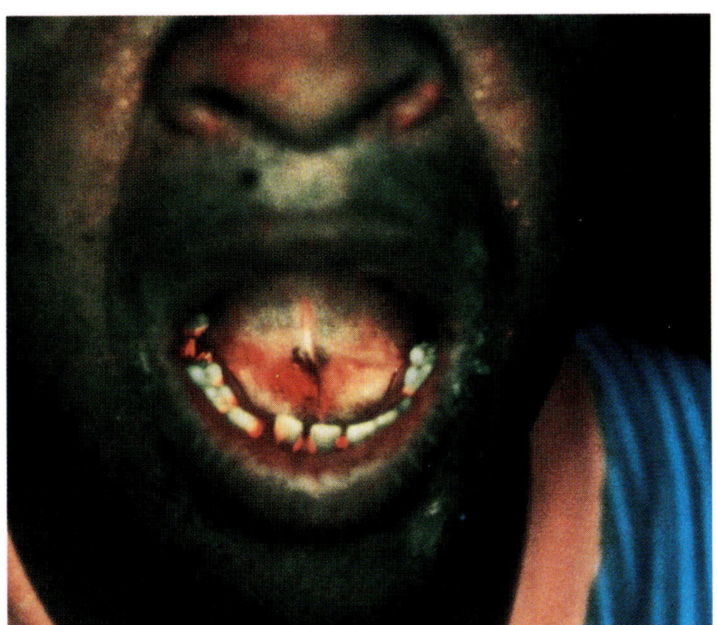

FIGURE 10–4. Intense fluorescence is noted in the area of cancer of the anterior floor of the mouth in Figure 10–3. This picture was taken 48 hours after the administration of DHE. (Courtesy of James Hill, M.D., deceased.)

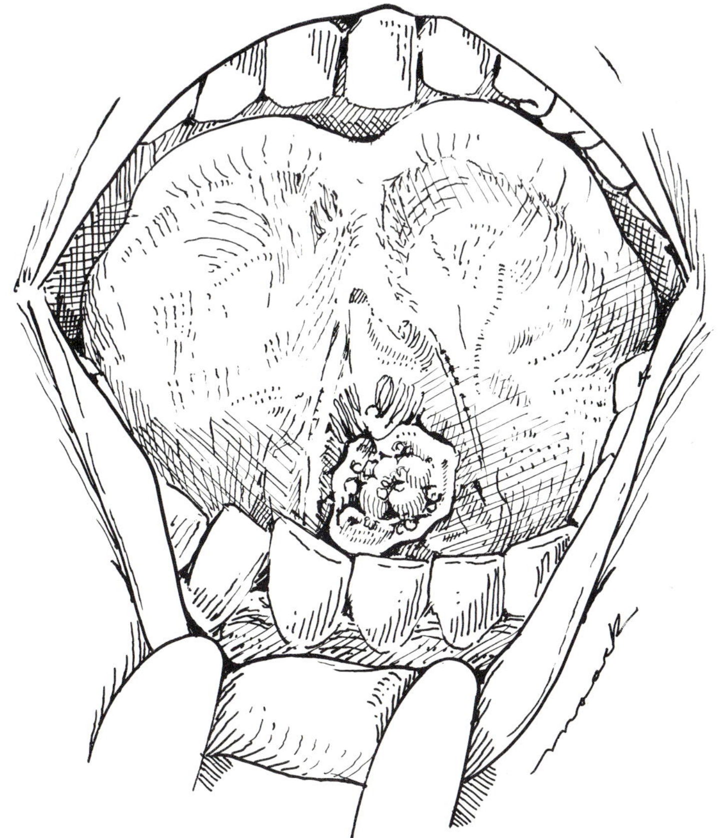

FIGURE 10–5. A T1 cancer is present on the anterior floor of the mouth. A circumferential cut has been accomplished with the CO_2 laser.

the laser is used to excise at the needed deep plane (Fig. 10–6). Frozen section biopsies can be taken at the edges of the excision as well as in the bed of the tumor excision.

Use of the operating microscope greatly facilitates the determination of the planes of excision. Typically, areas of concern can be seen under magnification afforded by the microscope and appropriate adjustments made in surgery. Obviously, confirmation of total excision depends on frozen section techniques.

Excellent work by Davidson and colleagues[12] has shown that the most accurate histologic techniques involve horizontal frozen sections patterned after the technique of Mohs. Although this certainly takes more time than conventional vertically placed frozen sections, the total area examined is significantly larger, which leads to greater precision in removal of the lesion.

Severe field cancerization as well as areas of known superficially invasive cancer can be treated by phototherapy. This is accomplished by injecting an appropriate photosensitizer, commonly DHE, 48 hours before surgery. Figure 10–7 shows three small areas of recurrent squamous cell cancer in a patient previously irradiated. Figures 10–8 and 10–9 show the lesions 1 week and 6 weeks, respectively, after phototherapy.

Figure 10–10 shows the technique of photoirradiating with the argon dye laser. The oral cavity is being treated with a diffusing beam attached to a quartz fiber. This technique has potentially great application in cases of severe field cancerization in which excision would remove large quantities of mucosa. Smaller lesions are probably better treated by excision without phototherapy. One of the advantages of phototherapy is that large areas can be treated and retreated as necessary.

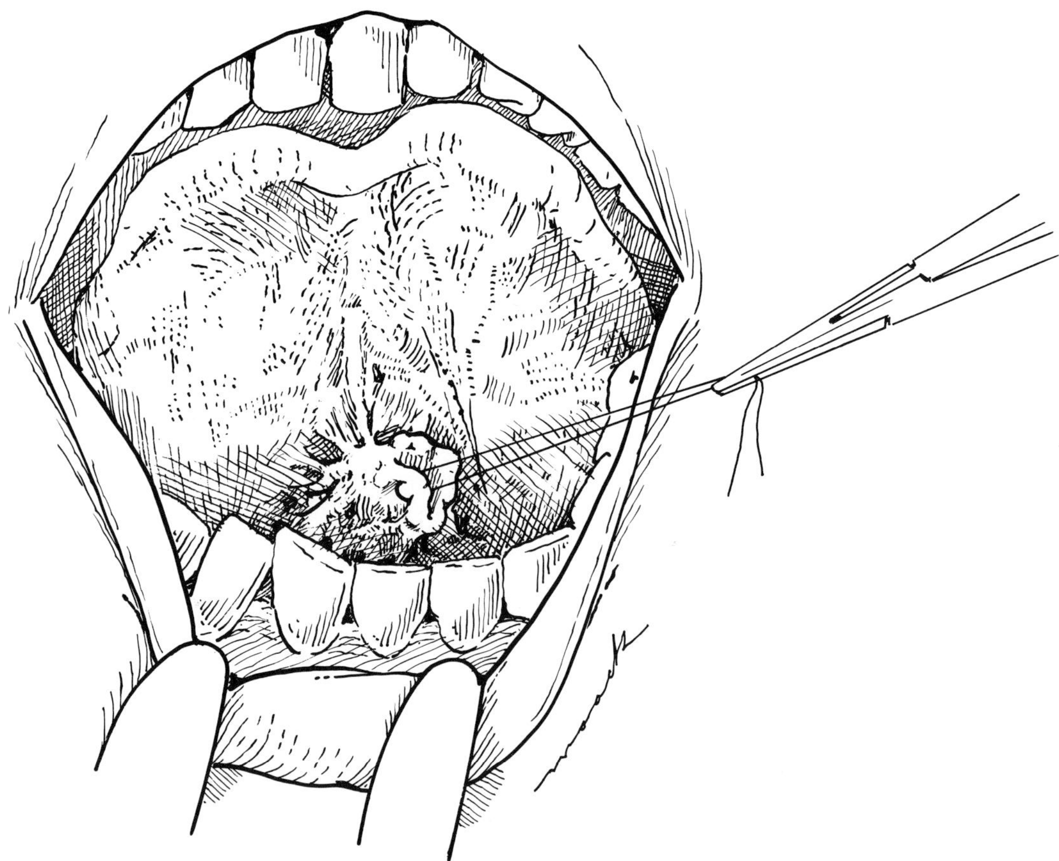

FIGURE 10–6. A traction suture has been placed to retract the specimen laterally. The CO_2 laser is used to excise at an appropriate depth. This incision is facilitated by the tension created with the traction suture.

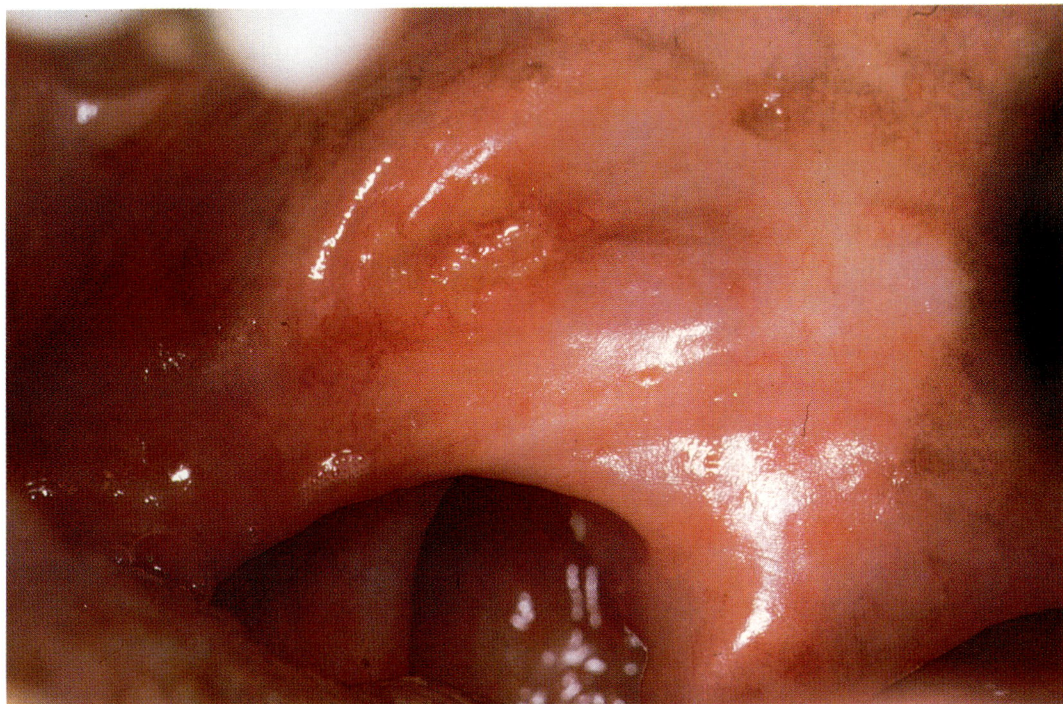

FIGURE 10–7. Three small areas of recurrence of squamous cell cancer on the palate of a patient treated earlier with radiation therapy.

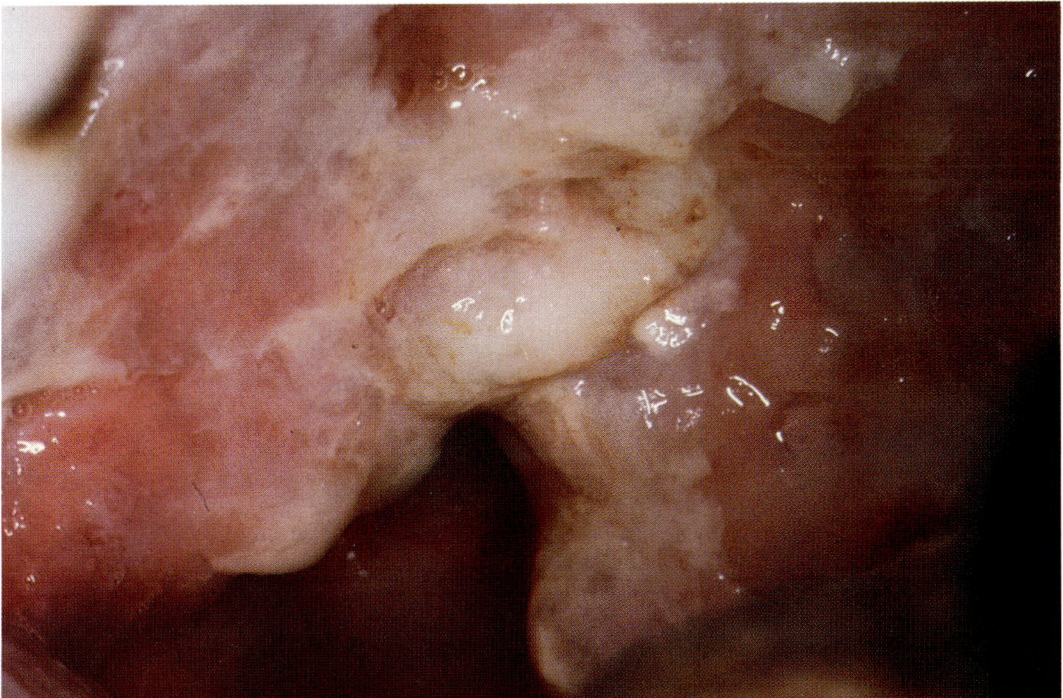

FIGURE 10–8. One week after photodynamic therapy for cancer in Figure 10–7, areas of dysplasia and early cancer are starting to slough.

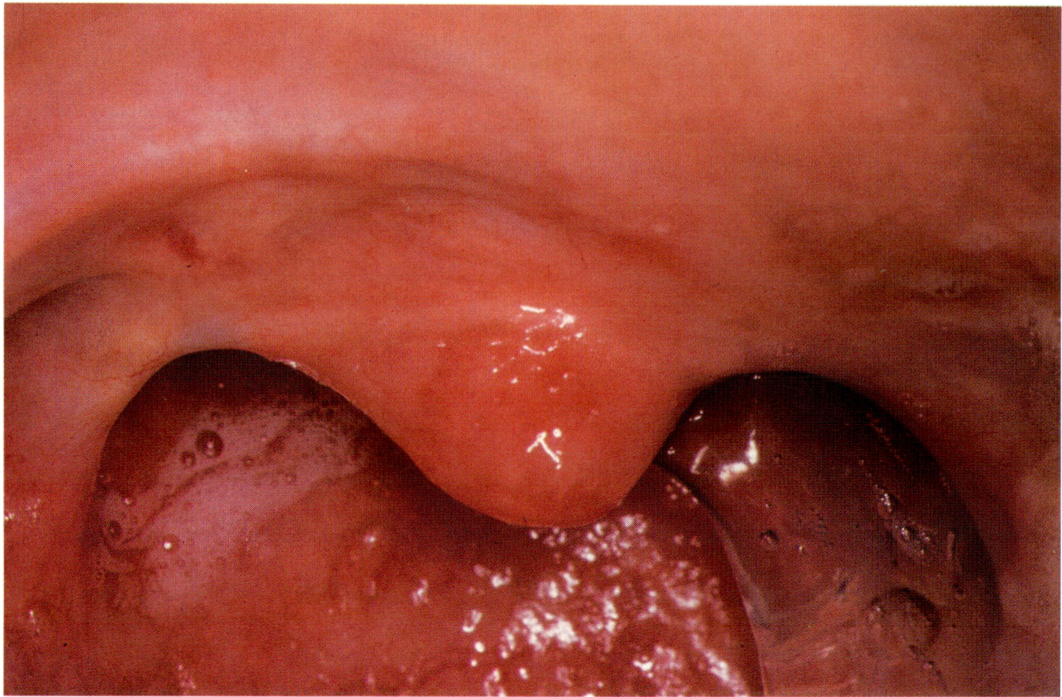

FIGURE 10–9. The well-healed palatine arch 6 weeks after photodynamic therapy for cancer in Figure 10–7.

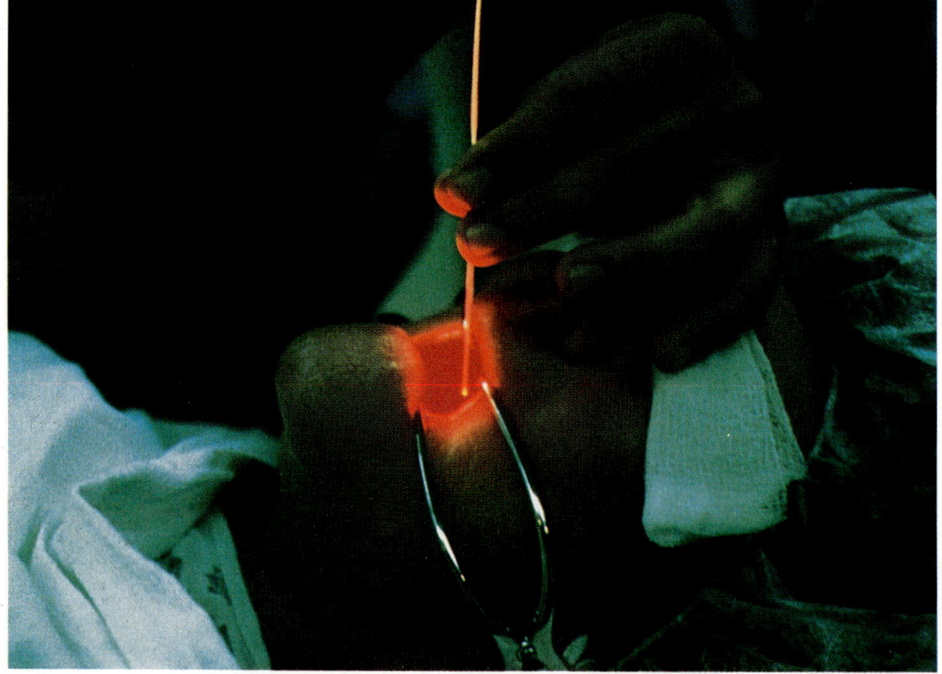

FIGURE 10–10. A patient is treated with photodynamic therapy utilizing the argon dye laser. Several different diffusing beams, which can be placed at the end of the treating fiber, can be used to treat more diffuse areas in the oral cavity.

Stage I Oral Cavity and Oropharyngeal Cancer

Stage I cancer (T1 lesions) of the floor of the mouth, the mobile tongue, the palate, and the palatine arch can be successfully treated with the CO_2 laser. The surgical technique in each of these locations is the same as that discussed above for therapy *by excisional biopsy*. The critical criterion in all of these cases is that excellent visualization must be gained.

It is normally possible to visualize the entire floor of the mouth. There is some difficulty when the tumor approaches the mandible. This is particularly difficult to view in dentulous patients. In these settings, the laser is used to outline the lesion in the soft tissues of the floor of the mouth. Incision is often necessary between the gingivae of the teeth and is best done using a cold knife technique. This incision is carried down and through the underlying periosteum, and the periosteum is reflected using appropriate elevators. If areas of potential tumor presence are suspected in the periosteum, these undergo biopsy. If the results of periosteal biopsies are abnormal, mandibulectomy (inner table or segmental) must be accomplished by standard technique. The CO_2 laser has little utility in the excision of bone. Indeed, use of the CO_2 laser leads to undue thermal damage and should not be undertaken. This same statement pertains to the use of the argon and neodymium:yttrium-aluminum-garnet (Nd:YAG) lasers in this setting. As lasers that confer less thermal damage are developed, their use could be contemplated. An example is the free electron laser, which cuts bone far more precisely than do current osteotomy techniques.

When the periosteum is removed down to the soft tissues in the floor of the mouth, the lines of laser incision can be connected to the periosteal incision lines and the specimen removed en bloc.

Surgery of the mobile tongue is effectively accomplished using the CO_2 laser. Traction is placed on the tongue, and an incision at a safe margin from the cancer is made with the laser as shown in Figure 10–11. After the initial incision, the area to be removed is grasped, and tension is placed on one side. This allows a clean laser cut. Figure 10–12 shows the surgical bed postoperatively. Glossectomy can be accomplished at high power density to facilitate removal. Electrocautery is selectively used to gain hemostasis of large vessels, thereby decreasing undue thermal energy.

An alternative to the CO_2 laser in such excision involves the use of the Nd:YAG laser with sapphire-tipped contact probes. These contact probes allow concentration of the laser energy in a precise manner without the deep penetration (''footprint'') seen when the Nd:YAG laser is used with a free fiber. This technique could become the treatment of choice, as better hemostasis is possible than with the use of the CO_2 laser. The potassium-titanyl-phosphate (KTP) laser may have some advantage in this regard. For any laser to confer an advantage, excision must be done with good hemostasis and less thermal damage than is possible with electrocautery excision alone.

After the tongue lesion has been excised, the defect can either be closed primarily or be allowed to granulate. Defects at the tip of the tongue or on the lateral mobile tongue are most often allowed to granulate.

Glossectomy by laser technique is difficult to accomplish posterior to the junction of the mobile tongue and the base of the tongue. In this case, visualization is difficult and standard techniques utilizing mandibulotomy for exposure should be added.

Resection of palate lesions and palatine arch lesions can be accomplished using the same laser techniques when excellent visualization can be obtained. Lesions that extend onto the base of the tongue from the palatine arch require better visualization than can be obtained using the CO_2 laser with the microscope.

Stage II Lesions

Stage II lesions (T2 N0 M0) of the floor of the mouth, the mobile tongue, the palate, and the palatine arch rarely should be approached with laser surgery. Floor of the mouth lesions that are of

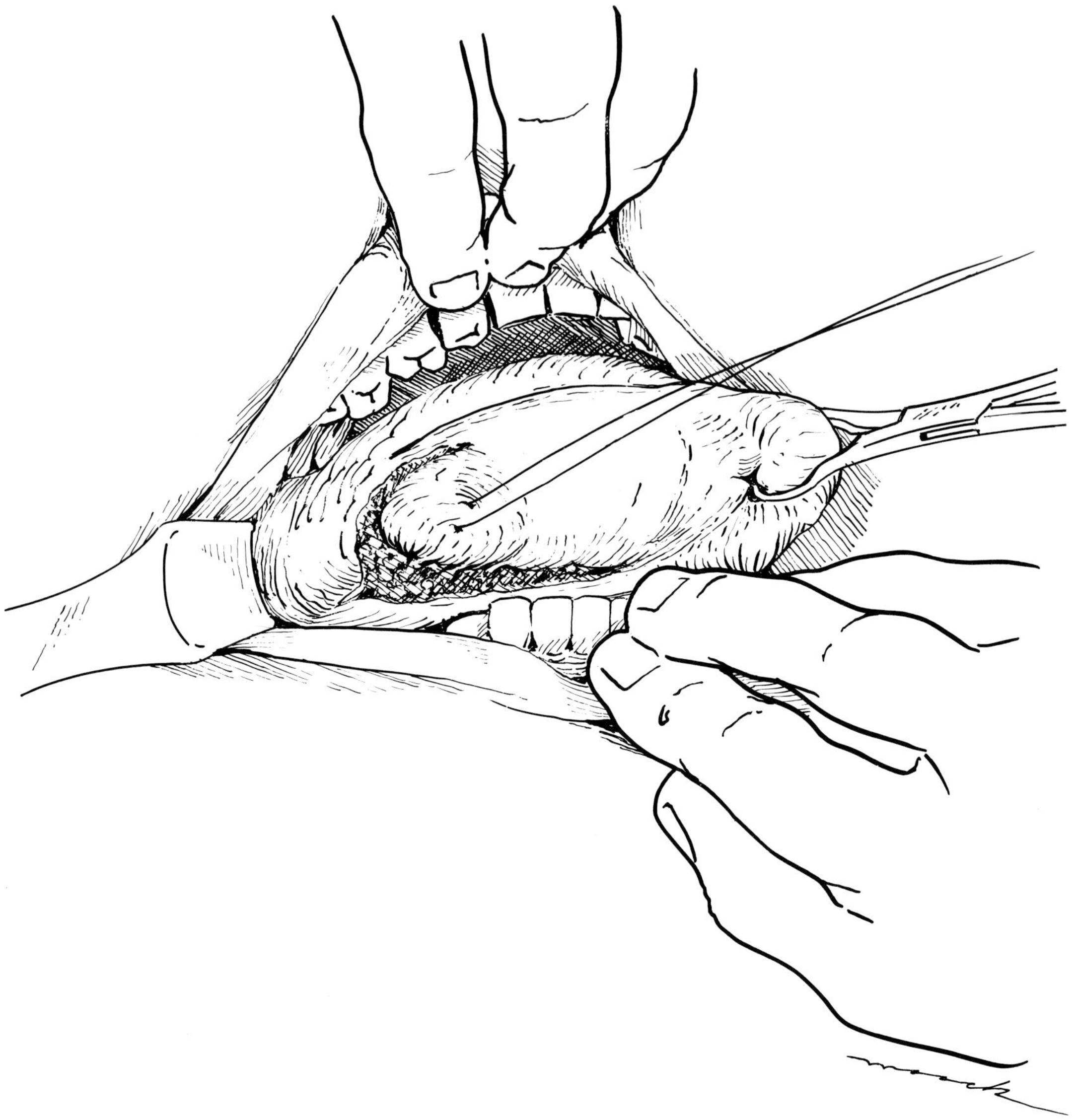

FIGURE 10–11. A traction suture is placed in the tongue to facilitate laser excision.

T2 size often involve periosteum of the mandible and need to be treated by standard open techniques, including mandibulectomy. Certainly (as mentioned above) these lesions have a great propensity for neck spread and necessitate treatment of the regional lymphatics. The only role of the CO_2 laser in the treatment of floor of the mouth neoplasia is to outline the area of excision with a careful margin of normal tissue. This can be extended deeply through the mucosa to help guide later pull-through procedures. The intraoral incision lines from the laser guide the through and through excision from the neck, which allows en bloc removal. This facilitates not violating the tumor and finding a safe margin of resection when an en bloc full thickness floor of the mouth excision is done.

T2 lesions of the mobile tongue can successfully be removed with the laser as the operative instrument. The same principles addressed for stage I lesions pertain. This is also true of lesions of the palate and the palatine arch. The same limiting principles pertain to these as to the stage I lesions.

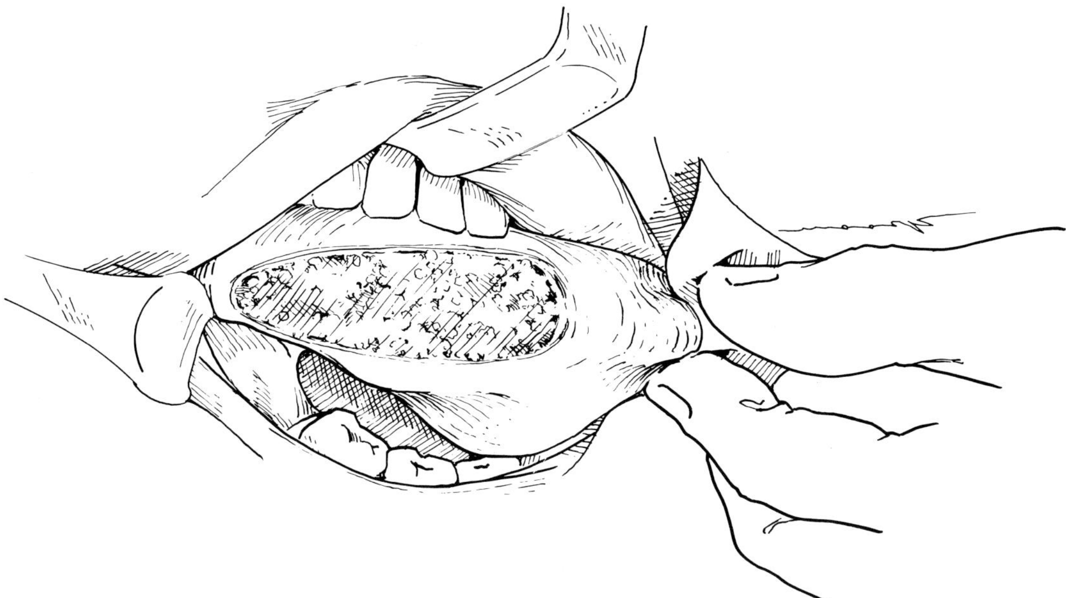

FIGURE 10–12. The postoperative surgical bed, which usually is left to granulate and mucosalize. In this circumstance, split thickness skin grafting confers no advantage.

T3 and T4 Oral Cavity Lesions

The only role of laser therapy in T3 and T4 lesions is the infrequently necessary outlining of such lesions prior to pull-through composite resection. This is rarely indicated, as mandibulotomy allows much better exposure than the pull-through technique.

Stage IV oral cavity cancer represents a devastating disease and poor survival rates with current standard therapy. Experimental protocols utilizing chemotherapy have made little difference in survival rates. Laser surgery is occasionally useful in the palliation of these lesions when other modalities have failed. When these lesions cannot be controlled, they typically cause severe pain, bleeding, and difficulty with local hygiene owing to tumor necrosis. Such lesions can be initially treated with the Nd:YAG laser to decrease vascularity followed by CO_2 laser ablation of the lesion. It often is necessary to retreat with the Nd:YAG laser on several occasions and to accomplish cytoreduction of the tumor carefully through CO_2 laser vaporization after Nd:YAG photocoagulation. After the tumor bulk has been greatly reduced, phototherapy could theoretically be added to gain deeper tumor control. This is rarely clinically indicated.

COMPLICATIONS

Laser-related complications of the oral cavity are extremely unusual if proper precautions are taken. The potential for endotracheal tube fire can be circumvented by using nasal intubation and by completely packing the tube away from the excision area in the anterior floor of the mouth. If laser surgery approaches the lateral tongue, a wrapped Rusch tube can be placed orally and protected on the opposite side of the mouth.

The major potential problem in laser excision comes from inadequate cancer excision in inappropriately selected patients. It must be carefully underscored that laser excision can only be done in cases of wide, clear visualization. Any malignant lesion that is situated at the base of the tongue primarily or that extends onto the tongue from the palatine arch should not be approached with laser excision. Benign lesions of the palatine arch and the base of the tongue can be treated with laser surgery (see Chapter 9).

As many blood vessels in the oral cavity are larger than 0.1 mm in diameter, these vessels must be controlled by standard nonlaser technique when utilizing the laser. Usually, when the laser is used with the operating microscope, large vessels can be seen as they come into the surgical field. These either are tied or are appropriately electrocauterized. In this method, the full thermal effects of total surgery by electrocautery can be avoided. If caution is not taken to secure hemostasis in these larger vessels, postoperative bleeding is a potential complication. In the author's experience, this is highly unusual when precautions are taken to gain hemostasis at surgery.

When working about the teeth, caution must be used to avoid laser damage to teeth. This is accomplished by careful attention at surgery and by appropriate protection of the teeth with moistened saline gauze and other measures. In general, thermal damage to bone is avoided by not treating bone with the CO_2 laser. Newer generations of CO_2 lasers and newer lasers such as the free electron laser may allow power densities high enough, spot sizes small enough, and superpulsed cutting modes to allow osteotomy without undue damage. At present, this is impractical for most medical centers.

Surgery in the anterior floor of the mouth often exposes Wharton duct (submandibular duct) on either side. The duct is simply transected if it is within the field of cancer excision. In the author's experience, less than 10 per cent of patients so treated have subsequently developed sialadenitis requiring any therapy. Less than 5 per cent of patients have required subsequent submandibular gland excision.

Most patients who undergo limited excisions of T1 carcinoma require no reconstruction of the surgical defect. The mucosa heals well, with minimal subsequent scar contracture, which would cause functional disability.

References

1. Strong MS, et al.: The role of the CO_2 laser in otolaryngology. Trans Am Acad Ophthalmol Otolaryngol 82:595, 1976.
2. Strong MS, Vaughan CW, Healy GB, et al.: Transoral management of localized carcinoma of the oral cavity using the CO_2 laser. Laryngoscope 89:897, 1979.
3. Platz H, Fries F, Hudec M, et al.: Carcinoma of the oral cavity: Analysis of various pretherapeutic classifications. Head Neck Surg 5:93, 1982.
4. Marks JE, Lee F, Smith PG, Ogura JH: Floor of mouth cancer: Patient selection and treatment results. Laryngoscope 93:475, 1983.
5. Newman AN, Rice OH, Ossoff RH, Sisson GA: Carcinoma of the tongue in persons younger than 30 years of age. Arch Otolaryngol 109:302, 1983.
6. Leipzig G, Cummings CW, Chung CT, et al.: Carcinomas of the anterior tongue. Ann Otol Rhinol Laryngol 91:94, 1982.
7. Holm LE, Lundquist PG, Ruden BI, et al.: Combined preoperative radiotherapy and surgery in the treatment of carcinoma of the anterior two-thirds of the tongue. Laryngoscope 93:792, 1983.
8. Yamamoto E, Kohama G, Sunakawa H, et al.: Mode of invasion, bleomycin sensitivity, and clinical course in squamous cell carcinoma of the oral cavity. Cancer 51:2175, 1983.
9. Slaughter DP: Multicentric origin of intraoral carcinoma. Surgery 20:133, 1946.
10. Strong MS, Vaughan CW, Incze JS: Toluidine blue in the management of carcinoma of the oral cavity. Arch Otolaryngol 87:527, 1968.
11. Hill JH, Plant RL, Harris DM, et al.: The nude mouse xenograft system: A model for photodetection and photodynamic therapy in head and neck squamous cell carcinoma. Am J Otolaryngol 7:17, 1986.
12. Davidson TM, Nahum AM, Haghighi P, et al.: The biology of head and neck cancer. Detection and control by parallel histologic sections. Arch Otolaryngol 110:193, 1984.

CHAPTER 11

Nasal and Paranasal Sinus Applications of Lasers

Leland P. Johnson

The development of the surgical carbon dioxide (CO_2) laser system in 1969, for initial use in the larynx, soon suggested other head and neck applications to those involved in early CO_2 laser research and surgery.[1,2] The CO_2 laser was used initially in the nasal cavity for lesions such as verrucous papilloma, turbinate hypertrophy in vasomotor rhinitis, and choanal atresia.[2-6] With the later introduction of the other two commonly used surgical lasers, the argon and neodymium:yttrium-aluminum-garnet (Nd:YAG) lasers with the wavelength specific property of red pigment absorption, their use was expanded to include the treatment of vascular lesions, such as the telangiectasias in hereditary hemorrhagic telangiectasia (HHT).[7,8] The more recent introduction of the 532 nm potassium-titanyl-phosphate (KTP-532) surgical laser with properties similar to those of the argon laser has also allowed many intranasal laser applications.[5] Photodynamic therapy utilizing the tunable dye laser may have a future role in treating intranasal malignancy.

This chapter discusses uses of the surgical lasers in the treatment of lesions of the nasal cavity and specifies when the laser offers an advantage to conventional techniques, an alternative to these techniques, or no advantage to present techniques. Surgical lasers in general, when compared with conventional techniques, offer a precision in vaporization or incision associated with decreased edema, decreased postoperative pain, improved healing, improved hemostasis, and decreased direct tissue contact and instrumentation. Specifically in nasal applications, the use of surgical lasers may avoid the need for nasal packing. Lasers also may be used in patients with bleeding disorders, in whom conventional surgical techniques would not be possible. The "no touch" (hands off) technique may also allow less extensive surgical approaches to be used. Decreased length of hospitalization and the ability to perform many procedures on an outpatient basis can also be benefits of surgical laser use.

Vaporization of tissue water by absorption of the CO_2 laser energy allows removal or incision of tissue. The CO_2 laser provides hemostasis by its ability to coagulate vessels up to 0.5 mm in diameter. The CO_2 laser spot size can be varied by focusing or defocusing the beam to provide a wider area of vaporization or a more precise point of tissue destruction.

The argon laser penetrates tissue more deeply than does the CO_2 laser and selectively photocoagulates vascular tissue. Vessels of 1 to 2 mm in diameter can be photocoagulated with the argon laser. A delayed tissue effect with the argon laser occurs such that the area finally affected is

30 per cent larger than the original visible treatment site. The argon laser commonly uses a 600 micron fiber, a power setting of 2 to 4 watts, and a distance of 0.5 cm from the treated tissue.

Still deeper tissue penetration and higher power densities are obtained with the Nd:YAG laser. Vessels less than 4 mm in diameter can be photocoagulated so that large vascular lesions would be indications for this laser's use. The combination of a 600 micron fiber, a power setting of 25 to 30 watts, and an operating distance of 1 cm from the treatment area are commonly used with the Nd:YAG laser. Unlike the CO_2 laser, which vaporizes the nasal mucosa, the argon and Nd:YAG lasers penetrate the mucous membrane to photocoagulate vessels with less disruption of the mucosal surface.

The use of surgical lasers in the nasal cavity, as well as on the external nose, requires careful attention to established laser safety principles. With the CO_2 laser, the patient's cornea and exposed skin surfaces are at risk for injury. The patient's eyes must be lubricated, taped shut, and covered by two thicknesses of saline-moistened sponges. All other exposed skin areas are likewise covered with moistened towels. The nasopharynx should be packed with saline-moistened cottonoids or sponges when performing procedures in the posterior nasal cavity. This maneuver avoids any potential damage to eustachian tube orifices or the skull base and also serves as a landmark to indicate when the nasopharynx is approached. All operating room personnel as well as the surgeon are required to wear clear glasses or goggles for use of the CO_2 laser. Standard means to protect an endotracheal tube, such as the use of a red rubber tube wrapped with metal foil, are utilized. Use of the argon, the Nd:YAG , or the KTP-532 laser necessitates the wearing of appropriately colored glasses by the surgeon, the operating room personnel, and the patient. Shapshay also uses crumpled aluminum foil as a protective barrier over the patient's exposed skin areas.[8] Selkin recommends the use of moist cotton work gloves to protect the surgeon's hands from laser injury.[9]

The choice of anesthesia for intranasal laser surgery is determined by the anticipated length of surgery, the bleeding expected, and the access to the nasal lesion. Small external or intranasal lesions can be treated with topical and local anesthesia. The standard topical anesthetic consisting of a 4 per cent cocaine solution and the local anesthetic consisting of 1 per cent lidocaine (Xylocaine) with 1:100,000 epinephrine are used. Spraying the nasal mucous membrane with a topical vasoconstrictor, such as phenylephrine (Neo-Synephrine) or oxymetazoline, can also be done prior to the administration of topical and local anesthesia. Longer surgical procedures or those in which significant bleeding can occur, such as the photocoagulation of telangiectasias, are better done with the patient under general anesthesia. With general anesthesia, muscle relaxation to avoid unexpected patient movement and possible laser injury is also possible.

INSTRUMENTATION

Presently available nasal and otologic surgical instruments lend themselves to the use of surgical lasers in the nasal cavity (Fig. 11–1). Exposure of intranasal lesions can be obtained with larger sized ear specula and the use of an ear speculum holder. Nasal specula with screw locks that can be stabilized to the operating table are also useful. Anodized black instruments to avoid glare from headlights or microscope lights make visualization much easier. It should be remembered that the laser beam can be reflected onto the metal speculum, and the heat generated can produce a burn of the nasal ala or vestibule. Periodic irrigation of the speculum with saline or the use of a pulsed versus continuous mode on the laser may prevent this heat generation. Placement of a rubber suction catheter in the nostril opposite the surgical site or in the nasopharynx for smoke evacuation can be helpful. A nasal speculum with a built-in suction for smoke evacuation has been developed by Selkin.[9] After the operative site has been visualized, the CO_2 laser (coupled with the surgical microscope using a 300 to 400 mm lens and the micromanipulator) is used in a fashion similar to that for microlaryngeal surgery. It is also possible to use the operating microscope with its magnification and illumination and a CO_2 laser handpiece. The argon laser can be coupled to the operating

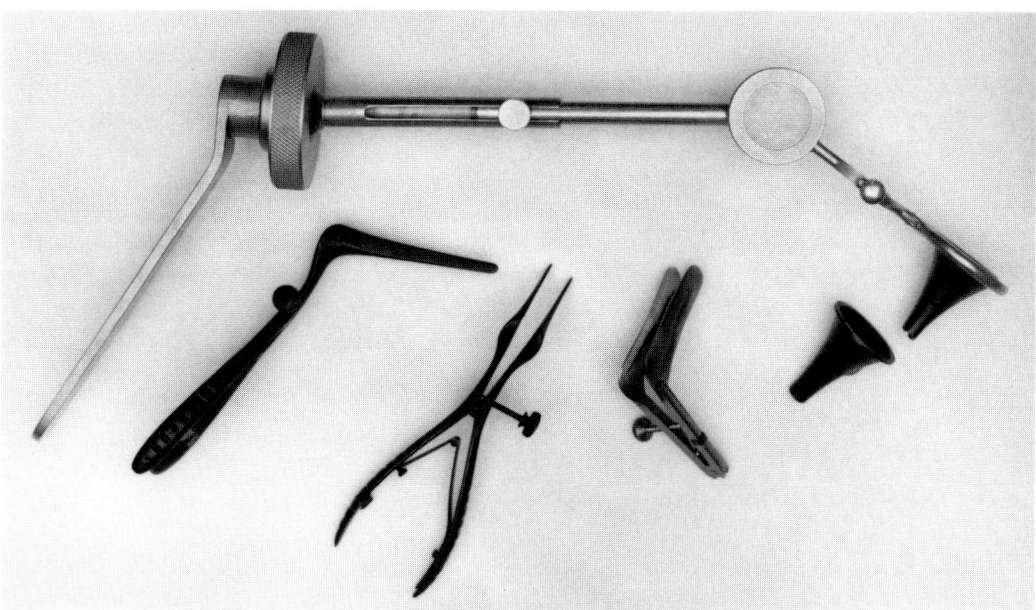

Figure 11–1. Nasal and ear specula with speculum holder used for intranasal laser surgery.

microscope, but is more often used in intranasal surgery by the surgeon's holding the transmission fiber directly or using a hand holder (Fig. 11–2). The Nd:YAG laser is also transmitted via a fiber and can be stabilized by passing it through a metal suction tip for control. The KTP-532 laser likewise is transmitted through a fiber, and a handpiece with an adjacent suction channel for smoke evacuation is available. Visualization can again be obtained using the operating microscope or the more recently available endoscopes. With use of the nasal endoscopes the eye safety filter is attached to the nasal endoscope for protection of the surgeon's eye. In procedures in which a large amount of smoke and tissue vaporization are expected, such as in the treatment of rhinophyma, the portable smoke evacuation system should be used.

The patient is positioned on the operating table in the standard fashion for nasal surgery, often with some Trendelenburg inclination for approach to the posterior nasal cavity. For anteriorly located lesions, the surgeon would be at the patient's side when using hand-held laser fibers or handpieces (Fig. 11–3). If the surgical microscope is used, it would extend over the patient's chest. When using the CO_2 laser for treatment of choanal atresia or rhinophyma, the surgeon and the operating microscope are located at the head of the operating table (Fig. 11–4).

Table 11–1 lists the extra- and intranasal lesions treated with the four currently available surgical laser systems.

METHODS OF LASER SURGERY

Choanal Atresia

Use of the CO_2 laser for correction of choanal atresia was first described by Healy and associates in 1978.[10] Because the CO_2 laser is able to incise and vaporize tissue, it would be an alternative treatment option and actually provide an advantage in treatment of a membranous choanal atresia. As up to 90 per cent of bilateral choanal atresias are bony, and the CO_2 laser is not effective for removing bone more than 1 mm in thickness, the use of an ear curette, a microrongeur, or a microdrill is still necessary with the laser technique for choanal atresia repair. Using the CO_2 laser

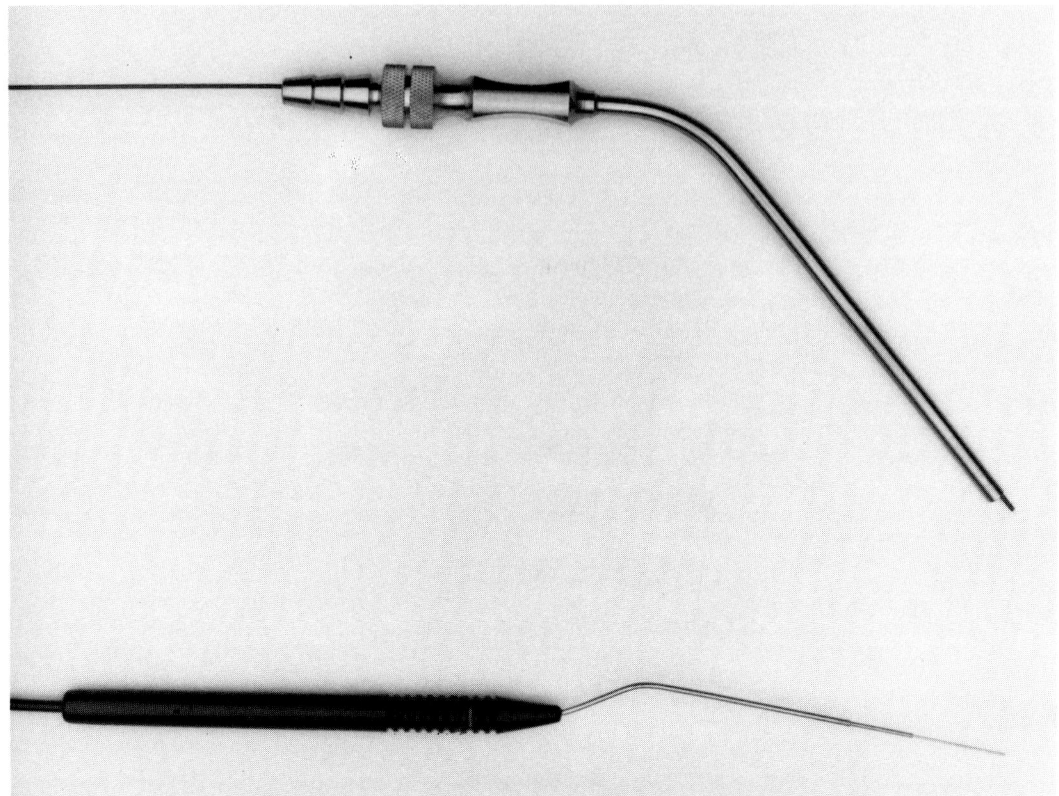

FIGURE 11–2. Fiber for the argon laser stabilized in a suction tip *(top)* and an argon laser handpiece *(bottom)*.

to vaporize bone results in overheating of the surrounding tissue, bone necrosis, sequestration, and excess scar formation.

Current nonlaser treatment of bilateral choanal atresia is by a transnasal microsurgical technique to create mucosal flaps from the anterior surface of the atresia plate and the use of the microdrill to remove the bony atresia plate. Dimethicone (Silastic) stenting is used in both techniques. With the decreased healing time claimed for experimental laser injuries, Healy and colleagues believed that a shorter period of stenting (i.e., 2 to 3 weeks) would be possible.[10] The restenosis rate in Healy and colleagues' report for bilateral choanal atresia was 33 per cent. After a second revision with the CO_2 laser, the patency rate was 83 per cent. Richardson and Osguthorpe reported a 36 per cent incidence of unilateral stenosis following microsurgical transnasal repair of bilateral choanal atresia.[11] The development of postoperative soft tissue stenosis or scarring after the bony atresia plate has been removed is ideally managed by the CO_2 laser.

The technique for repair of choanal atresia using the CO_2 laser utilizes transnasal exposure of the atresia plate with an appropriately sized ear speculum and speculum holder. The CO_2 laser is coupled to the operating microscope, and a power setting of 4 to 6 watts is used in a pulsed mode. The nasopharynx is packed with saline-moistened cottonoids or sponges. The mucous membrane overlying the anterior atresia plate is then vaporized to the level of the bony atresia plate, which is removed using ear curettes, a microrongeur, or a microdrill. The posterior membranous layer of the atresia plate is then vaporized, and the posterior choana is enlarged with removal of the posterior end of the nasal septum. Placement of a stent for 2 to 6 weeks is similar to that for nonlaser choanal atresia repair. In revision of restenosis with the CO_2 laser, or the removal of granulation tissue or scar formation, a stent is not routinely replaced.

Limitations to transnasal repair of choanal atresia are not unique to the use of the CO_2 laser and are detailed by Muntz.[12] Limited visualization due to turbinate enlargement or septal deform-

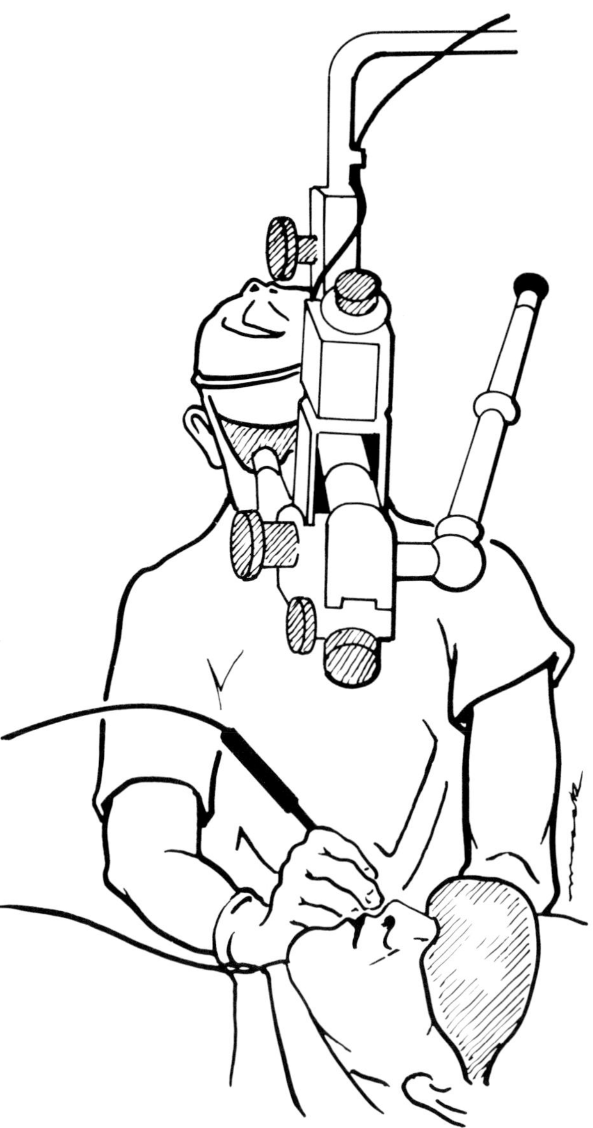

Figure 11–3. Position of the surgeon at the patient's side and use of the operating microscope for illumination.

ity, a high arched palate, and associated craniofacial disorders may require a later transpalatal repair or the use of a tracheostomy until midface advancement occurs or associated craniofacial disorders are corrected.

Hereditary Hemorrhagic Telangiectasia

Hereditary hemorrhagic telangiectasia (HHT), or Osler-Weber-Rendu disease, is a familial disease transmitted by a non–sex linked, autosomal dominant gene and characterized by a vascular malformation in which only an endothelial layer is present on a continuous basement membrane. The abnormal vessels are so fragile that minor trauma leads to bleeding. These telangiectasias are most common in the nasal mucous membrane, but can occur in multiple other sites, including the skin of the face, the fingertips, the toes, the nail beds, the gastric mucosa, the vaginal mucosa, the bladder, the uterus, the liver, the brain, the spinal cord, and the lungs. Severe, recurrent epistaxis

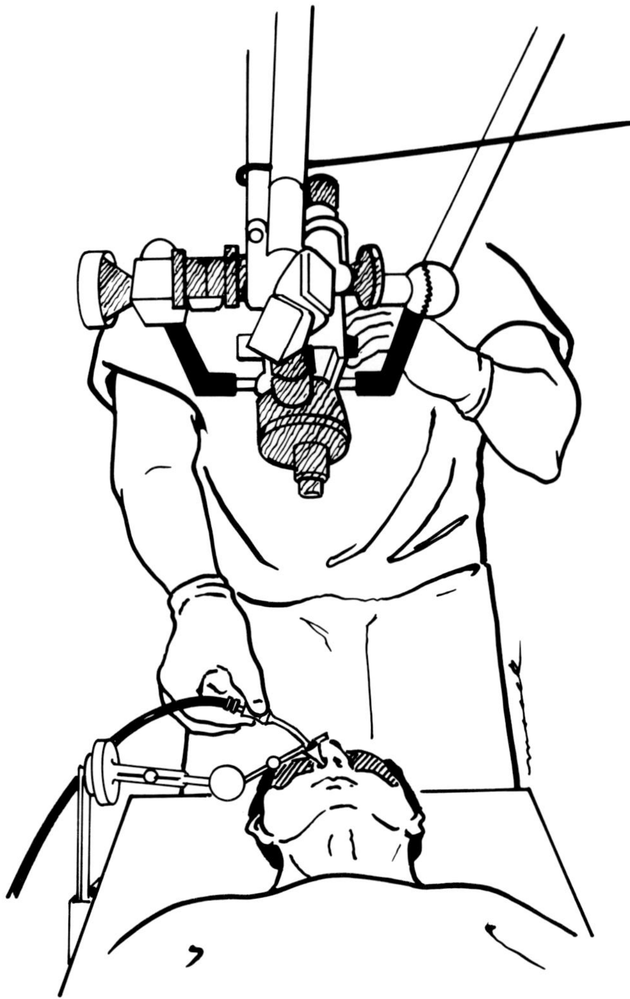

FIGURE 11–4. Position of the surgeon at the head of the operating table with use of CO_2 laser for the treatment of choanal atresia.

is the most common problem these patients experience, and its control has included chemical and electrical cautery, septal dermoplasty, arterial ligation and arterial embolization, and systemic estrogen therapy.

The use of the argon, Nd:YAG , and KTP-532 lasers to photocoagulate the telangiectasias in HHT before these bleed is an alternative to the treatment methods mentioned above. The benefit of laser treatment for HHT is reported to include a decreased severity of episodes of epistaxis, an increased interval between required treatments, and a decreased need for blood transfusion. Because the telangiectasias can reform in nontreated areas or even in areas of previous skin grafts, retreatment at 4 to 6 month intervals is often necessary.

For treatment, the nasal cavity is exposed using the nasal speculum with or without a speculum holder as detailed above. General anesthesia is recommended on the basis of earlier experiences using local anesthesia in which management of bleeding either from the telangiectasias or from coexisting nasal septal perforation edges became a problem in the awake patient. The fiber for the argon or the Nd:YAG laser is handheld or placed in a suction tip to act as a holder. The operating microscope can be used to provide illumination and magnification, or the standard headlight is used. The argon laser is used with a setting of 2 to 4 watts in a continuous mode with the fiber held 3 to 5 mm from the telangiectasia. The Nd:YAG laser settings are 20 to 25 watts at 0.3 to 0.5 second exposure with the fiber tip 1 to 2 cm from the telangiectasia.[16]

Table 11–1. INTRANASAL AND EXTERNAL NOSE LESIONS
TREATED WITH SURGICAL LASERS

Diagnosis	Surgical Laser Utilized
Adenocarcinoma of septum	CO_2 laser[6]
Angiomatous neoplasm	KTP-532 laser[5]
Choanal atresia	CO_2 laser[10]
Concha bullosa	KTP-532 laser[5]
Columellar cyst	CO_2 laser[9]
Papilloma	CO_2 laser,[3,6,9] KTP-532 laser[5]
Polyps (ethmoid, nasal, choanal)	CO_2 laser,[6,9] KTP-532 laser[5]
Port wine hemangioma	Argon laser[7]
Pyogenic granuloma	CO_2 laser[6]
Rhinophyma	CO_2 laser[6,13]
Sarcoid granuloma	CO_2 laser,[6] KTP-532 laser[5]
Sebaceous adenoma	CO_2 laser[6]
Septal hemangioma	CO_2 laser[9]
Septal spur	CO_2 laser[9]
Synechiae	CO_2 laser,[6,9] KTP-532 laser[5]
Telangiectasia (HHT), intranasal and cutaneous	CO_2 laser,[6,9] KTP-532 laser,[5] Nd:YAG laser[8]
Turbinate hypertrophy	Argon laser,[5] CO_2 laser,[4,9,16] KTP-532 laser[5]
Vestibular stenosis (postoperative, post traumatic, Wegener)	CO_2 laser,[9] KTP-532 laser[5]

Photocoagulation is started at the periphery of the main vessel and finally directed to the center of the telangiectasia to avoid the bleeding often caused with an initial central approach. All visible telangiectasias are treated at each treatment session. Many patients with HHT have septal perforations resulting from previous treatments, and the laser can be directed through the perforation to lesions in the opposite nostril to allow a more direct, less tangential angle of approach to the telangiectasias. Nasal packing is usually not needed postoperatively. Conventional suction and cautery are still needed if bleeding is not controlled with the argon or the Nd:YAG laser or if there is bleeding from the edge of existing septal perforations.

In addition to the use of the argon and Nd:YAG lasers in HHT, other intranasal vascular lesions such as hemangiomas can be treated in a similar fashion. Especially when using the Nd:YAG laser with its deeper tissue penetration, simultaneous treatment on opposite sides of the nasal septum should be avoided to prevent the development of nasoseptal perforation. Telangiectasias of the nasal and facial skin can be treated with the argon laser in a similar fashion after management of the intranasal lesions.

Rhinophyma

Rhinophyma is the end stage of acne rosacea; there is hypertrophy of the sebaceous elements of the skin of the nose and the adjacent cheek, resulting in a cosmetic nasal deformity. Treatment has included near total excision of the hypertrophic nasal skin with skin grafting or partial excision with dermabrasion of the thickened tissue. With the partial excision techniques, reepithelization is then possible from remnants of the glandular epithelium. All techniques require care not to expose the nasal cartilages and not to disrupt the continuity of the nasal alar rim.

Use of the CO_2 laser to vaporize the hypertrophic tissue in rhinophyma was described by Shapshay and coworkers in 1980.[13] In this technique the operating microscope is coupled to the

CO_2 laser to better identify the remaining sebaceous glands and to be certain that excision is at an appropriate depth. The use of the CO_2 laser is more precise and provides an almost bloodless operating site, especially when compared with the previous techniques of partial excision and dermabrasion. The bloodless field obtained with the CO_2 laser gives this technique of rhinophyma treatment a distinct advantage over prior methods. In general, the operating time is longer than with nonsurgical techniques. The postoperative results are similar for the CO_2 laser and nonlaser methods.

The rhinophyma tissue is removed in layers to sculpt the nose, with care being taken to preserve an intact nasal rim and not to expose cartilage. The depth of excision is monitored by the presence of the sebum coming from the remaining sebaceous ducts. Excision is completed when only a small amount of sebum is produced by pressure on the nasal skin. The laser excision can be extended at a more superficial level onto the cheeks to feather the excision of the tissue involved by rhinophyma. The laser setting described is 10 to 50 watts in a continuous mode.[13] Postoperatively, the surgical site is coated with an antibiotic ointment, with reepithelization occurring within 3 to 4 weeks.

A complication of CO_2 laser excision of rhinophyma consisting of extensive tissue loss and scarring has been reported; this emphasizes the need to avoid too deep an excision with the loss of all glandular epithelial elements for resurfacing the nose[14] (Figs. 11–5 to 11–7).

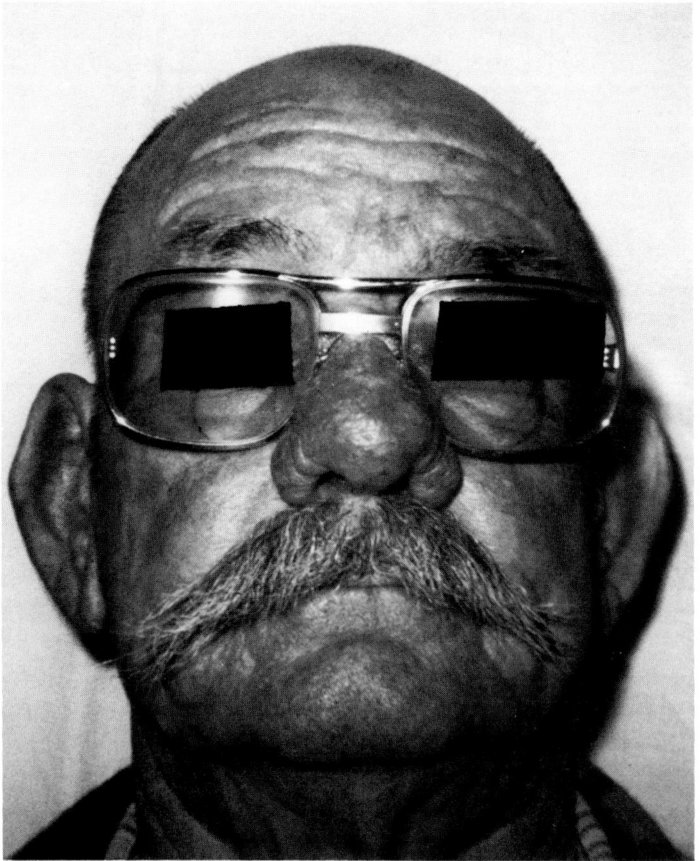

FIGURE 11–5. Preoperative appearance of a patient with rhinophyma.

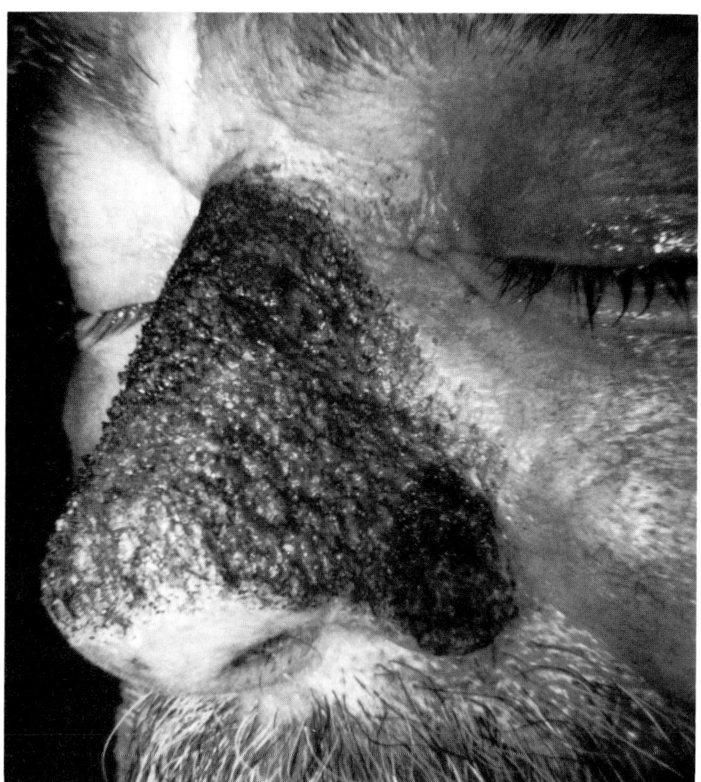

Figure 11–6. Intraoperative view of patient in Figure 11–5.

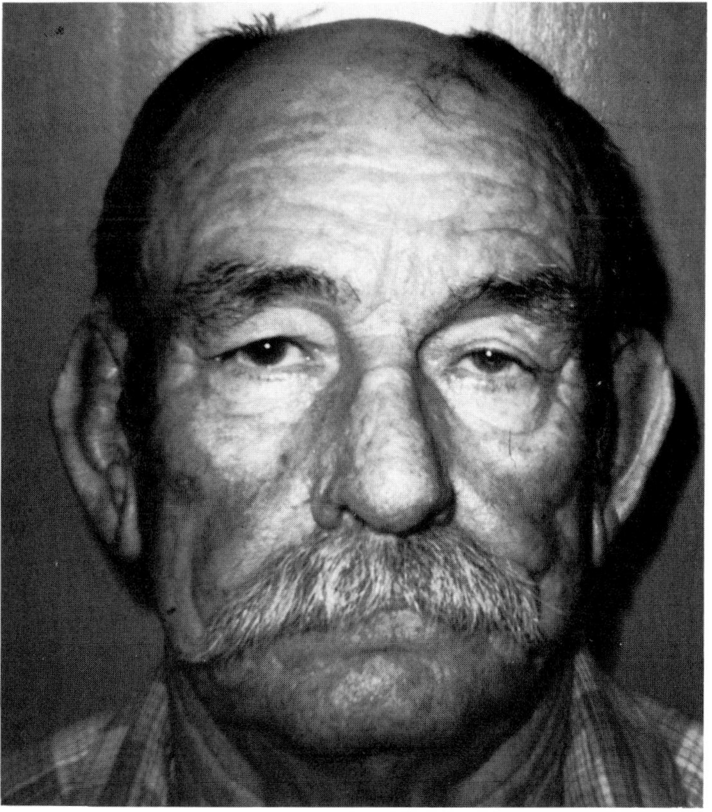

Figure 11–7. Postoperative result after CO_2 laser excision of rhinophyma shown in Figures 11–5 and 11–6.

Hypertrophic Turbinate Mucosa

The hypertrophic turbinate mucosa developing in allergic rhinitis, vasomotor rhinitis, and compensatory turbinate hypertrophy with septal deformities has been surgically treated by reducing the size and bulk of the inferior turbinate and occasionally the middle turbinate. The CO_2 laser with its ability to vaporize tissue with simultaneous hemostasis offers some advantages over treatment techniques such as classic submucous resection of the inferior turbinate. Lenz first used the argon laser for decreasing the size of the inferior turbinate.[15] Since then the use of the CO_2 laser as well as the KTP-532 laser for reduction of turbinate size has been described.[4,5,16,17]

The surgical technique involves the previously described methods for exposure of the lateral nasal wall. Treatment is confined to the anterior one third to one half of the inferior turbinate. Fukutake and colleagues developed a modified CO_2 handpiece to better approach the surfaces of the inferior turbinate.[4] They recommend using a defocused beam of 20 to 30 watts in a continuous mode. Argon laser surgery as described by Lenz[15] or the KTP-532 laser technique described by Levine[5] utilizes the fiber in a holder. Visualization is obtained with a standard headlight, the operating microscope, or nasal endoscopes. With any of these techniques, there is some sloughing of the mucosa of the turbinate, but healing occurs in 3 to 4 weeks. Some of the decreased turbinate size may result from development of submucosal scarring.

The long-term results of the treatment of turbinate hypertrophy using surgical lasers in terms of recurrent turbinate swelling are not different from those achieved with nonlaser techniques. The advantage would be improved hemostasis and often the avoidance of the need for nasal packing. If the turbinate hypertrophy is also related to an enlarged inferior conchal bone, the bone should be removed by conventional methods in combination with use of the laser for treatment of the mucosal hypertrophy.

Other Intranasal Lesions

A variety of other intranasal lesions have been treated with the various surgical lasers. Selkin used the CO_2 laser for removal of small nasoseptal spurs in which vaporization was confined to the mucosa and bone on one side of the septum only.[9] If this nasoseptal spur is a component of a more extensive nasoseptal deformity, traditional surgical techniques for nasoseptal reconstruction would be preferred. Selkin,[9] using the CO_2 laser, and Levine,[5] using the KTP-532 laser, described the removal of nasal, ethmoid, and antral choanal polyps. Because of the increased time required for removal of extensive nasal or ethmoid polyps, the use of the laser provides no advantage over traditional surgical methods. With the present increased use of endoscopic techniques for sinus surgery and the availability of laser probes for both the argon and KTP-532 lasers, their use for nasal polyp surgery may be expanded. Other lesions treated by the various surgical lasers include sarcoid granulomas in the nose, nasal granulation tissue due to cocaine abuse, nasal papillomas, and intranasal scar at the vestibule or in the area of the middle meatus related to prior ethmoid sinus surgery or as a consequence of nasal packing.

The surgical laser offers an advantage in palliation of recurrent nasal and nasopharyngeal tumors if airway obstruction occurs and surgical treatment for cure is not possible. Levine described the use of the KTP-532 laser for treating small recurrent inverting papillomas.[5] Because of the known biologic behavior of inverting papilloma, close follow-up would certainly be needed to monitor any recurrence. The CO_2 laser has been used to maintain a nasal airway in a patient with an inverting papilloma who refused the recommended surgery of medial maxillectomy.

Paranasal Sinus Applications

The limited use of the surgical lasers for nasal, ethmoid, and antral choanal polyps was mentioned above. Likewise, the laser application for paranasal sinus neoplasms for palliation when surgical treatment for cure is unavailable was established. The various surgical lasers could be used to vaporize maxillary sinus retention cysts. These are well managed with current surgical or endoscopic approaches. Brightwell[18] mentioned the creation of a nasoantral window by Lenz[15] using the argon laser in an experimental model. Again, at present, even if this technique were available for the patient, no clear advantage exists over previous surgical methods. The CO_2 laser has been used by Williams to perform a vidian neurectomy for treatment of vasomotor rhinitis.[19] Twelve patients were included in his series; the CO_2 laser was used for the creation of the opening through the anterior and posterior walls of the maxillary sinus, as well as for vaporization of the vidian nerve. His report showed comparable results for control of vasomotor rhinitis to those obtained with prior surgical methods.[19]

With the increased endoscopic and nasal sinus surgical experience and the development of newer surgical laser systems, more applications in the paranasal sinuses may be developed.

References

1. Jako GJ: Laser surgery of the vocal cords. Laryngoscope 82:2204, 1972.
2. Strong MS, et al.: Laser surgery in the aerodigestive tract. Am J Surg 126:529, 1973.
3. Crockett DM, Healy GB, McGill TJ, Friedman EM: Benign lesions of the nose, oral cavity and oropharynx in children: Excision by carbon dioxide laser. Ann Otol Rhinol Laryngol 94:489, 1985.
4. Fukutake T, Yamashita T, Tomoda K, Kumazawa T: Laser surgery for allergic rhinitis. Arch Otolaryngol Head Neck Surg 112:1280, 1986.
5. Levine HL: The KTP-532 laser. Rhinologic Surgery, KTP-532 Clinical Update, Number 11, April 1988.
6. Simpson GT, Shapshay SM, Vaughan CW, Strong MS: Rhinologic surgery with the carbon dioxide laser. Laryngoscope 92:412, 1982.
7. Parkin JL, Dixon JA: Laser photocoagulation in hereditary hemorrhagic telangiectasia. Otolaryngol Head Neck Surg 89:204, 1981.
8. Shapshay SM, Oliver P: Treatment of hereditary hemorrhagic telangiectasia by Nd:YAG laser photocoagulation. Laryngoscope 94:1554, 1984.
9. Selkin S: Pitfalls in intranasal laser surgery and how to avoid them. Arch Otolaryngol Head Neck Surg 112:285, 1986.
10. Healy GB, McGill T, Strong MS, Jako GJ, Vaughan CW: Management of choanal atresia with the carbon dioxide laser. Ann Otol Rhinol Laryngol 87:658, 1978.
11. Richardson MA, Osguthorpe JD: Surgical management of choanal atresia. Laryngoscope 98:915, 1988.
12. Muntz H: Pitfalls to laser correction of choanal atresia. Ann Otol Rhinol Laryngol 96:43, 1987.
13. Shapshay SM, et al.: Removal of rhinophyma with the carbon dioxide laser. Arch Otolaryngol Head Neck Surg 106:257, 1980.
14. Amedee RG, Routman MH: Methods and complications of rhinophyma excision. Laryngoscope 97:1316, 1987.
15. Lenz H: Endonasal laser surgery. *In* Koebner HK (ed): Lasers in Medicine. Boston, Wiley, 1980.
16. Mittleman H: CO_2 laser turbinectomies for chronic obstructive rhinitis. Lasers Surg Med 2:29, 1982.
17. Selkin S: Laser turbinectomy as an adjunct to rhinoseptoplasty. Arch Otolaryngol Head Neck Surg 111:446, 1985.
18. Brightwell AP: The role of lasers in nasal surgery. *In* Carruth JAS, Simpson GT (eds): Lasers in Otolaryngology. Chicago, Year Book Medical Publishers, 1988.
19. Williams JD: Laser vidian neurectomy. Ann Otol Rhinol Laryngol 92:281, 1983.

Lasers in Facial Plastic and Reconstructive Surgery

Milton Waner

Scott Dinehart

CUTANEOUS VASCULAR MALFORMATIONS

Laser Development Perspective

Since the pioneering work of Goldman and Rockwell some 20 years ago,[1] laser photocoagulation of cutaneous vascular malformations has finally come of age. The chemical content of skin, its optical properties, and the judicious use of yellow light (577 nm) have finally made real the possibility of coagulating subcutaneous vascular tissue through an intact, unaffected epidermis. Further refinements in the laser devices used, as well as the techniques of treatment, will no doubt lead to the attainment of this intriguing goal.

The first laser developed, a ruby laser (1960), emitted light in the visible spectrum at 694.4 nm. This brilliant red light found its first medical application in the treatment of retinal detachments.[2] Ruby laser light was absorbed by the pigmented tissue of the chorioretinal layer, causing a chorioretinal scar. The detached retina was thus "welded" to adjacent tissue. Between 1966 and 1968, two independent groups began experimenting with an argon laser, at Stanford University and at the Harkness Eye Institute. The blue-green light of an argon laser (490 and 514 nm) was found to be well absorbed by hemoglobin as well as various other pigmented tissues. This additional property meant that an argon laser could be used to coagulate vascular tissue. The possibility of treating diabetic retinopathies thus became a reality. The first published data were those of L'Esperance (1968).[3] Soon after this Goldman and Rockwell reported on their experiences with these lasers in cutaneous diseases.[1] Although early results were encouraging, technical problems with delivery of light from the device to the affected area often resulted in inadequate treatment. Only linear capillary hemangiomas appeared to respond well.[3]

By 1976, argon lasers had replaced ruby lasers for the treatment of capillary hemangiomas.[4,5] The blue-green light from an argon laser was thought to be selectively absorbed by hemoglobin, resulting in thermal coagulation, thrombosis, ablation of vascular tissue, and hence a lightening in color of port wine stains. Although a wide range of treatment variables and techniques have been described,[6–10] the results are essentially the same.[9] About 10 per cent of patients with port wine stains experienced complete disappearance of their lesion. In a further 80 per cent good fading was noted, whereas about 5 per cent experienced only slight fading, and an additional 5 per cent of patients experienced no improvement. The incidence of hypertrophic scarring remained at approximately 4 per cent.[8]

Histologic studies of areas treated with argon lasers have shown nonspecific epidermal and dermal destruction as well as vessel destruction.[11–14] This probably occurs because, although 490 nm light is absorbed by oxyhemoglobin, it is also well absorbed by melanin. Furthermore, neither the 490 nm nor the 514 nm band corresponds to a peak in the absorption spectrum of oxyhemoglobin. More appropriate therapeutic wavelengths are at 540 and 577 nm (Fig. 12–1). These wavelengths correspond to two of the absorption peaks of oxyhemoglobin. Because light at 577 nm penetrates biologic tissue to deeper levels than does light at 540 nm, experimental work using lasers that emitted light at 577 nm began.

Theoretic and experimental considerations led to the use of both pulsed and continuous wave tunable dye lasers at 577 nm.[14,15] Pulsed tunable dye lasers or flashlamp pumped dye lasers have been shown experimentally and clinically to produce selective vascular photocoagulation while sparing the overlying epidermis.[15–17] The continuous wave argon ion pumped dye laser, used in a chopped or gated mode, was also found to ablate subcutaneous vascular tissue with less damage to the overlying epidermis than was evident with a blue-green argon laser. It would seem, therefore, that the pulsed tunable dye laser is the laser of choice for the treatment of port wine stains. This, however, has not been proved. Although pulsed tunable dye lasers appear to be more selective, in the experience of the author, they are less efficacious in the treatment of nodular or cavernous-capillary hemangiomas and telangiectasia.

More recently, the development of a copper vapor laser added further confusion. This laser also emits pulsed light at 578 nm. The pulse characteristic is considerably different from that of the flashlamp pumped dye laser (tunable dye laser) mentioned above (Figs. 12–2 to 12–4). The copper vapor laser emits nanosecond pulsed light, whereas the flashlamp pumped dye laser emits micro-

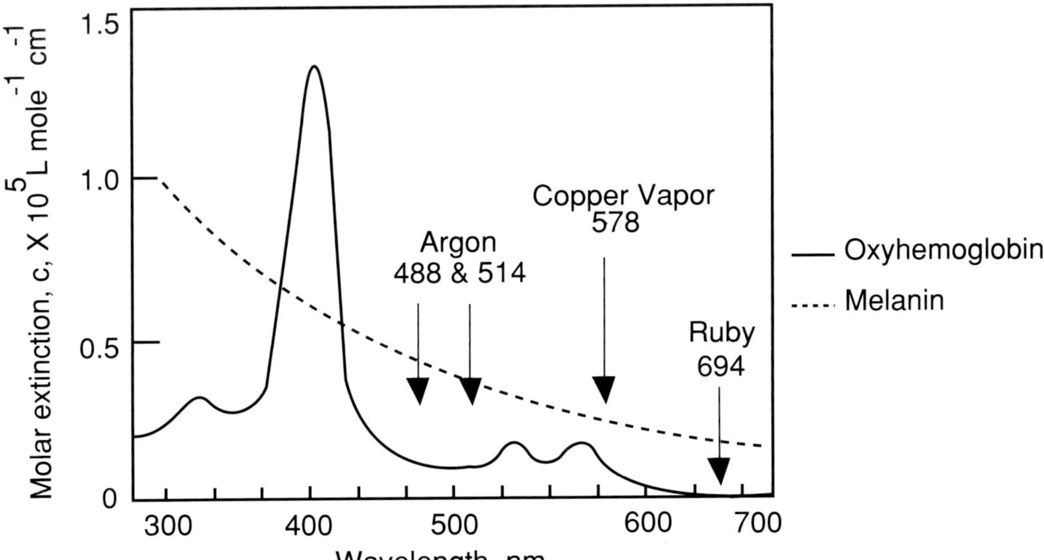

FIGURE 12–1. The absorption spectra of oxyhemoglobin and melanin and the emission wavelengths of argon, copper vapor, and ruby lasers.

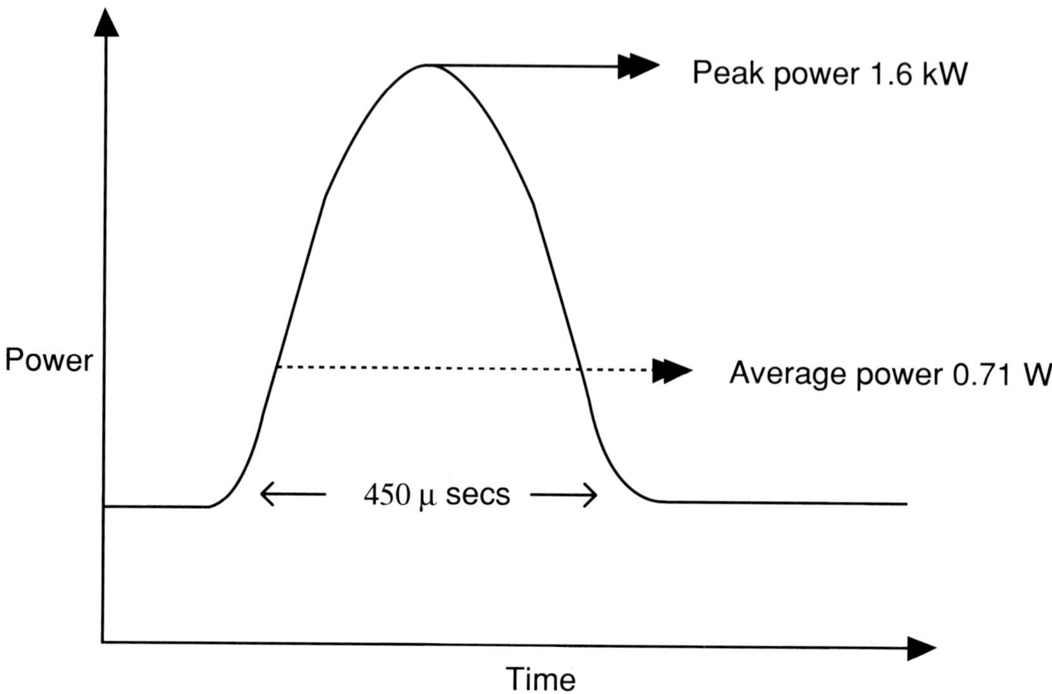

Figure 12–2. The power profile of a microsecond (μsec) pulsed flashlamp pumped dye laser.

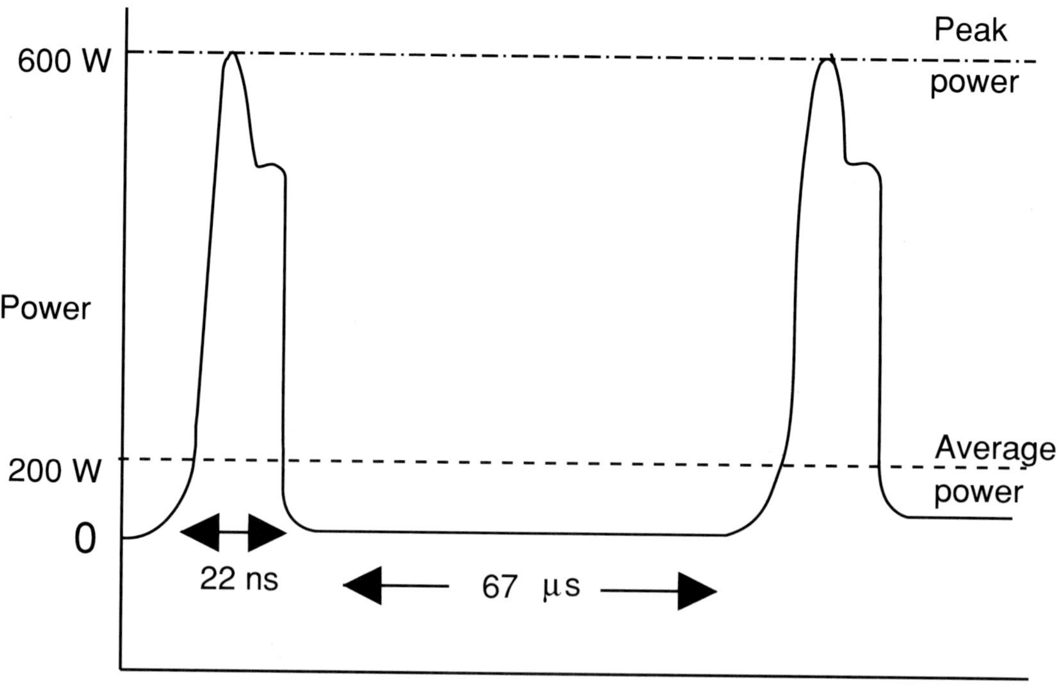

Figure 12–3. The power profile of a nanosecond (nsec) pulsed copper vapor laser.

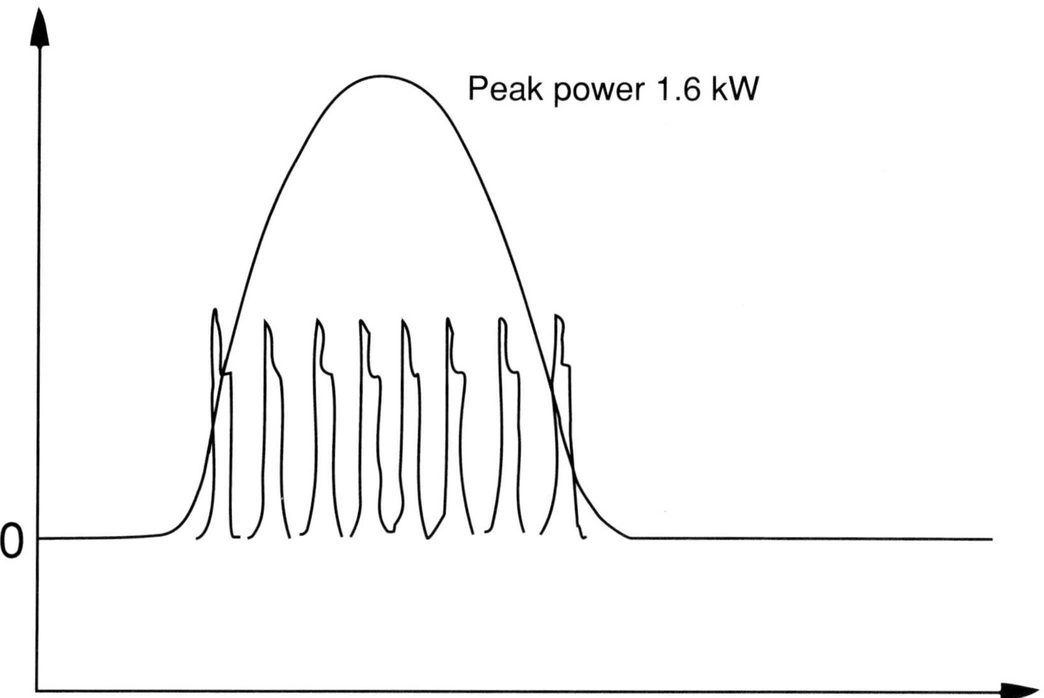

Figure 12–4. Comparison of the power profiles of a flashlamp pumped dye laser and a copper vapor laser.

second pulsed light. The peak powers are therefore considerably different. The mode of action also appears to be different. The author has found this device to be reliable, and the results of the treatment of cavernous or nodular port wine stains as well as telangiectasia have been excellent. These devices are not, however, effective in the treatment of pink to light red port wine stains.

Biophysics

A thorough understanding of the interaction between light and skin is essential to understanding laser photocoagulation. Light incident on a skin surface may be reflected, transmitted to deeper layers, scattered, or absorbed within any layer (Fig. 12–5). However, only the absorbed portion of light has any effect.

About 4 to 7 per cent of incident light in the visible spectrum is reflected.[19] In addition to this, a significant portion of visible light is scattered. Scattering, in general, is a function of wavelength. The shorter the wavelength, the greater is the scattering.[19] Scattering increases the average distance light must travel to reach the deeper structures of the skin. Therefore, the shorter the wavelength (of visible light), the less the depth of penetration is. Visible light is thus attenuated by skin. The amount of light diminishes with increasing depth. This is illustrated by the following examples:

At 500 nm only 50 per cent of the light reaches 0.16 mm and only 10 per cent of the light reaches 0.53 mm.

At 600 nm only 50 per cent of the light reaches 0.38 mm and only 10 per cent of the light reaches 1.27 mm.[19]

Present within biologic tissue are certain substances capable of absorbing light; these substances are termed chromophores (Table 12–1). Chromophores contained within skin include hemoglobin, oxyhemoglobin, beta carotene, and collagen in the dermis and melanin in the epidermis. Each of these substances has a different absorption spectrum, which in turn is determined by its chemical structure.

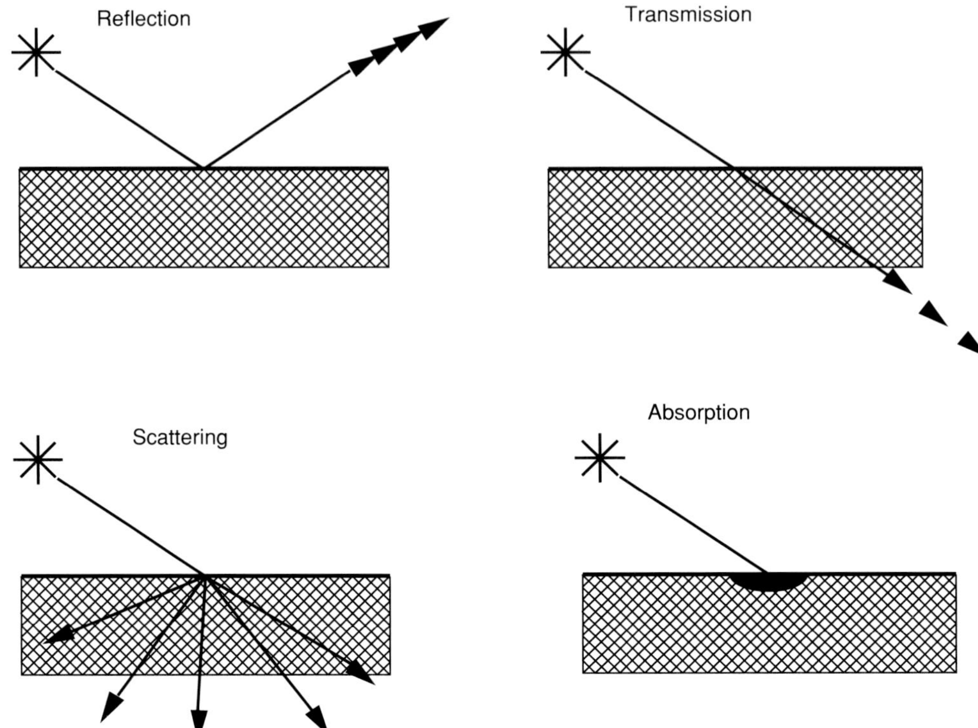

FIGURE 12–5. Mechanisms of interaction of light and biologic tissue.

Light absorbed by a chromophore is converted to heat. In this way, the effects of most laser applications are accomplished. In general, tissues heated to 60°C coagulate, whereas tissues heated to 100°C vaporize. Because oxyhemoglobin is the dominant form of hemoglobin and is entirely vascular, it is the logical chromophore target when treating vascular malformations. Similarly, melanin would be the logical target when treating pigmented malformations. The absorption peaks of oxyhemoglobin are at 418, 542, and 577 nm (see Fig. 12–1). As mentioned above, each wavelength has a finite effective depth of penetration. When selecting the appropriate wavelength, one must therefore also consider the depth of the target. The mean vessel depth is 0.365 to 0.665 mm.[20] Taking these factors into consideration (i.e., the oxyhemoglobin absorption spectrum and the mean vessel depth), it would seem logical that 577 nm is the wavelength of choice. Although good results have been obtained with argon lasers (488 and 514 nm), quite clearly these

Table 12–1. LASERS AND THEIR WAVELENGTHS AND
CHROMOPHORES

Laser	Wavelength	Chromophore
CO_2	10,600 nm	Water
Copper vapor	511 and 578 nm	Melanin (oxyhemoglobin)
	1578 nm	Oxyhemoglobin (melanin)
Flashlamp pumped dye	585 nm	Oxyhemoglobin
Argon dye	587 nm	Oxyhemoglobin
Nd:YAG	1060 nm	Water (poorly absorbed)

wavelengths do not respond to an absorption peak of oxyhemoglobin nor do they penetrate deeply enough. The mechanism of action of an argon laser with respect to vascular malformations, therefore, appears to be attributable to a more generalized thermal damage rather than selective vascular coagulation. This has been confirmed histologically.[11–14]

Three lasers being used are capable of producing yellow light (577 nm). These are a copper vapor laser, an argon ion pumped dye laser, and a flashlamp pumped dye laser.

Copper Vapor Lasers

Copper vapor lasers produce pulsed yellow light at 578 nm. The pulse width is 25 nsec, and the pulsed repetition rate 15 kHz. The interval between pulses is therefore 67 μsec (see Fig. 12–3). Because the thermal relaxation time for blood vessels of the diameter typical of a port wine stain is in the region of 0.1 to 10 msec, the theoretic advantage of using a short nanosecond pulse should ensure selective vascular damage.[19] This, however, does not appear to be the case. When used in the continuous mode, the high pulse repetition rate causes thermal transmission beyond the confines of the vessels. The net thermal effect produced is cumulative, and the laser should, therefore, be regarded as a quasicontinuous wave device. The high peak powers (10 kW at an average power of 200 mW), however, result in a more efficient photocoagulation of oxyhemoglobin and hence a more efficient ablation of vascular tissue. This is especially good for the treatment of more cavernous port wine stains. Furthermore, when using a small spot size, one can ensure complete destruction of the ectatic vessels seen in the various forms of facial telangiectasia. Perivascular damage and consequent perivascular fibrosis are desirable. This ensures a substantially decreased vessel diameter after healing of the treated area (see Fig. 12–5). Although some destruction of the overlying epidermis results, the amount of destruction incurred appears to be far less than that seen with a continuous wave laser at the same wavelength (argon dye laser).

Using a small spot size technique (100, 150, and 200 microns) no cases of hypertrophic scarring have been seen in over 1000 patients treated at five centers (Waner, Sydney, Australia; Bekhor and associates, Melbourne, Australia; Grossman, Southport, Australia; Studniberg and colleagues, Sydney, Australia; Liu, Hong Kong). The only adverse reaction seen was postinflammatory hyperpigmentation (4 per cent of cases). This was treated with a 4 per cent hydroquinone cream and responded in all cases. No evidence of hyperpigmentation was present 8 weeks after the commencement of hydroquinone application.

Argon Ion Pumped Dye Laser

This laser emits continuous wave light at 577 nm. The theoretic advantage of yellow light (577 nm) was mentioned above. Limited experience with these lasers used in the chopped or gated mode has been favorable. An incidence of hypertrophic scarring of less than 1 per cent has been reported, and the efficacy with various vascular malformations has been reported to be superior to that of a conventional argon laser.[18,21] The only disadvantage of this laser is its low efficiency and difficulty of maintenance. The recent entry into the market of a fixed wavelength copper vapor laser should allow replacement of argon dye lasers in this application.

Flashlamp Pumped Dye Lasers

Although judicious use of the 577 nm waveband ensured as selective a reaction as possible, further attempts at reducing the amount of thermal transmission of heat outside the target vessel were undertaken by Anderson and Parrish.[14,15] They accomplished this by using a laser that emitted pulsed light in which the pulse width was shorter than the thermal relaxation time of the vessels typically found in vascular malformations (0.1 to 10 msec). This was found to be possible with a flashlamp pumped dye laser. Using a pulse width of 1 μsec, selective thermal injury of vascular tissue was histologically confirmed.[14,15,22] Further work showed that a more desirable outcome could be accomplished with a wider pulse width.[23] This study showed selective nonhemorrhagic vascular necrosis at pulse widths of 20 μsec or greater. A pulse width of 300 μsec has also been used with a favorable clinical outcome.[16] The flashlamp pumped dye laser currently used at most institutions has a pulse width of 450 μsec! (see Figs. 12–2, 12–3). A more gentle heating of the vessels is achieved with these wider pulse widths, and no microvascular rupture or hemorrhage is evident. Instead, an intravascular coagulum is formed, and subsequent vascular necrosis is seen histologically.[23] To accomplish this, however, a higher power density is required. As a consequence of this wider pulse width and higher power density, some evidence of epidermal damage was noted in the biopsy material taken. This epidermal damage, however, appeared to be minimal.

Clinical results with this laser have been extremely encouraging. Excellent results have been obtained in the treatment of fine pink to red port wine stains, but, as mentioned above, thick cavernous port wine stains appeared to respond less favorably.

A flashlamp pumped dye laser is therefore an extremely useful addition to the lasers used in the treatment of vascular malformations. Its principal use is in the treatment of fine pink to red port wine stains, for which it is indispensable.

It should be apparent that no single laser currently being used is ideal for *all* vascular malformations. The type of practice one conducts determines the type of laser that is necessary. In the experience of the author, the vast majority of patients are referred for the treatment of telangiectasia. Only 20 per cent of patients are referred for port wine stains, and a smaller percentage of these are light pink to red. A copper vapor laser is therefore the basic laser used for most applications. However, to offer a comprehensive facility, a flashlamp pump dye laser is essential. In addition to providing the effective treatment of lighter port wine stains, it can also be used to treat the residual redness sometimes present after treatment with a copper vapor laser.

Clinical Considerations

Capillary Hemangiomas (Port Wine Stains)

Port wine stains are members of a larger group of congenital vascular malformations, termed nevus flammeus, which are present in 75 per cent of newborns.[24] These lesions are uniformly macular pink to red at birth and usually disappear by the end of the first year. Port wine stains, unlike the rest of these lesions, persist. Port wine stains can sometimes be confused with strawberry nevi because they are of a similar color and indeed have a similar appearance in the neonatal period. Eventually, however, a strawberry nevus becomes raised, bulky, and compressible.[25] Furthermore, 70 per cent of strawberry nevi have involuted by age 7 years, and 90 per cent by age 12.[25] Port wine stains, on the other hand, do not disappear.

Histologic sections of port wine stains in early childhood show few abnormalities, whereas in adults these lesions consist of masses of postcapillary venules in the upper 0.5 mm segment of the dermis. These lesions are therefore believed to represent a progressive ectasia of postcapillary venules.[26] This accounts for the increased intensity of color and thickness found with advancing age (Figs. 12–6 to 12–8). This important point is often not well explained to patients. Patients must therefore be counseled that the birthmark will grow thicker and darker with age.

Port wine stains most commonly appear on the face and neck but may be found on any part of the body.[27] The incidence of these lesions is believed to be less than 1 per cent.[28] Port wine stains are initially light pink and flat. Following puberty, the lesion appears to darken from pink to deep red or purple. Fifty to 60 per cent of facial lesions begin to undergo a nodular or cavernous change

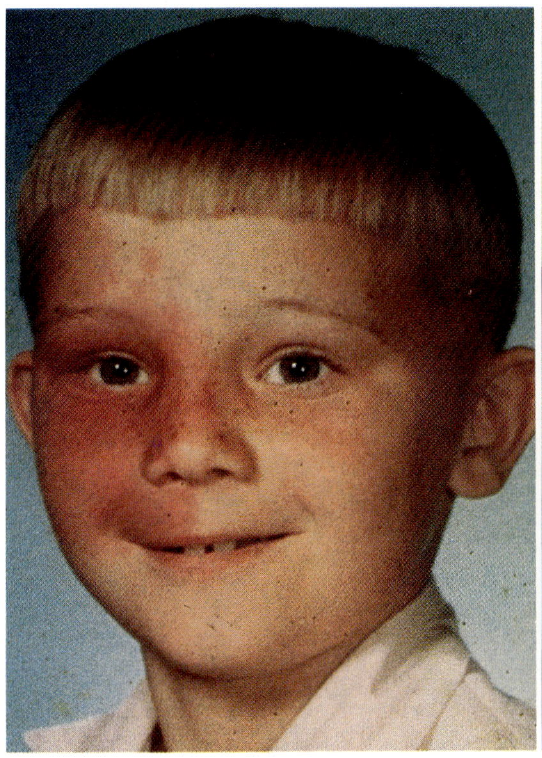

Figure 12–6.

Figure 12–7.

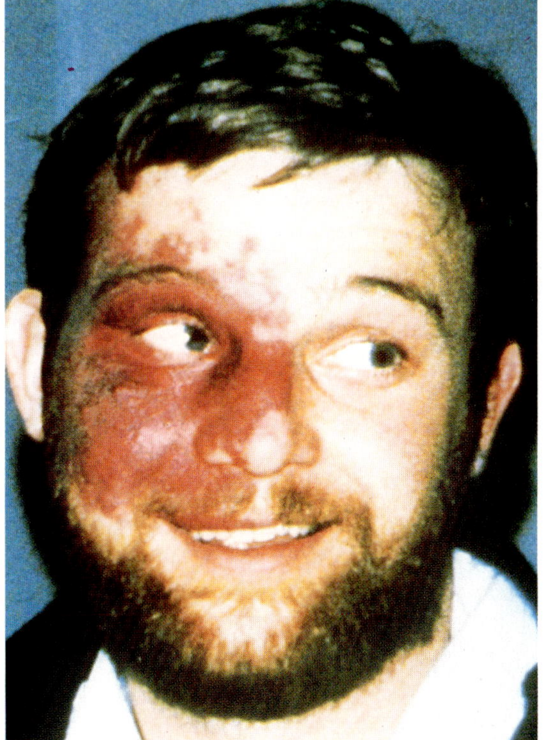

Figure 12–8.

Figure 12–6. A facial port wine stain on the right side in a 6 year old boy.

Figure 12–7. The patient in Figure 12–6 at age 16, showing darkening and thickening of the lesion.

Figure 12–8. The patient in Figures 12–6 and 12–7 at 28 years of age. Note the thickness and nodularity of the lesion.

after the age of 30 years.[28] These nodules protrude 2 to 3 mm above the surface of the skin and eventually tend to sag. These changes are due to progressive ectasia of the vessels as well as degeneration of the supportive structures of the skin.

To date, no satisfactory, uniformly acceptable means of classifying these lesions exists. Color coding of port wine stains using various standards has been employed in the past, but is too subjective.[29] The author uses a classification based on the degree of ectasia of the vessels. Accordingly, port wine stains are divided into four grades (Fig. 12–9):

- *Grade 1:* These are light pink lesions made up of small vessels. These lesions, when transilluminated with yellow light at 578 nm and viewed with 6 × magnification, show discrete end on vessels appearing like grains of sand. These vessels are small and fairly sparse (Fig. 12–10).

- *Grade 2:* These lesions are somewhat darker (dark pink to light red) and when viewed under similar circumstances show discretely larger vessels with much less normal skin between them (Fig. 12–11).

- *Grade 3:* These lesions seem to be made up of discrete ectatic vessels almost touching each other (Fig. 12–12).

- *Grade 4:* A homogeneous mass of vessels is seen, some more elevated than others. No normal-appearing skin is seen between these vessels (Fig. 12–13).

- *Grade 5:* This is used to describe nodular lesions (Fig. 12–14).

When treating a port wine stain using a small spot size method (100 to 150 microns), one can often see regression through these grades.

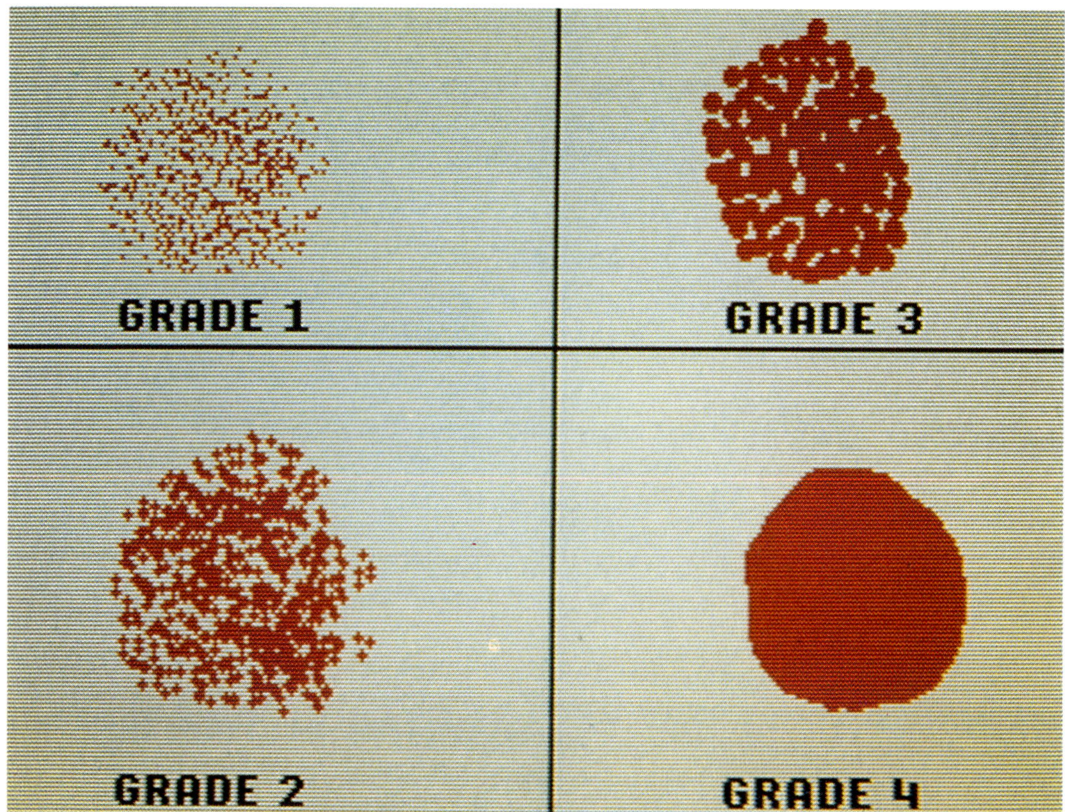

FIGURE 12–9. The grades of port wine stains according to the degree of ectasia of the vessels.

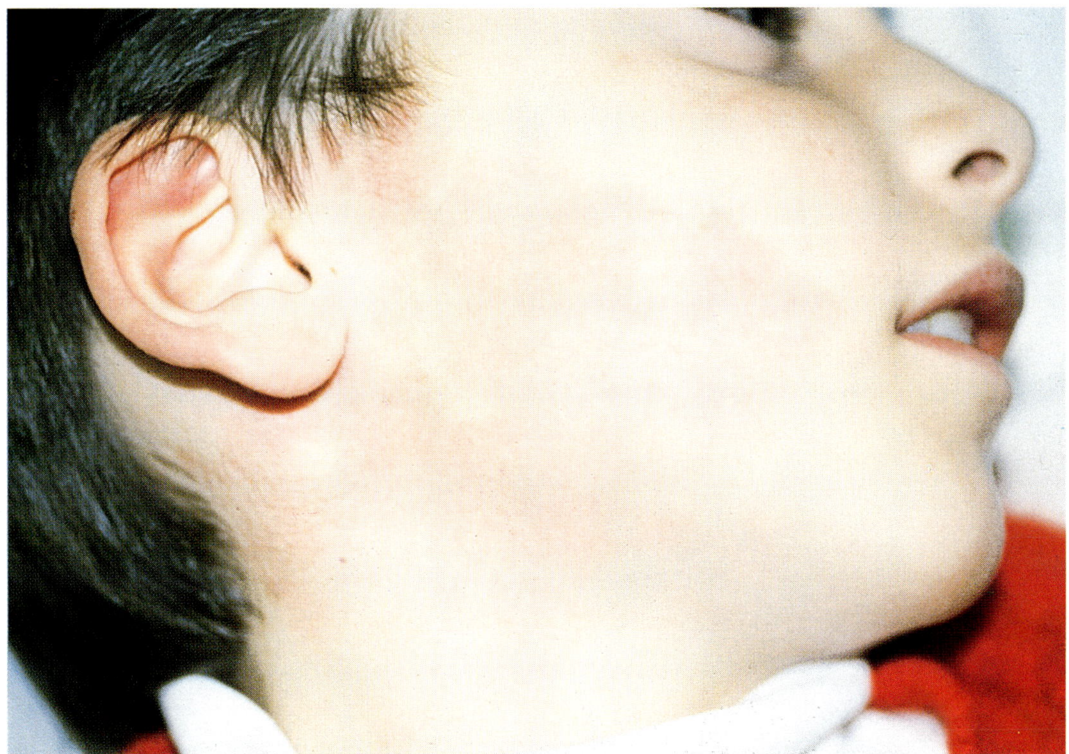

Figure 12–10. A patient with a grade 1 port wine stain.

Prior to the advent of lasers, port wine stains were treated in many ways. These included partial or total excision with skin grafting or flap rotation; dermabrasion and grafting; cauterization; irradiation; ligation of the blood supply; and use of sclerosing agents, carbon dioxide snow, liquid nitrogen, cortisone, protamine, or heparin (both locally and systemically). An attempt was often made to reduce the visual impact of the port wine stain by tattooing flesh-colored pigments into the skin overlying the lesion. Two problems were encountered with this latter technique: these were

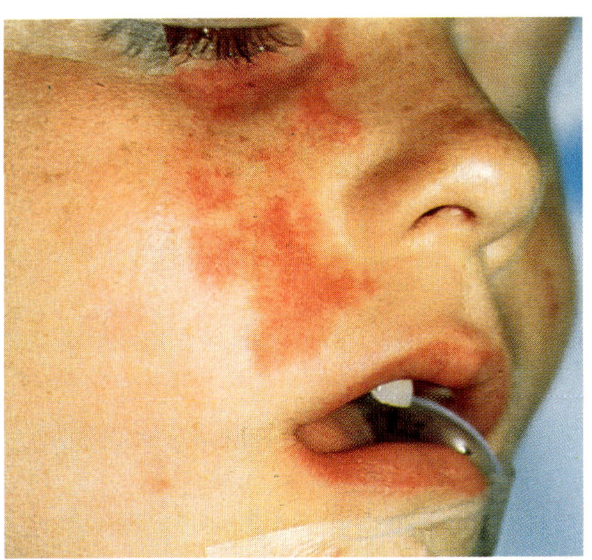

Figure 12–11. A patient with a grade 2 port wine stain. Note the increased intensity of the color.

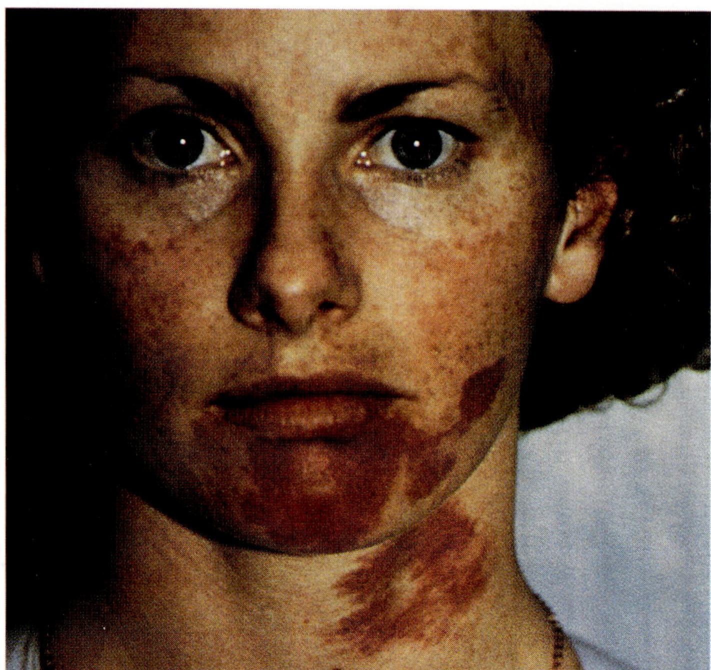

FIGURE 12–12. A patient with a grade 3 port wine stain.

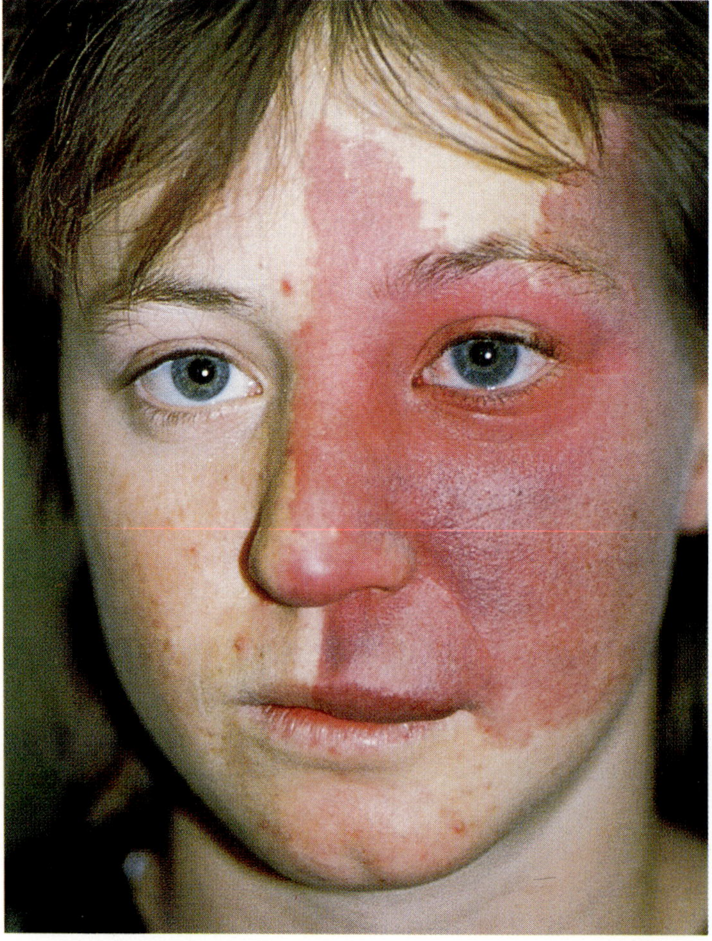

FIGURE 12–13. A patient with a grade 4 port wine stain. Note the increased thickness and intensity of the color.

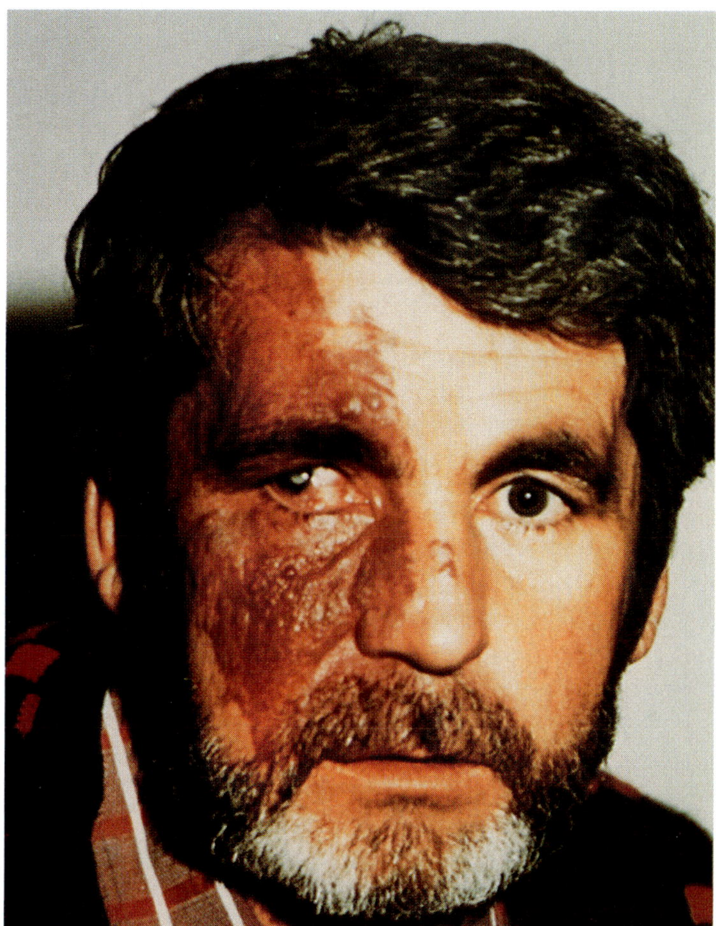

FIGURE 12–14. A patient with a grade 5 port wine stain. Note the obvious nodules over the right cheek.

difficulty in matching skin tones and migration of the pigment with progressive ectasia of the lesion. Tattooing is thus not a satisfactory form of treatment. A further attempt at visual reduction can be undertaken with the application of various cosmetics. Fine light pink to red port wine stains can be relatively easily masked. Thicker, more cavernous and cobblestoned lesions, however, cannot be adequately disguised.

Lasers have undoubtedly become the treatment of choice. The treatment of port wine stains with a copper vapor laser is discussed because the author believes that this is the best method for most lesions. The technique described is based on the excellent work of Scheibner,[30] an innovator in the field of laser photocoagulation of vascular malformations. This technique was originally reported for argon lasers and, more recently, argon ion pumped dye lasers. This technique has been modified for use with a copper vapor laser.

All treatments begin with a test patch. One should select a representative area of the port wine stain and, if possible, a relatively inconspicuous area. An inconspicuous area is chosen because, in the extremely unlikely event of scarring, the offending area is much less noticeable. The rationale for doing a test patch treatment is multifold (Table 12–2). From the surgeon's point of view, the degree of response to a single treatment can be ascertained. One is also able to determine the likelihood of complications; these include scarring (hypertrophic or atrophic) and pigmentation changes (hyperpigmentation or hypopigmentation). It must be stated, however, that the correlation of test patch result to final outcome is not absolute. One should therefore view the test patch as a less than perfect indicator. From the patient's point of view, he or she gets an idea of the discomfort associated with treatment, the type of skin reaction to be expected, the healing time, and the degree of response.

Table 12–2. RATIONALE FOR TEST PATCH

Physician	Patient
Power setting	Expectations
Response	Pain
Fading	Scabbing
Pigment changes	Healing time
Scarring	Result
Number of treatments	Number of treatments

After having chosen a representative, inconspicuous site, the area (usually about 1 cm^2) is outlined with a fine-tipped surgical marker. One per cent lidocaine without epinephrine is infiltrated subcutaneously if desired. Suitable eye protection is necessary for both the patient and the surgeon (at 578 nm, the most appropriate eye protection for the surgeon is a BG36 Shott-Glass filter; the patient's eyes are protected by simply covering them with green gauze, which is firmly taped down so to prevent them from opening). Using a 6 × magnifying loupe, a handpiece, and a 100 micron spot size focus, the lesion within the test patch area is treated.

Two methods of blanching port wine stains are used:

- *Vessel blanch:* For grade 1, 2, and 3 lesions, in which individual vessels are clearly visible, the focused point of the laser beam is moved from vessel to vessel. The end point one looks for is complete disappearance of the vessel before moving on to the next vessel. The speed at which one moves depends on how soon the end point is reached, which in turn depends on the power setting being used.

- *Field blanch:* With Grade 4 and 5 lesions and those for which previous treatments have taken place, in which few or no individual vessels are distinguishable, the field or area being treated is blanched by moving the focused point of the laser beam from area to area, watching for blanching as one proceeds. Again, the speed depends on the power setting being used.

The power setting varies with the grading of the port wine stain and the age of the patient. In general, 90 to 140 mW is used for children under the age of 12 years; 120 to 180 mW, for children aged 12 to 18 years; and 180 to 260 mW for patients over the age of 18. Alternatively, when dealing with adults the grade of the lesion determines the power density (Table 12–3). In achieving the end point mentioned above, one may see either erythema of the overlying skin when lower power settings are used (Figs. 12–15, 12–16) or mild to moderate blanching with higher power settings (Figs. 12–17, 12–18). Usually, the thicker the lesion, the more blanching one accepts.

The test patch is evaluated after 6 to 8 weeks. One may even wait longer with olive-skinned patients because postinflammatory pigmentation may take longer to develop (Figs. 12–19, 12–20). By this time the patient is more able to fully understand the implications of further

Table 12–3. DETERMINING POWER SETTING FROM GRADE
OF PORT WINE STAIN IN ADULTS*

Grade of Port Wine Stain	Power Setting (mW)
Grade 1	160
(rare in adults)	
Grade 2	160–190
Grade 3	190–220
Grade 4	220–240
Grade 5	240–260

*Older than 12 years of age.

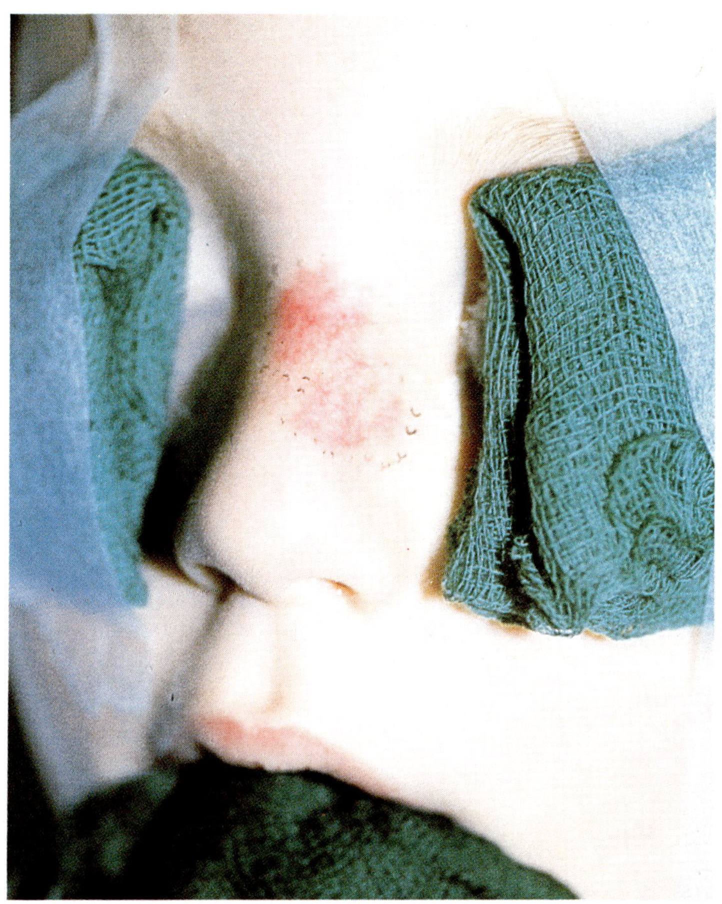

FIGURE 12–15. A grade 2 port wine stain prior to treatment. The outline of the lesion was marked with a fine-pointed surgical marker.

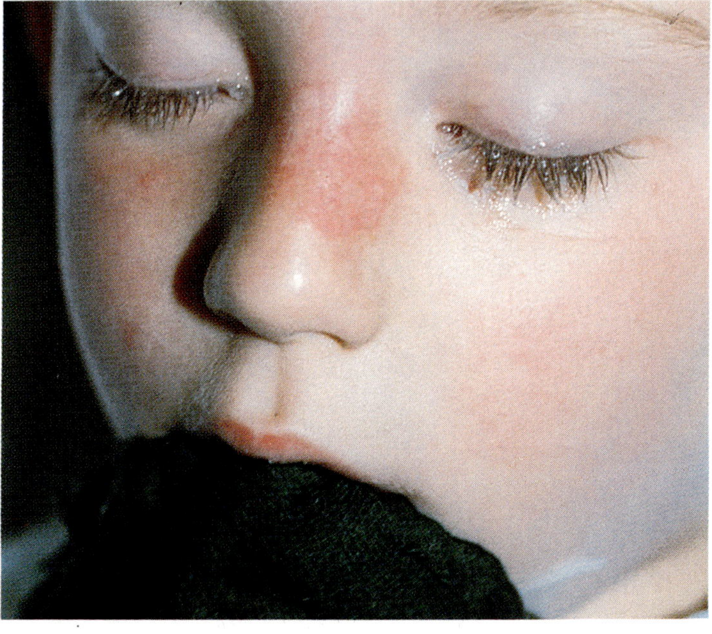

FIGURE 12–16. The lesion in Figure 12–15 immediately after treatment. Note the disappearance of the vessels and the erythema of the overlying skin.

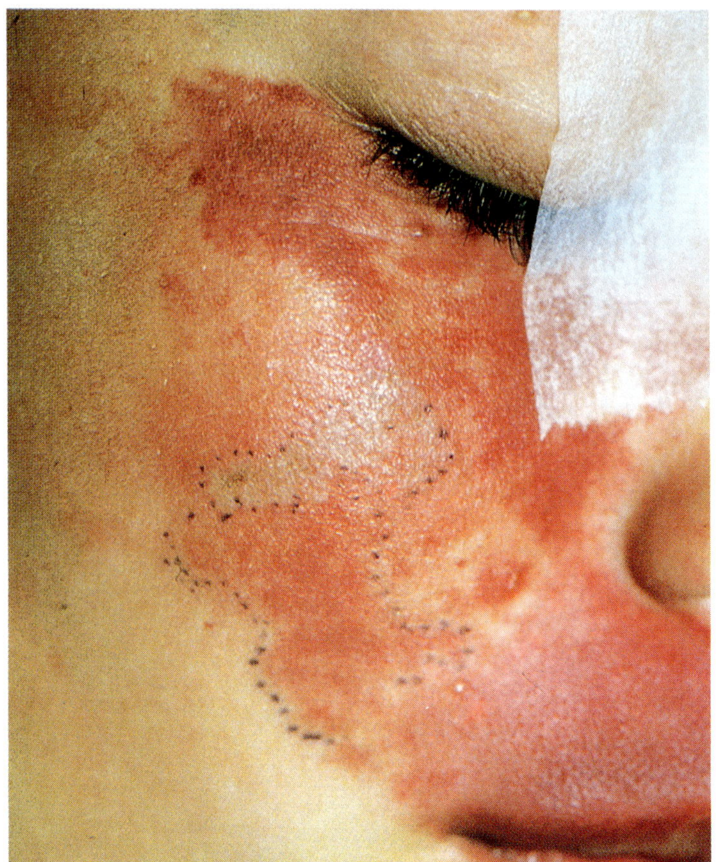

FIGURE 12–17. A grade 3 port wine stain during treatment. The outline of the port wine stain was marked with a fine-pointed surgical marker. A small area over the malar eminence was treated. Note the blanching of the overlying skin.

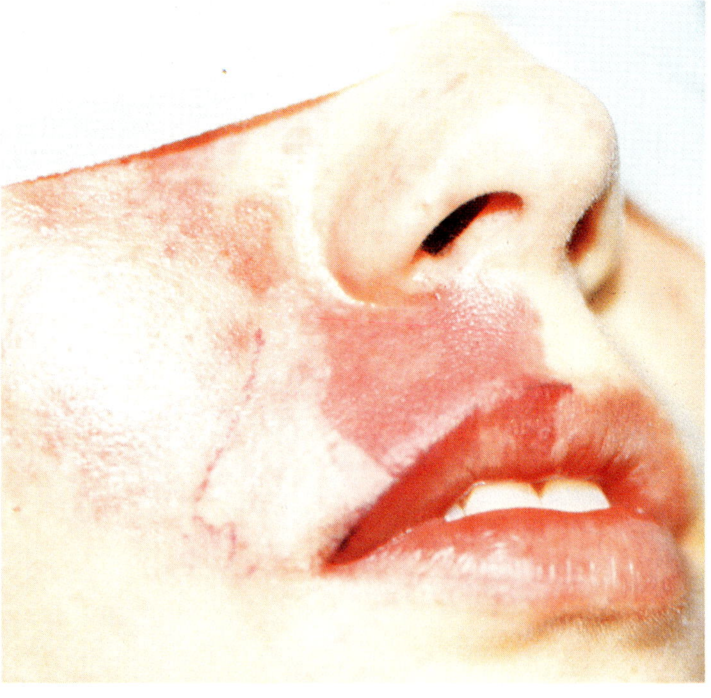

FIGURE 12–18. The patient in Figure 12–17 after most of the cheek and the lateral third of the upper lip were treated. The treatment was conducted up to the vermilion border. Note the blanching of the overlying skin.

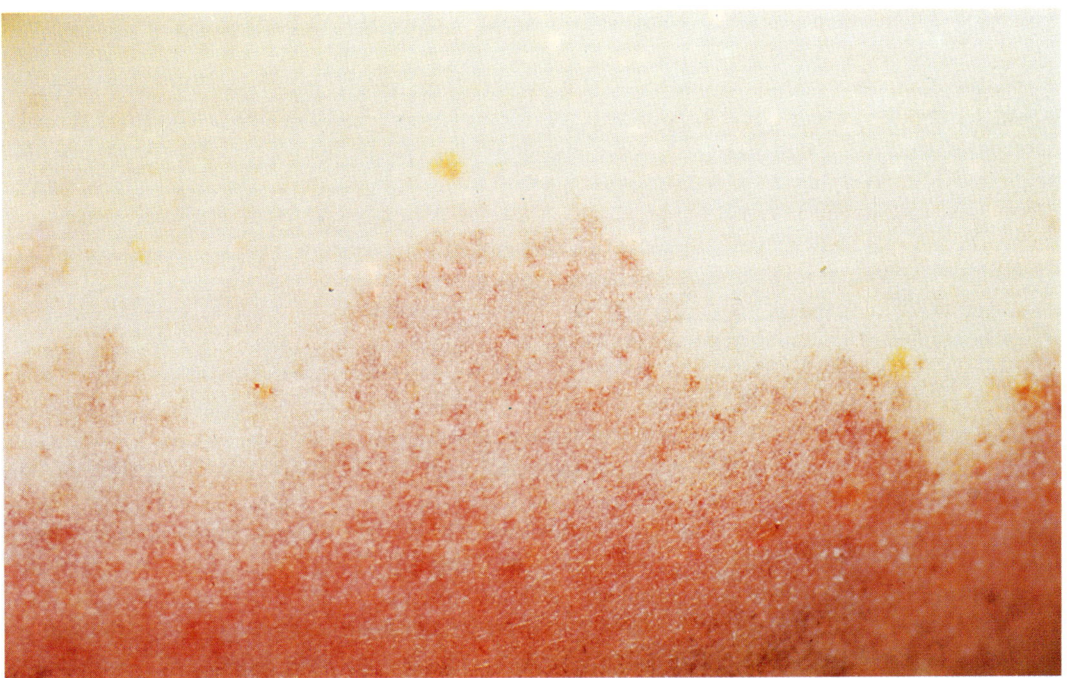

FIGURE 12–19. A grade 2 port wine stain prior to the performance of a test patch treatment.

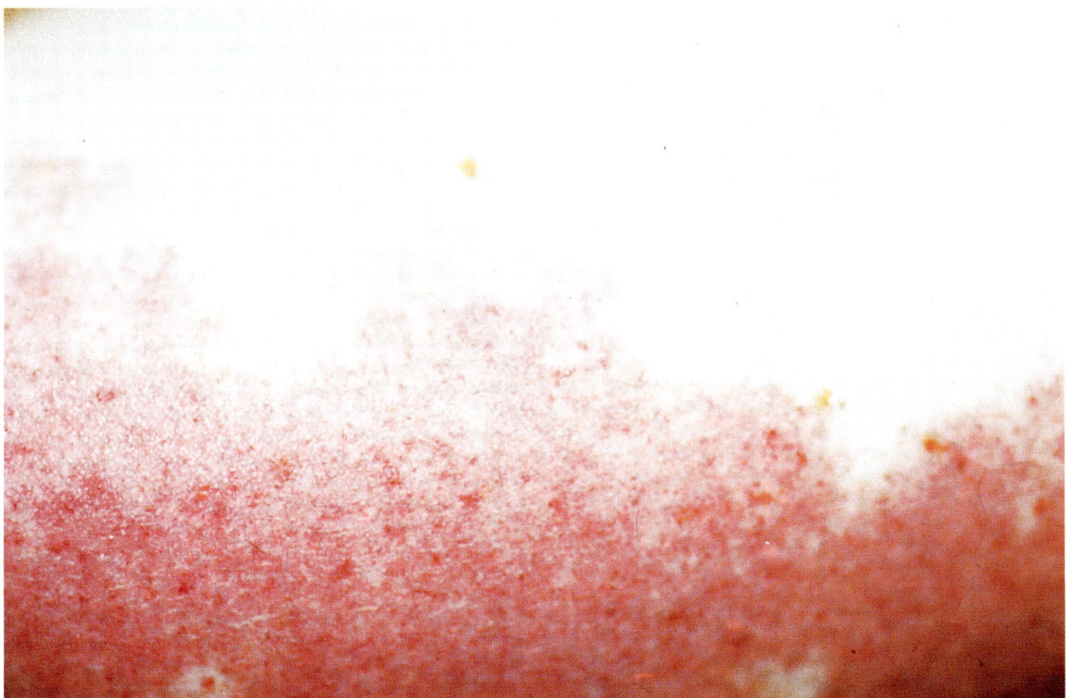

FIGURE 12–20. Three weeks after the treatment of a test patch of port wine stain in Figure 12–19. Note the presence of postinflammatory hyperpigmentation. This hyperpigmentation disappeared spontaneously within 6 weeks after the test patch treatment.

treatment. This is then discussed with the patient, and, if agreed on by both doctor and patient, further treatment is carried out.

Using the power setting for the test patch, modified by the test patch reaction, an appropriate power setting is selected. Local anesthetic in the form of 1 per cent lidocaine is infiltrated subcutaneously, if required, and treatment is commenced. With a fine-pointed surgical marker the area to be treated is divided into 2 cm squares with a dotted line. Each square is then treated as described previously, making sure to treat the area underneath the dotted line as well. The total surface area treated in one session depends on the level of tolerance of the patient as well as that of the surgeon. The author prefers to restrict each treatment session to 30 minutes. Occasionally, treatment is prolonged if the patient has traveled a long distance for treatment or, alternatively, if the treatment is being administered under general anesthesia.

Using the technique described above, successive areas are blanched during one or more sessions until the entire lesion has been treated. The patient is then reevaluated at 2 weeks, 3 months, and 6 months. Retreatment of the lesion is usually carried out at 6 months, and as many times thereafter as is necessary (at 6 month intervals) to obtain either significant lightening of the lesion or complete disappearance. If the port wine stain progressively lightens with each treatment, the treatments are continued. Both the surgeon and the patient, through discussion, determine when a satisfactory end point has been accomplished. Figures 12–21 to 12–26 show examples of patients who have been treated in this way.

Although children can be treated with heavy sedation in a consulting room, the author prefers to administer these treatments under general anesthesia in an operating theater. The necessity for anesthetic depends on the tolerance of the child. Most children under the age of 10 years require general anesthesia. However, at least two patients of 8 years old have been treated under local anesthesia. Although most practitioners have shied away from treating children owing to the reputed increased incidence of hypertrophic scarring, the author treats children 4 years of age or older. At least two other workers have recently demonstrated the safety of treating children.[31,32]

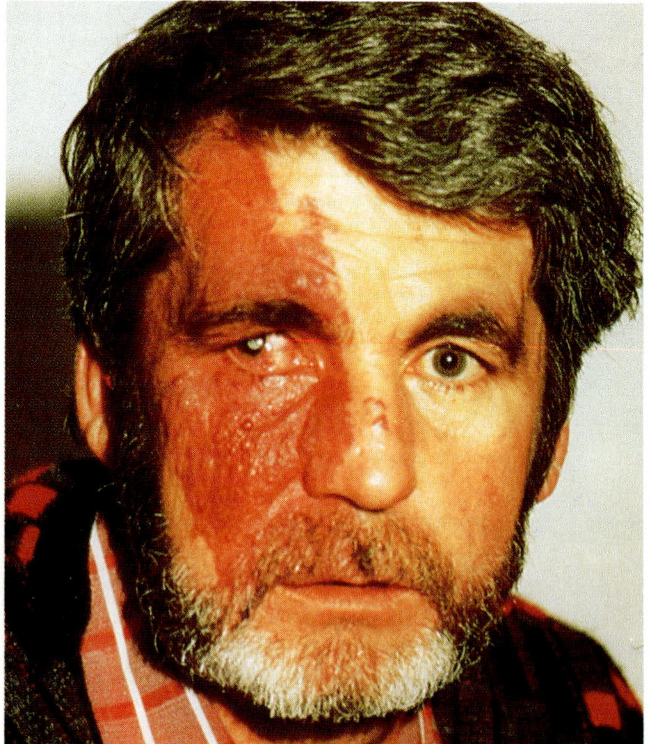

Figure 12–21. A patient with a grade 5 port wine stain prior to treatment.

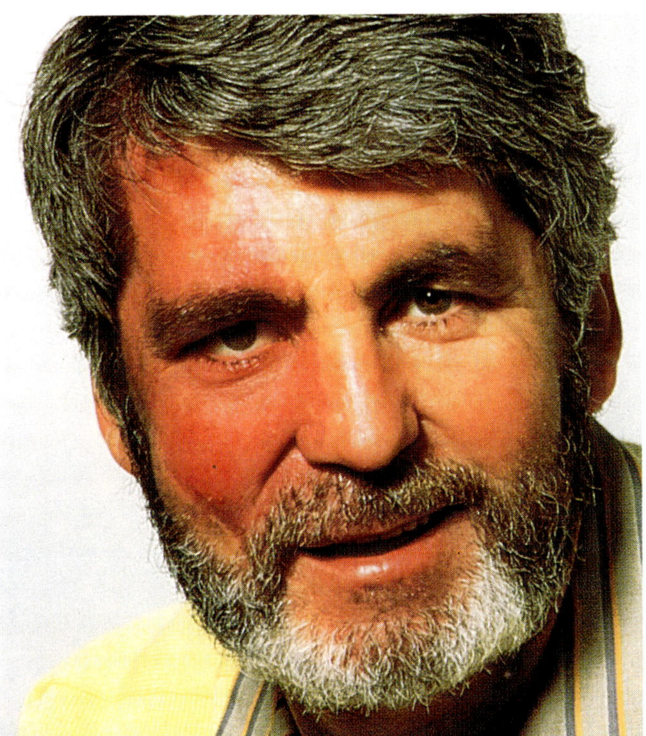

FIGURE 12–22. The patient in Figure 12–21 after four complete treatments. Note the complete disappearance of the nodules, a marked decrease in the intensity of the color, and the presence of normal skin contours.

Telangiectasia

The term telangiectasia is used to describe a superficial vessel of the skin that is visible to the naked eye. These vessels may represent an expanded venule, capillary, or arteriole and vary between 0.1 and 1 mm in diameter. In general, telangiectasias originating from the arterial side of a capillary loop tend to be bright red and small. Telangiectasias originating from the venous side of a capillary loop tend to be blue and wide and often protrude above the surface of the skin. Occasionally, an ectatic vessel arising from a capillary loop may be red at first, but with time may become blue as a result of increasing hydrostatic pressure and backflow from the venous side of the capillary loop. Varicose veins, on the other hand, are dilated veins arising in vessels larger than venules and measuring more than 1 mm in diameter. Telangiectasias have been classified into four types: sinus, or simple; arborizing; spider, or star; and punctiform. This classification is based on their clinical appearance[33] (see Fig. 12–6).

Telangiectasias are believed to be the end result of a release or activation of vasoactive substances.[34,35] Release of these substances may be caused by anoxia, infection, hormones, chemicals, and physical injuries. The result is capillary or venular ectasia.

The most common forms of facial telangiectasia are linear and arborizing. These vessels usually start out as linear vessels and with time arborize extensively. They are commonly seen over both cheeks and across the dorsum of the nose. The alar grooves are also commonly affected. These ectasias arise from persistent arteriolar dilation due to a weakness in the vessel wall, as well as a decrease in the elastin content of the surrounding connective tissue[36] and chronic sun exposure. Facial telangiectasias are also frequently seen in people of a fair complexion.

Spider telangiectasias (spider nevi) usually consist of a central vertical AV fistula in the dermis.[37] The central vessel varies from less than 1 mm to 3 mm or more in diameter and frequently protrudes above the surface of the skin (Fig. 12–27). Punctiform or papular telangiectasis is frequently seen in Osler-Weber-Rendu syndrome or associated with collagen vascular diseases.

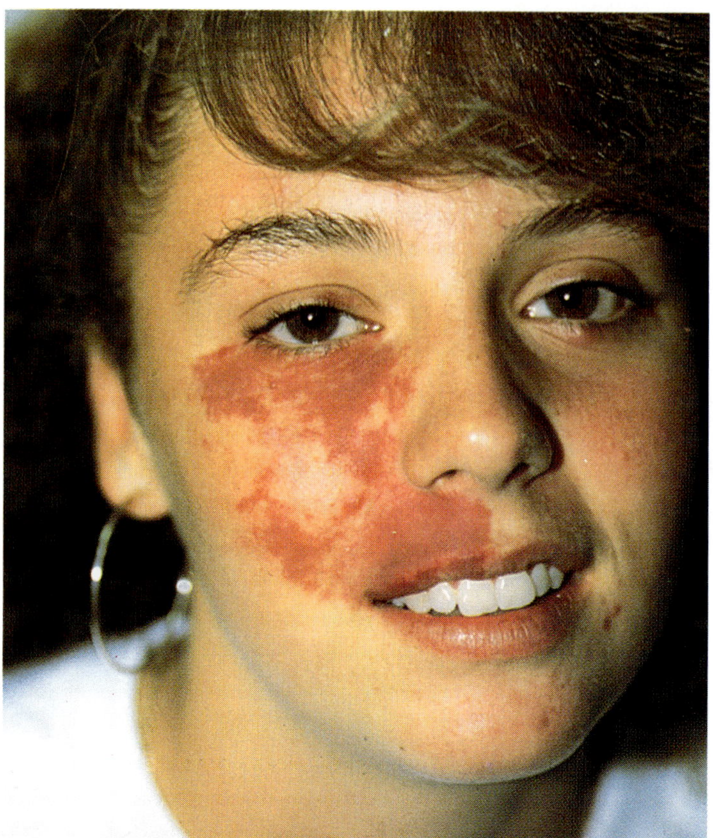

Figure 12–23. A 16 year old girl with a port wine stain of her right cheek and upper lip.

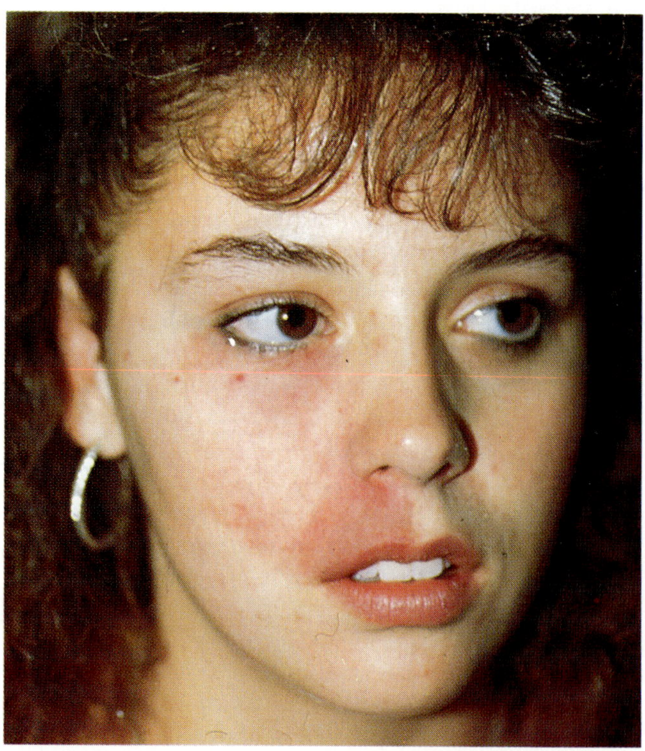

Figure 12–24. The patient in Figure 12–23 after three complete treatments of her cheek and upper lip.

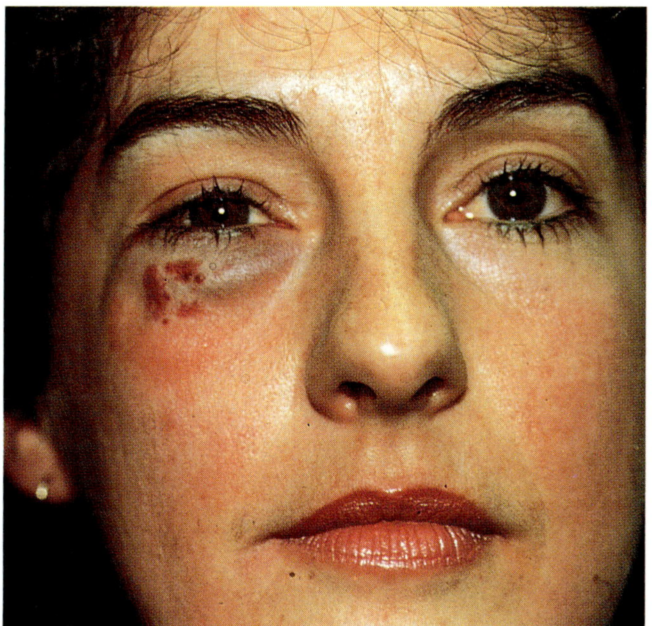

FIGURE 12–25. A patient with a nodular port wine stain of the right lower eyelid prior to treatment.

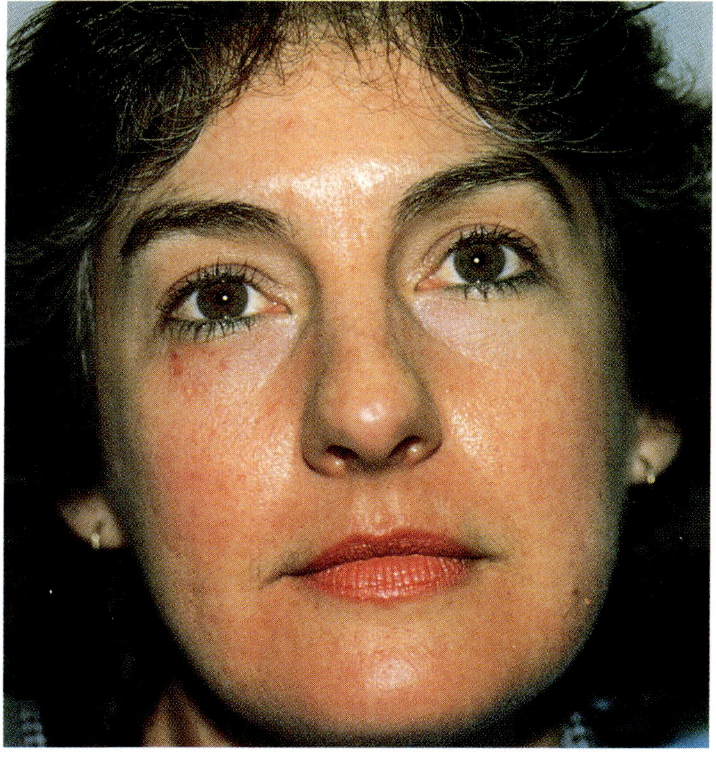

FIGURE 12–26. The patient in Figure 12–25 after treatment. There are a small number of residual vessels. These can be removed at a subsequent treatment if desired.

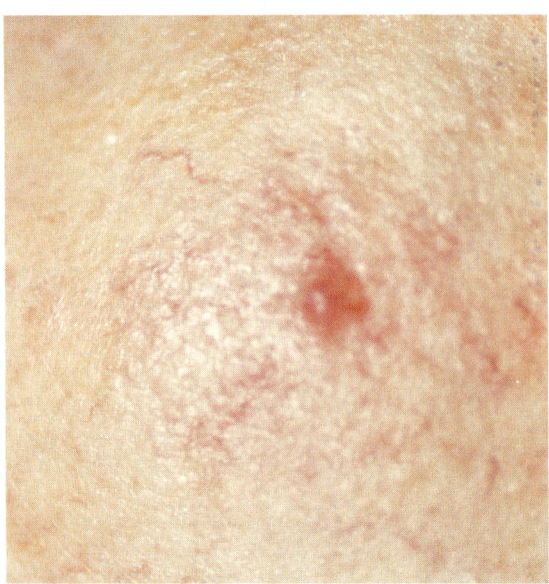

FIGURE 12–27. A spider nevus of the left cheek with a large central vessel.

Because the vast majority of these vessels are within 1 to 2 mm from the surface of the skin, they are amenable to laser photocoagulation. The mechanism of action of laser photocoagulation in these instances is similar to that described above. Intravascular heat generated from the absorption of yellow light by oxyhemoglobin results in intravascular coagulation of the blood vessels. Thermal transmission invariably radiates outward and may damage the overlying epidermis. If the spot size used is small, the amount of epidermal damage is minimal, and scarring is therefore highly unlikely.[38] In the vast majority of cases, the author has used a 150 micron spot size and a power setting of between 200 and 400 mW. Fine vessels can be adequately treated with a 100 micron spot size at power settings between 180 and 260 mW.[38,39] Occasionally, large ectatic vessels may require a 200 micron spot size and power settings of up to 600 mW.[38,39] The appropriate end point one should aim for is a complete blanching of the vessel. Ideally, the overlying skin should not blanch; however, this is not always possible to avoid. A small amount of epidermal blanching is acceptable.

Using 6 × magnification, the vessel is traced from the thinnest point, or distal end, to the origin. Second and third generation branches should be coagulated first, followed by the trunk of the vessel. The power setting should be adjusted to achieve complete blanching of the vessel with a single pass. Subsequent passes are more difficult because coagulation of melanin has taken place with the first pass, and a small amount of edema is present, thus preventing adequate treatment of the vessel. Patients with extensive networks of telangiectasia should be treated over two or three sessions. Because treatment of these patients frequently requires considerable power, which may result in blanching of the overlying skin, one should avoid large confluent areas of blanching. Every second or third vessel is therefore treated, with the remaining areas coagulated at a subsequent treatment session. Although this method may seem tedious, one is able to treat a patient with extensive telangiectasia in 2 or 3 half-hour sessions (Figs. 12–28 to 12–31).

Immediately after treatment, minimal discomfort is experienced. Occasional blistering may result; however, this is not common. If an extensive area has been treated, swelling commences about 24 hours postoperatively. This lasts 3 to 4 days and gradually subsides. Application of ice packs immediately after treatment often reduces the swelling. Eschar formation is usually found at approximately 4 to 5 days posttreatment. These eschars are usually thin and linear and follow the course of the vessel treated. Between 10 and 14 days after treatment they separate, leaving mildly erythematous skin behind. This erythema subsides during a further 1 to 2 weeks. Occasional areas

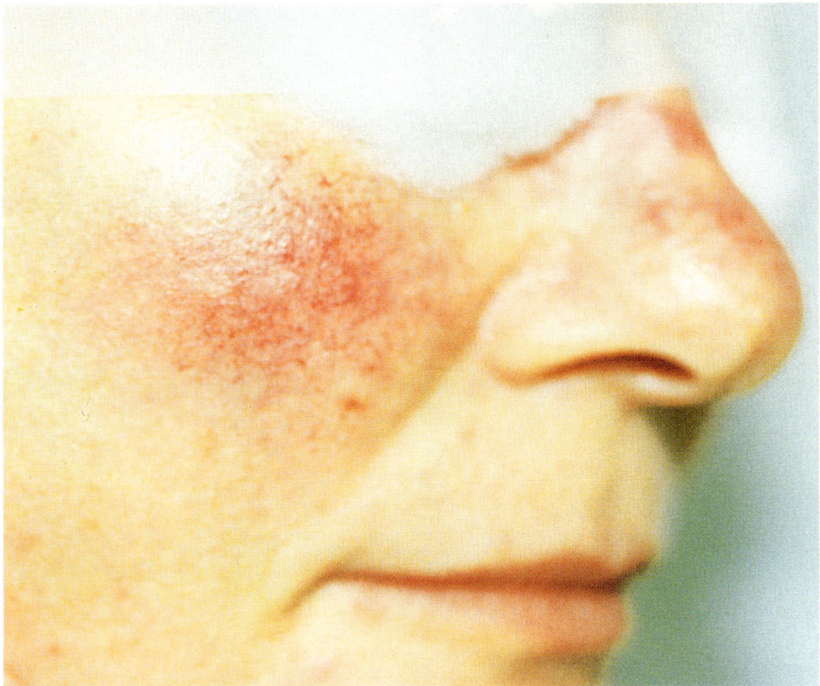

FIGURE 12–28. A patient with extensive telangiectasia involving the right cheek and dorsum of the nose.

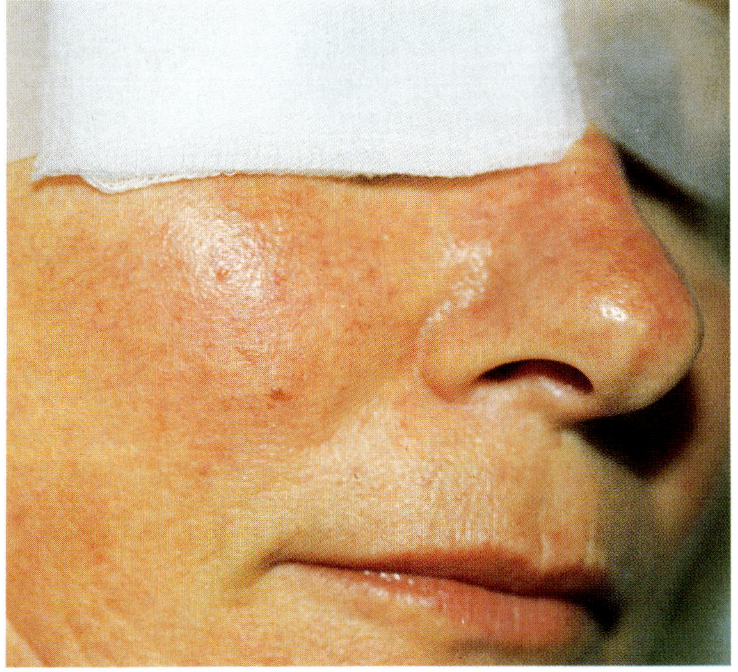

FIGURE 12–29. The patient in Figure 12–28 after treatment.

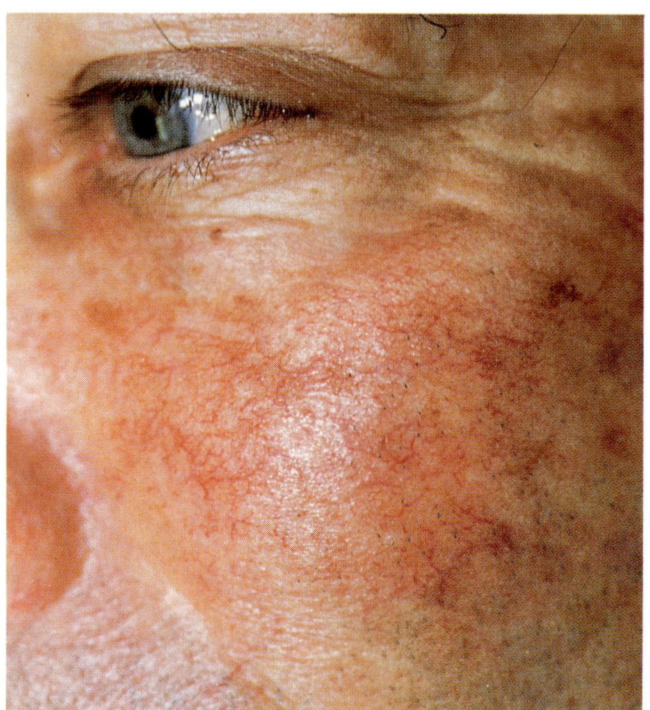

FIGURE 12–30. A patient with marked telangiectasia of the left cheek.

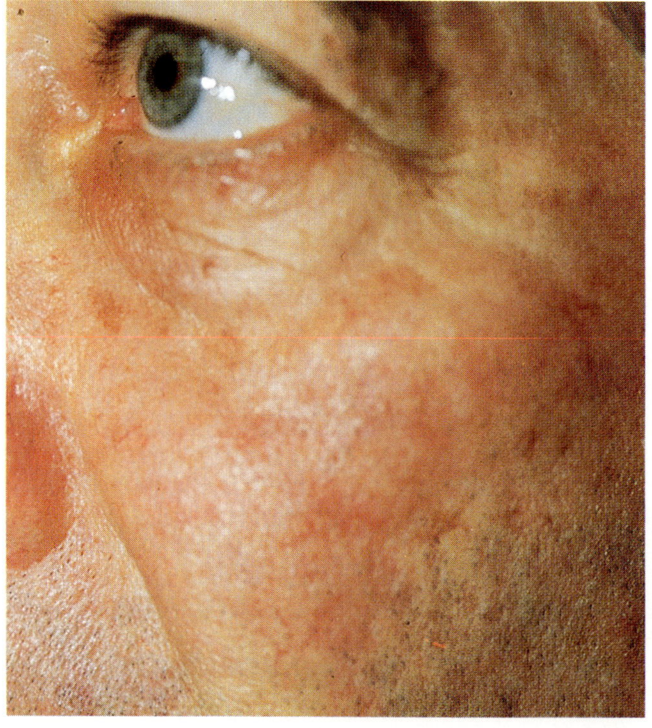

FIGURE 12–31. The patient in Figure 12–30 after treatment.

of pitting are seen, but these are usually mild and fill out adequately within 3 to 6 months. This, however, is not common and is occasionally found when one has used a 200 micron spot size in the alar grooves. A frequent complication is postinflammatory hyperpigmentation. This may occur in up to 4 per cent of patients and is frequently associated with posttreatment sun exposure.[38] It is also more common in olive-skinned patients. Hyperpigmentation is usually noticed within 4 to 8 weeks of a treatment. It responds well to topical 4 per cent hydroquinone cream and always subsides. The author has not seen any cases of permanent hyperpigmentation.

Spider nevi are treated in a slightly different manner. The central AV malformation has in the past frequently recurred following simple blanching; vaporizing the central feeding vessel with a 100 micron spot size and a power setting of 500 mW prevents recurrence. This is accomplished by first carefully marking the central vessel with a fine-pointed surgical marker, coagulating the peripheral vessels in the standard way, and then finally increasing the power to approximately 500 mW and vaporizing the central vessels to a depth of 1 to 2 mm.[39] The central AV malformation is thus destroyed and is replaced by scar tissue. However, using a 100 micron spot size in this manner prevents extensive damage to the epidermis and thus prevents visible scarring[36] (Figs. 12–32, 12–33).

Cherry Hemangiomas (Campbell De Morgan Spots)

These lesions are ectasias of the superficial vascular plexus. They are bright red, dome-shaped papules and are exceedingly common in middle-aged patients[37] (Fig. 12–34). Although they are found more frequently on the trunk, Campbell De Morgan spots may also be seen on the neck and face.

These lesions are treated with a 150 micron spot size at a power setting of approximately 300 to 400 mW. The entire hemangioma is coagulated until a uniform graying of the lesion appears. This heals in the conventional manner, with scab formation and usually complete resolution.

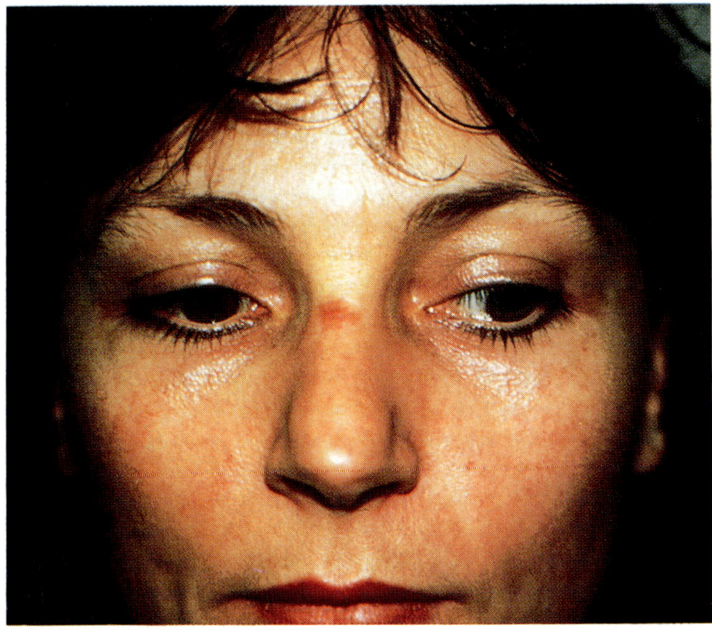

FIGURE 12–32. A spider nevus on the bridge of the nose.

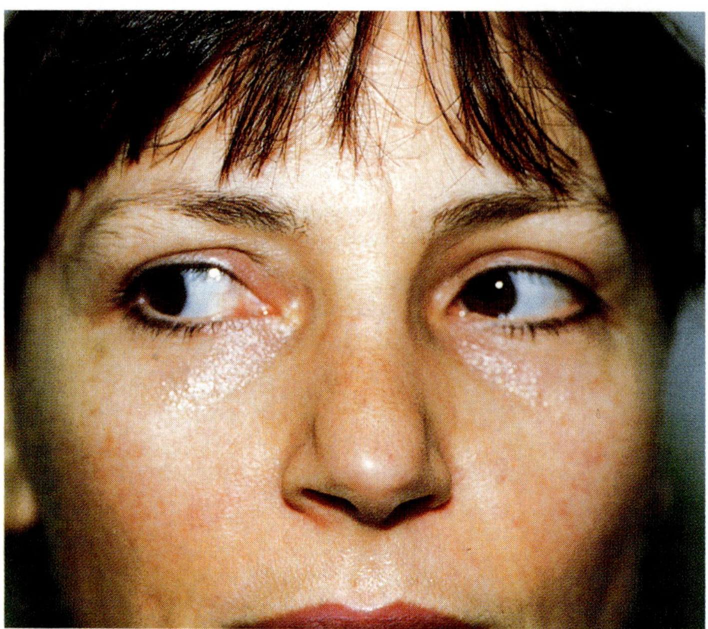

FIGURE 12–33. The patient in Figure 12–32 after treatment.

Venous Lakes

Venous lakes are ectasias of the superficial venous plexus and are commonly found in elderly patients.[37] They usually affect the upper lip, are frequently multiple, and measure between 1 and 6 mm in diameter. Venous lakes are believed to result from trauma and excessive sunlight exposure.[40] These lesions may be bothersome in that they bleed with relatively mild trauma.

Because these lesions represent extensive ectasia of the venous plexus, it is necessary to compress the lake using a glass slide. A 200 micron spot size, at a power setting of about 500 mW, is then used to uniformly blanch the lesion. By compressing the vascular walls, sufficient thermal

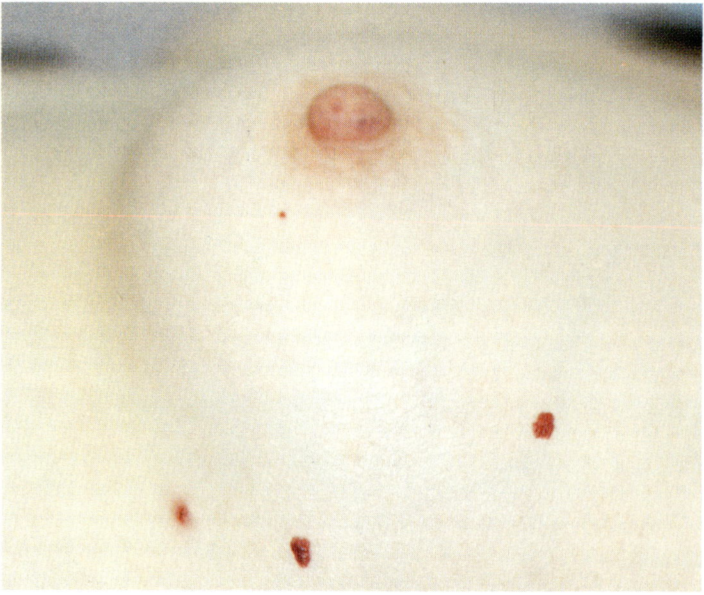

FIGURE 12–34. Cherry hemangiomas on the chest of a patient.

energy can be generated within the lesion to completely coagulate it. If the lake is treated without compression, the amount of energy generated may be insufficient to completely eradicate it with one treatment. These lesions heal in much the same way as Campbell De Morgan spots, and an excellent result can be expected.

Pyogenic Granuloma

Pyogenic granulomas classically arise fairly rapidly after minor localized trauma or during pregnancy. They are considered to be a form of benign reactive vascular hyperplasia and represent a proliferation of granulation tissue.[37]

Smaller lesions respond to laser photocoagulation using a 200 micron spot size and 500 to 600 mW of power. The lesion is blanched and heals as mentioned above. Larger lesions may need to be partially vaporized, and the remaining 2 mm of tissue above the skin surface can then be blanched.

PIGMENTED MALFORMATION

Biophysics

The epidermal melanocyte, of neuroectodermal origin, migrates during fetal life to its normal position in the basal layer of the epidermis. Each melanocyte has several cytoplasmic dendritic processes, which communicate with adjacent keratinocytes. The exact ratio of epidermal melanocytes to surrounding basal cells is about 1:10 and varies with body site, past history of sun exposure, and possibly the age of the patient.[41,42] Consequently, this ratio is higher on sun exposed areas, such as the face, the arms, and the dorsal surfaces of the hands. Histologically, melanocytes appear as relatively clear cells on hematoxylin and eosin staining, but can be well visualized with special staining. Epidermal melanocytes synthesize the pigment melanin and distribute it via the dendritic processes to surrounding keratinocytes. The combination of one melanocyte and its dependent keratinocytes constitutes an epidermal melanin unit.[43] Interestingly enough, the number of melanocytes is similar in matching sites in Caucasian and Negroid skins, but the melanin is synthesized more rapidly in colored-skinned individuals, and the size of the melanin granules is larger.[44]

From the absorption spectrum shown in Figure 12–1 one can see that the absorbance of melanin decreases with increasing wavelength. To prevent permanent scarring, the melanin targeted for destruction should be in the epidermis and in the papillary dermis. Light at 500 nm is attenuated by 50 per cent at a depth of 0.16 mm.[19] Because the epidermis is 0.065 mm thick, it would appear that 500 nm would be the optimal wavelength to selectively coagulate melanin, as a target chromophore, without causing extensive damage.

Three lasers are capable of producing light at about 500 nm. These include

- *Argon lasers:* Argon lasers produce light at 490 and 514 nm. This blue-green light is optimal for the treatment of pigmented malformation.

- *Argon ion pumped dye lasers:* By deactivating the dye laser, one is able to use the argon laser in the same way as a conventional argon laser. Furthermore, a flashlamp pumped dye laser may be tuned at 500 nm. Because vascular malformations are selectively coagulated at 578 nm, a separate dye would have to be used.

- *Copper vapor lasers:* Because copper vapor lasers emit light at 511 and 578 nm, they are ideal for the treatment of both pigmented and vascular malformations. By simply switching filters, one is able to change from yellow light for vascular malformations (578 nm) to green light for pigmented malformations (511 nm). Furthermore, the pulsed nature of copper vapor laser light probably results in a more efficient photocoagulation of melanin.

■ Although the author has had experience with all three lasers for the treatment of pigmented malformations, the most recent experience was with copper vapor lasers, which were found to be the most convenient.[35]

■ When treating pigmented malformations, the maxim used should be that any lesion requiring biopsy should not be treated with a laser. This would therefore exclude many lesions. The common ephelis (freckle) or a lentigo is, on the other hand, amenable to treatment.

Clinical Considerations

Ephelis

With ultraviolet stimulation, some melanocytes produce larger amounts of melanin than others. This increased production results in a clinically visible freckle. Freckles vary greatly in size and occur histologically as an irregular increase in melanin granules within the basal layer of the epithelial cells.[43]

The first step in treating these lesions is to mark carefully the outline of the freckle with a fine-tipped surgical marker. Approximately 1 mm of normal skin should be left between the surgical markings and the perimeter of the lesion. This helps in identifying the lesion and ensures that the lesion is coagulated in its entirety because, when using the conventional orange filter (for 511 nm light), lighter pigmented lesions are less easily seen than are darker ones. Using a 100 micron spot size, 511 nm light, and a power setting of 160 to 240 mW, the entire lesion is coagulated. The end point is determined by how intensely pigmented the lesion was initially. With darker freckles a more intense darkening of the lesion is seen (Figs. 12–35 to 12–37). Lighter freckles, on the other hand, should be coagulated until the appearance of tiny bubbles under the surface of the skin is noted. These bubbles are from melanin that has been vaporized. A faint crackling sound is sometimes heard during treatment. This is from bursting keratinocytes.

Although only pigmented keratinocytes are targeted, melanocytes in the area are also destroyed. This should prevent repigmentation (Figs. 12–38, 12–39). If melanocytes are present in hair follicles or sweat glands, however, partial repigmentation may result.

Within 3 to 4 days of treatment, a thin eschar appears over the surface of the lesion that is being treated. This eschar separates over 7 to 12 days, leaving slightly scaly erythematous skin behind. The scaliness soon settles, as does the erythema. The erythema may persist for several

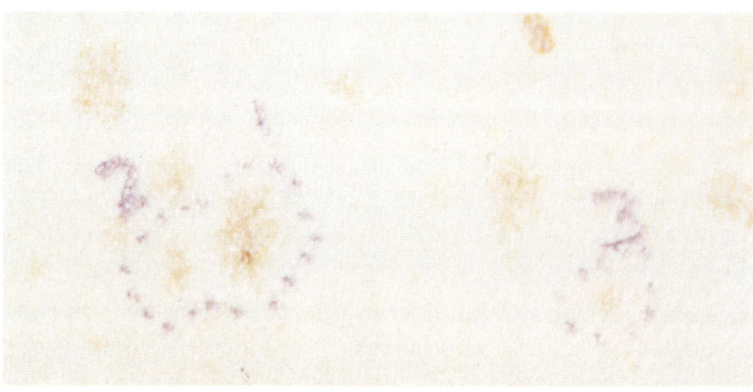

FIGURE 12–35. Freckles on the chest of a patient prior to treatment. Note that the freckles have been outlined clearly with a fine-pointed surgical marker.

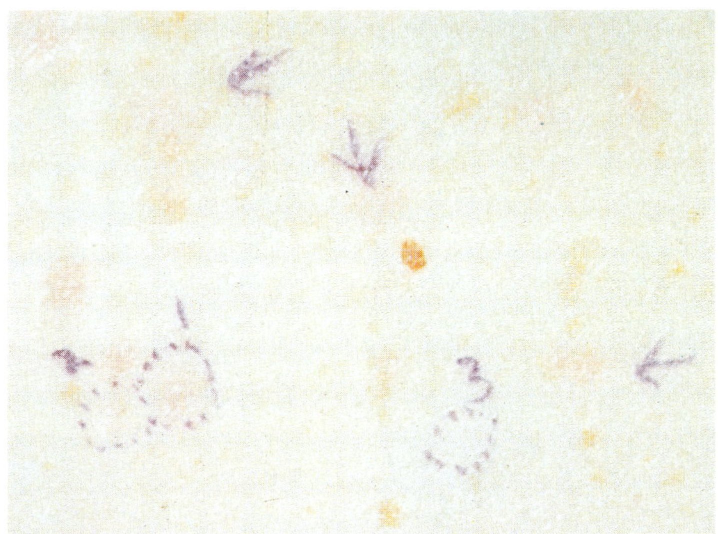

FIGURE 12–36. The lesions shown in Figure 12–35 immediately after treatment. Note the slight darkening of the freckles. This is especially well seen in lesion 1.

weeks after treatment. Postinflammatory hyperpigmentation is sometimes seen. This can be treated conservatively or with 4 per cent hydroquinone in a sorbiline base, applied twice daily. In both instances, the pigmentation resolves within 8 weeks. After extensive experience with this technique, no complications have been seen.[38] However, the potential of producing hypopigmentation must always be kept in mind. This is especially so when treating lesions on the neck.

Lentigo

Lentigines result from the replacement of normal basal cells by melanocytes. This, in turn, results in a greatly increased amount of pigment in the overlying keratinocytes.[43] Lentigines are commoner in older individuals and are etiologically related to excessive ultraviolet light exposure. There is no migration of melanocytes upward through the epidermis or downward into the papillary dermis.[43] These lesions are therefore completely benign and are easily treated (Figs. 12–40, 12–41). The principles and outcome of the treatment of lentigines are the same as those for freckles.

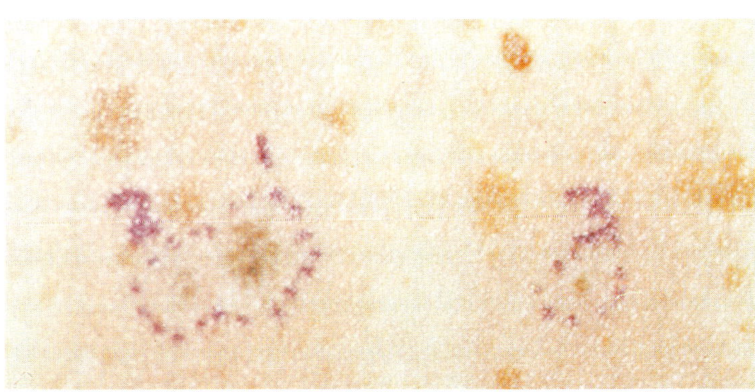

FIGURE 12–37. The lesions in Figures 12–35 and 12–36 approximately 3 weeks after treatment. Some erythema is still present. This will disappear within a few weeks. The additional arrows point to several other lesions that had been treated about 2 weeks previously.

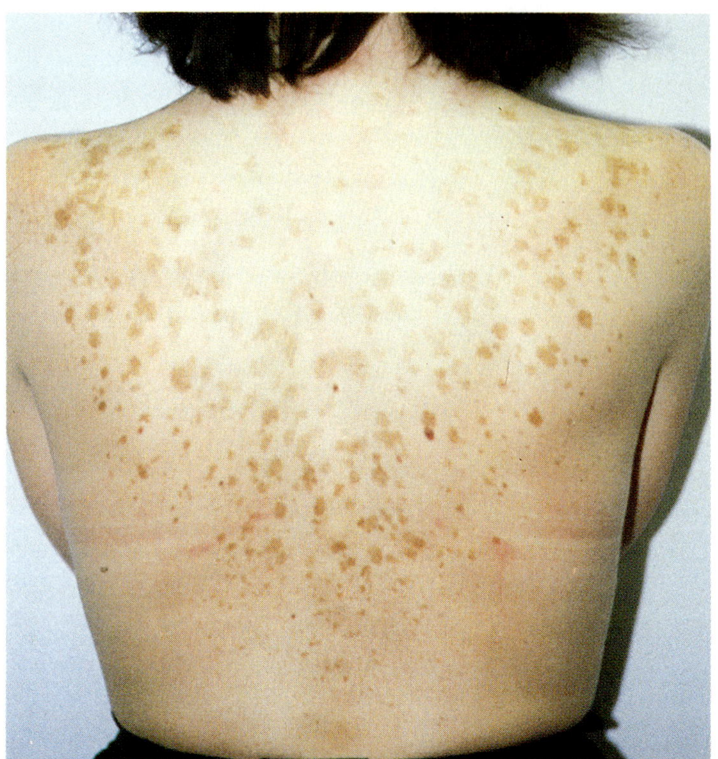

FIGURE 12–38. Freckles on the back of a patient.

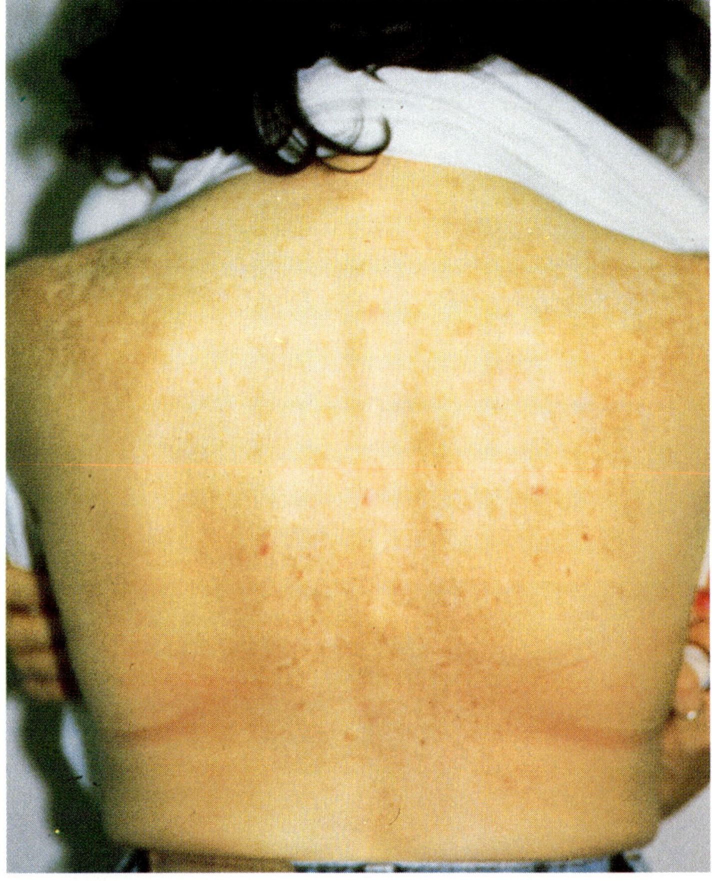

FIGURE 12–39. The patient in Figure 12–38 6 months after treatment.

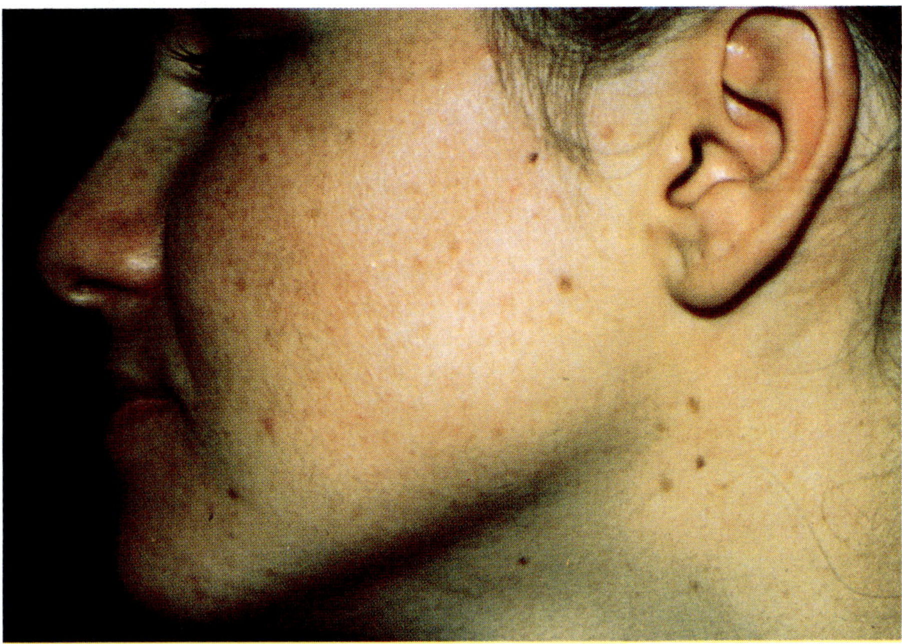

FIGURE 12–40. Lentigines on the face and neck of a patient.

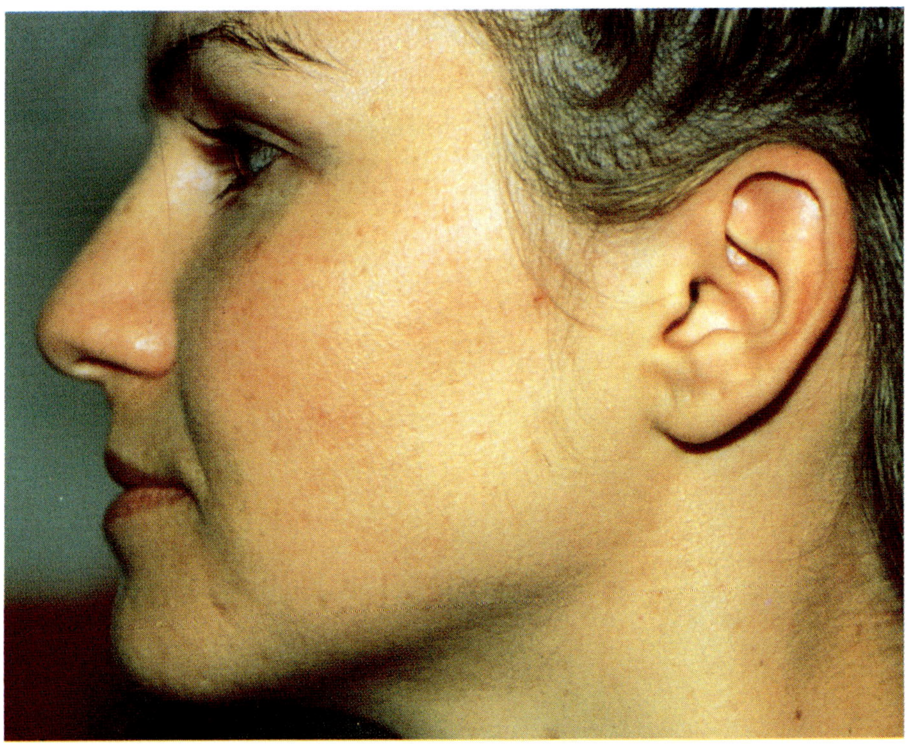

FIGURE 12–41. The patient in Figure 12–40 after treatment.

CARBON DIOXIDE LASER IN FACIAL COSMETIC SURGERY

Biophysics

Unlike the argon and yellow light lasers, which were designed to provide selective ablation of specific chromophores within tissue, the CO_2 laser functions as a nonspecific vaporizer of tissue. This laser's invisible beam is emitted in the far infrared spectrum of light at 10,600 nm and shows no selective color absorption. The major chromophore in this region is water.

Several qualities make the CO_2 laser useful for selective applications in facial and cosmetic surgery. The CO_2 laser can be used in a sharply focused, excision mode to incise tissue or it can be used in a defocused, vaporization mode to remove tissue in thin layers. The handpiece or lens system does not need to be changed to allow the operator to go from a focused beam to a defocused beam. All that is required is for the operator to move the handpiece farther from the operating surface to defocus the beam. In contrast to the case with electrosurgical instruments, there is minimal damage to adjacent tissues through conduction of heat.[45] Many operations can be performed in a hemostatic environment because blood vessels of up to 0.5 mm in diameter are sealed by the CO_2 laser as tissue is vaporized.[46]

Clinical Considerations

Benign Lesions

The CO_2 laser is most useful when nonspecific ablation or sculpting of a variety of benign cutaneous processes is desired. A number of common and unusual conditions can be treated in this manner (Table 12–4). Results vary only slightly with the type of disease process being treated but vary greatly with regard to the anatomic location of the various lesions. Results of CO_2 laser ablation are most pleasing when lesions are located in anatomic areas where second intention healing produces good results (Figs. 12–42 to 12–44). Anatomic areas that generally yield excellent results include the lip (actinic cheilitis),[47] the concha of the ear (trichoepitheliomas),[48] the alar groove (adenoma sebaceum),[49] and the periorbital area (xanthelasma, syringomas).[50] Some inves-

Table 12–4. COSMETIC AND FACIAL CONDITIONS TREATED BY CO_2 LASER

Tattoos[63]
Verruca vulgaris (warts)[64]
Granuloma faciale[65]
Xanthelasma[70]
Tuberous sclerosis[49]
Lymphangioma circumscriptum
Benign familial pemphigus[68]
Rhinophyma[60–62]
Epidermal nevi
Lentigines
Glomus tumor[69]
Eruptive vellus hair cyst[70]
Trichoepithelioma[48]
Keloid[72]
Syringoma[73]
Acne keloidalis[73]
Neurofibroma[74]

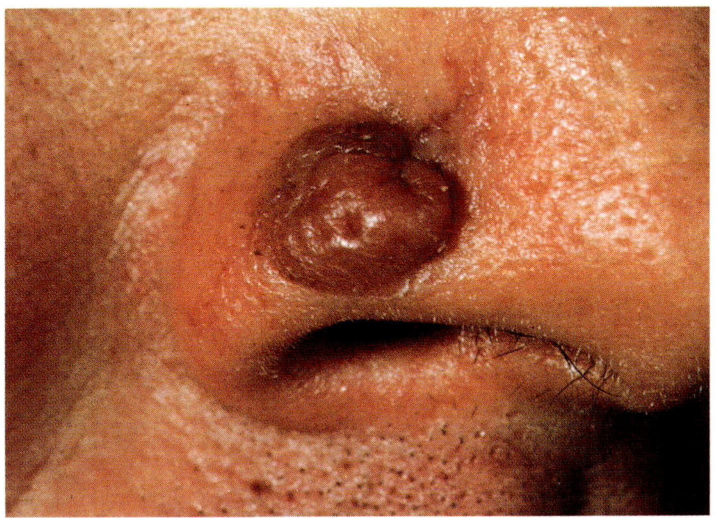

Figure 12–42. Nodular lesion of granuloma faciale. This is an uncommon benign cutaneous condition of unknown cause, which is often unresponsive to nonsurgical treatment. Histologic examination shows a dermal infiltrate of neutrophils and eosinophils separated from the epidermis by grenz.

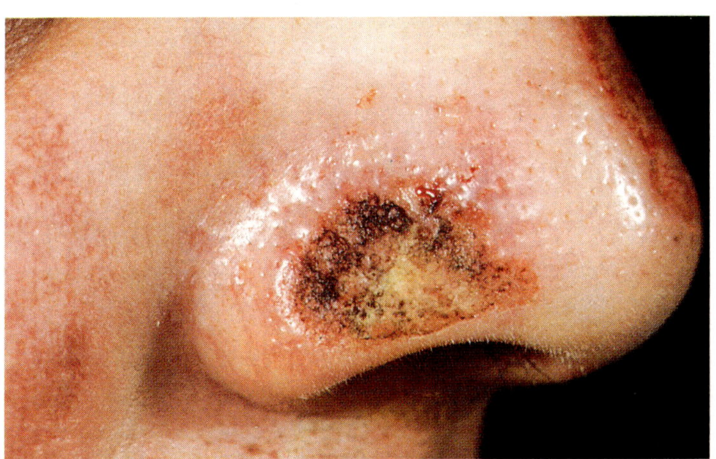

Figure 12–43. Lesion in Figure 12–42 shortly after treatment by CO_2 laser vaporization. Note that the lesion is located in an anatomic area (the nasal ala) where second intention healing historically has given good results.

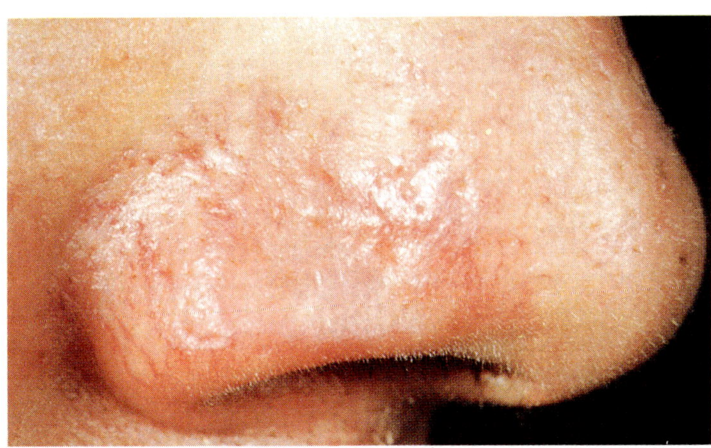

Figure 12–44. Improved cosmetic appearance 6 weeks after treatment of lesion in Figures 12–42 and 12–43 with CO_2 laser. Results are similar to those achieved with CO_2 laser treatment of other benign nodular lesions found in this anatomic area, such as adenoma sebaceum, trichoepitheliomas, and rhinophyma.

tigators have suggested that port wine stains and other vascular lesions can be successfully treated with this laser.[51] Theoretically, the nonselective qualities of the CO_2 laser increase the chance of textural changes and scarring when compared with the yellow light lasers.[52,53] In the author's clinical experience yellow light lasers are therapeutically superior to the CO_2 laser for treatment of vascular lesions.

Malignant Lesions

Despite predictions that CO_2 laser modification of Mohs micrographic surgery would be widely adapted,[54] the scalpel and scissors are still the mainstay of almost all who practice this highly specialized type of skin cancer removal. The CO_2 laser can be used as an important adjunctive tool to conventional Mohs surgery when removal of bone is necessary. Used in the focused excision mode, this laser is powerful enough to cut through bone and can be of assistance in removing specimens for histologic examination. Other useful applications of the CO_2 laser for malignant lesions include the removal of superficial skin cancers in the small number of patients in whom electrosurgery is contraindicated because of the presence of a pacemaker.[55] The CO_2 laser has also found application in precipitating granulation tissue formation over areas of exposed bone. Despite selected use in these instances, the majority of cutaneous malignancies are best treated by conventional methods, such as surgical excision, cryotherapy, or electrodesiccation and curettage.

Other Cosmetic Applications

Several cosmetic procedures performed with the CO_2 laser deserve special comment. Blepharoplasty performed with a scalpel by an experienced operator yields excellent results in most cases. Less bleeding and less postoperative ecchymosis are reported advantages of CO_2 laser blepharoplasty.[56,57] An innovative use of the CO_2 laser to revise full thickness skin grafts has been described.[58] The CO_2 laser has also been effective in more evenly aligning and blending some healed grafts with the surrounding skin.[59]

Both CO_2 laser surgery and electrosurgery are effective methods for surgical treatment of rhinophyma,[60–62] a type of benign sebaceous gland hyperplasia, which results in an enlargement and disfiguration of the nose. Electrosurgery is faster and less expensive, but CO_2 laser has less risk of scarring because it provides for pinpoint accuracy without additional damage from transfer of heat. In the treatment of this condition by either method it is important not to remove so much tissue that sebaceous material or pores cannot be seen. Removal of tissue by either method to a level of deep dermis or cartilage often results in unacceptable scarring and distortion of the nose.

Clinical Technique

Although a number of conditions can be treated successfully with the CO_2 laser, the treatment of actinic cheilitis best illustrates the technique. This premalignant condition occurs clinically as a scaly crusted appearance of the lower lip. Actinic cheilitis is caused by chronic unprotected exposure to the sun and is most prominent on the lower lips of affected individuals. A shave biopsy specimen shows changes similar to those of an actinic keratosis. In the past, total lip shaves, cryotherapy, and vermilionectomy were suggested treatments. The highly favorable results seen in treating this condition with the CO_2 laser have made it the author's method of choice. Patients are warned before the procedure that eating rough or spicy foods immediately after surgery may be unpleasant. Prior to scheduling the procedure, shave biopsy of the thickest or most hyperkeratotic part of the lesion is taken to exclude squamous cell carcinoma. Areas of clinical involvement of the lip are marked with a fine-pointed surgical marker, and the vermilion border of the lip is also outlined. Although a test patch treatment is not routinely performed in actinic cheilitis, it is suggested when treating lesions located in anatomic areas where uniformly successful results are not as common or when multiple lesions are to be treated. A moist gauze sponge is placed between the lip and the patient's teeth to prevent inadvertent laser injury to adjacent tissue. Moist towels are also draped around the patient's neck. Carbon dioxide laser vaporization of the involved area is performed after first obtaining local anesthesia with 1 per cent lidocaine with 1:2000,000 epinephrine. The author most commonly uses local infiltration of anesthetic in the form of a field block, but nerve blocks can also be used. The laser is used in a defocused mode with irradiances of 12,700 to 19,100 watts/cm^2. The 0.2 mm spot size is preferred. One pass over the lower lip using a continuous setting is generally sufficient to remove the epidermis. The resulting black, charred tissue is removed with a cotton swab that has been dipped in 3 per cent hydrogen peroxide. A second pass, or touch-ups to specific areas, ensures complete extirpation of all atypical epithelium. An end point of complete removal of the epidermis with little destruction of the dermis is desired. Care is taken not to cross the vermilion border of the lip; however, vaporization can approach this important cosmetic boundary. Wounds are dressed with antibiotic ointment alone, and patients are instructed to apply the ointment as many times as needed per day to keep the area moist. Postoperative wound care includes twice daily cleaning with 3 per cent hydrogen peroxide. Scabbing and crusting of the wound is discouraged, as it slows healing and generally makes the patient more uncomfortable. Patients are seen in 1 week to ensure that proper care and healing are taking place. Complete healing takes 4 to 6 weeks. Sensory changes may persist for several months, but are not a problem in most patients. This method of treatment is superior to other conventional therapies.

References

 1. Goldman L, Rockwell RJ Jr: Lasers in Medicine. New York, Gordan and Breach, 1971.
 2. Zavet MM, Ripps H, Siegel IM: Breinin laser photocoagulation of the eye. Arch Ophthalmol 69:97, 1963.
 3. L'Esperance F: Argon laser photocoagulation system. Design construction and laboratory investigations. Trans Am Ophthalmol Soc 66:827, 1968.
 4. Goldman L, Dreffer R, Rockwell JR Jr: Treatment of port wine stains by an argon laser. J Dermatol Surg 2:385, 1976.
 5. Apfelberg DB, Maser MR, Lash H: Argon laser management of cutaneous vascular deformities. A preliminary report. West J Med 124:99, 1976.
 6. Apfelberg DB, Morton R, Maser MD, et al.: The argon laser for cutaneous lesions. JAMA 245:2073, 1981.
 7. Carruth JAS, Shakespeare P: Toward the ideal treatment for the port wine stain with the argon laser. Better prediction and an ''optimal'' technique. Lasers Surg Med 6:2, 1986.
 8. Dixon JA, Gilbertson JJ: Argon and neodymium YAG laser therapy of dark nodular port wine stains in older patients. Lasers Surg Med 6:5, 1986.
 9. Arndt K: Argon laser therapy of small cutaneous vascular lesions. Arch Dermatol 118:220, 1982.
10. Cosman B: Experience in the argon laser therapy of port wine stains. Plast Reconstr Surg 65:119, 1980.
11. Summerman H, Doldman L, Henderson B: Histopathology of the laser treatment of port wine lesions. J Invest Dermatol 50:141, 1968.
12. Apfelberg DB: Histology of port wine stains following argon laser treatment. Br J Plast Surg 32:232, 1979.
13. Greenwald J, Rosen S, Anderson RR, et al.: Comparative histological studies of the tunable dye (at 577 nm) laser and argon laser: Specific vascular effects of the dye laser. J Invest Dermatol 77:305, 1981.
14. Anderson RR, Parrish JA: Microvasculature can be selectively damaged using dye lasers: A basic theory and experimental evidence in human skin. Laser Surg Med 1:263, 1981.
15. Anderson RR, Parrish JA: Selective photothermolysis: Precise microsurgery by selective absorption of pulsed radiation. Science 220:524, 1983.
16. Morelli JG, Tan OT, Garden J, et al.: Tunable dye laser (577 nm) treatment of port wine stains. Lasers Surg Med 6:91, 1986.
17. Tan OT, Carney JM, Margolis R, et al.: Histologic responses of port wine stains treated by argon, carbon dioxide, and tunable dye lasers. Arch Dermatol 122:1016, 1986.
18. Cotterill JA: Preliminary results following treatment of vascular lesions of the skin using a continuous wave tunable dye laser which emits at 577 nm. Clin Exp Dermatol 11:628, 1986.
19. Parrish JA, Anderson RR: Considerations of selectivity in laser therapy. In Arndt KA, Noe JM, Rosen S (eds). Cutaneous Laser Therapy: Principles and Methods. New York, John Wiley & Sons, 1983.
20. Rosen S: Nature and evolution of port wine stains. In Arndt KA, Noe JM, Rosen S (eds): Cutaneous Laser Therapy: Principles and Methods. New York, John Wiley & Sons, 1983.

21. Keller GS, Doiron DR, Keller RS: The treatment of vascular lesions with a CW yellow dye laser—initial trials. Otolaryngol Head Neck Surg 95:527, 1986.
22. Tan OT, Kerschmann R, Parrish JA: The effect of epidermal pigmentation on selective vascular effects of pulsed laser. Lasers Surg Med 4:365, 1984.
23. Garden JM, Tan OT, Kerschmann R, et al.: Effect of dye laser pulse duration on selective cutaneous vascular injury. J Invest Dermatol 87:653, 1986.
24. Caro WH: Tumors of the skin. *In* Moschella S, Pillsbury D, Hurley H: Dermatology. Philadelphia, WB Sanders Co, 1975.
25. Bowers RE, Graham E, Tomlinson K: The natural history of the strawberry nevus. Arch Dermatol 82:59, 1960.
26. Van Gemert M, Welch AJ: Is there an optimal laser treatment for port wine stains? Laser Surg Med 6:76, 1985.
27. Hobby LW: Treatment of port wine stains and other cutaneous lesions. Contemp Surg 18:22, 1981.
28. Jacobs HA, Walton RG: The incidence of birth marks in the neonate. Pediatrics 58:218, 1976.
29. Dixon JA: Argon laser treatment of port wine stains. *In* Arndt KA, Noe JM, Rosen S (eds): Cutaneous Laser Therapy: Principles and Methods. New York, John Wiley & Sons, 1983.
30. Scheibner A, McCarthy WH: Argon laser treatment of superficial blood vessel malformations on the trunk and extremities in adults and on the face in children (abstract). Lasers Surg Med 6:244, 1986.
31. Hobby LW: Argon laser treatment of superficial vascular lesions in children. Lasers Surg Med 6:16, 1986.
32. Brauner GJ, Schliftman A: Laser surgery for children. J Dermatol Surg Oncol 13:178, 1987.
33. Redisch W, Pelzer RH: Localized vascular dilatations of the human skin: Capillary microscopy and related studies. Am Heart J 37:106, 1949.
34. Noe JM, Finley J, Rosen S, Arndt KA: Postrhinoplasty "red nose": Differential diagnosis and treatment by laser. Plast Reconstr Surg 67:661, 1981.
35. Merlen JF: Red telangiectasias, blue telangiectasias. Soc Franc Phlebol 22:167, 1970.
36. Goldman MP, Bennett RG: Treatment of telangiectasia: A review. J Am Acad Dermatol 17:167, 1987.
37. Gilchrest BA, Rosen S: Predicting the utility of argon laser therapy for vascular lesions of the skin. *In* Arndt KA, Noe JM, Rosen S (eds): Cutaneous Laser Therapy: Principles and Methods. New York, John Wiley & Sons, 1983.
38. Waner M, Woods C: The treatment of facial capillary telangiectasia with pulsed yellow light. Lasers Surg Med 8:189, 1988.
39. Murdoch L, Waner M, Griffin E: The treatment of vascular and pigmented malformations with a copper vapor laser (abstract). Lasers Med Sci 462, 1988.
40. Wheeland RG: Lasers in Skin Disease. New York, Thieme Medical Publishers, 1988.
41. Szabo G: The number of melanocytes in human epidermis. Br Med J 1:1016, 1954.
42. Gilchrest BA, Blog FB, Szabo G: Effects of aging and chronic sun exposure on melanocytes in human skin. J Invest Dermatol 73:141, 1979.
43. Mackie RN: Disorder of the cutaneous melanocyte. *In* Milne: Dermatopathology. Edward Arnold, 1984.
44. Toda K, Pathak MA, Parrish JA, Fitzpatrick TV: Alteration of racial differences in melanosome distribution in human epidermis after exposure to ultraviolet light. Nature 236:143, 1972.
45. Ben-Bassat M, Kaplan I: A study of the ultrastructural features of the cut margin of skin and mucous membrane specimens excised by carbon dioxide laser. J Surg Res 21:77, 1976.
46. Slutzki S, Shafir R, Bornstein LA: Use of the carbon dioxide laser for large excisions with minimal blood loss. Plast Reconstr Surg 60:250, 1977.
47. David L: Laser vermilion ablation for actinic cheilitis. J Dermatol Surg Oncol 11:1004, 1985.
48. Sawchuk WS, Heald PW: CO_2 laser treatment of trichoepithelioma with focused and defocused beam. J Dermatol Surg Oncol 10:905, 1984.
49. Wheeland RG, Bailin PL, Kantor GR, et al.: Treatment of adenoma sebaceum with carbon dioxide laser vaporization. J Dermatol Surg Oncol 11:861, 1985.
50. Apfelberg DB, Maser MR, Lash H, White DN: Treatment of xanthelasma palpebarum with the carbon dioxide laser. J Dermatol Surg Oncol 13:149, 1987.
51. Ratz JL, Bailin PL: The case for use of the carbon dioxide laser in the treatment of port wine stains. Arch Dermatol 123:74, 1987.
52. Tan OT, Carney JM, Margolis R, et al.: Histologic responses of port wine stains treated by argon, carbon dioxide and tunable dye laser. Arch Dermatol 122:1016, 1986.
53. Van Gemert MJC, Welch AJ, Tan OT, Parrish JA: Limitations of carbon dioxide lasers for treatment of port wine stains. Arch Dermatol 123:71, 1987.
54. Bailin PL, Ratz JL, Lutz-Nagey L: CO_2 laser modification of Mohs' surgery. J Dermatol Surg Oncol 7:621, 1981.
55. Wheeland RG, Bailin PL, Ratz JL, Roenigk RK: Carbon dioxide laser vaporization and curettage in the treatment of large multiple superficial basal cell carcinomas. J Dermatol Surg Oncol 13:119, 1987.
56. David LM, Sander G: CO_2 laser blepharoplasty: A comparison to cold steel and electrocautery. J Dermatol Surg Oncol 13:110, 1987.
57. David LM: The laser approach to blepharoplasty. J Dermatol Surg Oncol 14:741, 1988.
58. Wheeland RG: Revision of full-thickness skin grafts using the carbon dioxide laser. J Dermatol Surg Oncol 14:130, 1988.
59. Wheeland RG, Bailin PL: Scalp reduction surgery with the carbon dioxide laser. J Dermatol Surg Oncol 10:565, 1984.
60. Roenigk RK: CO_2 laser vaporization for treatment of rhinophyma. Mayo Clin Proc 62:676, 1987.
61. Greenbaum SS, Krull EA, Watnick K: Comparison of CO_2 laser and electrosurgery in the treatment of rhinophyma. J Am Acad Dermatol 18:363, 1988.
62. Wheeland RG, Bailin PL, Ratz JL: Combined carbon dioxide laser excision and vaporization in the treatment of rhinophyma. J Dermatol Surg Oncol 13:172, 1987.

63. Levine H, Bailin PL: Carbon dioxide laser treatment of cutaneous hemangiomas and tattoos. Arch Otolaryngol Head Neck Surg 108:236, 1982.
64. McBurney E, Rosen D: Carbon dioxide laser treatment of verrucae vulgaris. J Dermatol Surg Oncol 10:45, 1984.
65. Wheeland RG, Ashley JR, Smith DA, et al.: Carbon dioxide laser treatment of granuloma faciale. J Dermatol Surg Oncol 10:730, 1984.
66. Bailin PL, Kantor GR, Wheeland RG: Carbon dioxide laser vaporization of lymphangioma circumscriptum. J Am Acad Dermatol 14:257, 1986.
67. Eliezri YD, Sklar JA: Lymphangioma circumscriptum: Review and evaluation of carbon dioxide laser vaporization. J Dermatol Surg Oncol 14:357, 1988.
68. Don PC, Carney PS, Lynch WS, et al.: Carbon dioxide laserabrasion: A new approach to management of familial benign chronic pemphigus (Hailey-Hailey disease). J Dermatol Surg Oncol 13:1187, 1987.
69. Dover JS, Smoller BR, Stern RS, et al.: Low-fluence carbon dioxide laser irradiation of lentigines. Arch Dermatol 124:1219, 1988.
70. Barnes L, Estes SA: Laser treatment of hereditary multiple glomus tumors. J Dermatol Surg Oncol 12:912, 1986.
71. Huerter CJ, Wheeland RG: Multiple eruptive vellus hair cysts treated with carbon dioxide laser vaporization. J Dermatol Surg Oncol 13:260, 1987.
72. Kantor GR, Wheeland RG, Bailin PL, et al.: Treatment of earlobe keloids with carbon dioxide laser excision: A report of 16 cases. J Dermatol Surg Oncol 11:1063, 1985.
73. Kantor GR, Ratz JL, Wheeland RG: Treatment of acne keloidalis nuchae with carbon dioxide laser. J Am Acad Dermatol 14:263, 1986.
74. Roenigk RK, Ratz JL: CO_2 laser treatment of cutaneous neurofibromas. J Dermatol Surg Oncol 13:187, 1987.

CHAPTER 13

OTOLOGIC APPLICATIONS OF LASER SURGERY

James L. Parkin

David R. Nielsen

Proper and judicious application of laser energy to the solution of surgical problems is an exciting challenge to all surgeons, including otolaryngologists. The laser is a new surgical tool with rapidly expanding applications in virtually every area of surgical therapy. The laser can accomplish many functions, but there are also problems unsolved by its use. The laser does not replace sound surgical principles, but does refine them.

The potential advantages of laser surgery of specific interest to the otologic surgeon include selective absorption by different tissues, the ability to transmit laser energy through flexible fiber-optic systems, the minimization of tissue traction and contact, the reduction of vibratory ossicular manipulation, and increased ambulatory surgery with reduced hospitalization and reduced total treatment costs. Disadvantages include high initial cost of laser acquisition, special requirements for electrical circuitry and plumbing in operating rooms, the potential hazards to patients and medical personnel from inadvertent laser exposure, the large size and nonportability of some laser systems, the complex maintenance requirements of laser equipment, the necessity for special training of surgeons and other operating room personnel, and the temptation to justify the cost of the equipment through inappropriate and unnecessary use.

The applications of lasers in otologic and neuro-otologic surgery are increasing. Limitations have also been indentified. The proper understanding and use of laser energy allow the surgeon to coagulate vessels for improved bleeding control, to incise tissue with reduced manipulation of surrounding structures, and to vaporize tissue to enhance visualization and remove pathologic conditions.

Power density and laser wavelength determine the laser effectiveness in accomplishing these functions. Vessel photocoagulation is best accomplished with lasers in the visible light spectrum, such as the argon, neodymiumyttrium-aluminum-garnet (Nd:YAG), and 532 nm potassium-titanyl-phosphate (KTP-532) lasers. Limited photocoagulation of small vessels can be performed with the CO_2 laser if the spot size is large and the power setting is low. Tissue incisions are most effectively performed at high power densities (i.e., small spot size and high power settings). Tissue vaporization is generally performed with larger spot size but mid to high power settings.

Power density is defined as the amount of power per unit area (watts per square centimeter). The power density can be increased by increasing the power output of the laser or by decreasing the spot size. This is an important principle to understand in the applications of lasers in otologic surgery. For example, if a hand-held fiber is used with the argon laser, the laser energy is diverging

192

as it leaves the fiber. This means that the closer the tip of the fiber is held to the tissue being treated, the smaller is the spot size and the higher is the power density (Fig. 13–1).

When the laser energy is being focused through the microscope lens system, the power density can be decreased either by decreasing the energy output from the laser tube or by defocusing the microscope and thereby increasing the spot size. This principle also represents a safety factor when the laser is used through a microscope because the tissue that lies beyond the area being treated is receiving defocused energy of lower power density. Hence, if the footplate of the stapes is being treated, defocused energy of lower power density is being experienced by the structures of the vestibule. The same is true of the hand-held probe because of the divergence of the beam after it leaves the fiber. The farther the probe end is from the tissue, the lower the power density is (Fig. 13–1).

Each of the different lasers has advocates for otologic use. The argon laser has historically been used most frequently in the development of otologic techniques. The CO_2 laser has some advantage in the dissection and vaporization of poorly pigmented tissue, but has the disadvantage of being a poor blood vessel coagulator. The KTP-532 laser has become more popular in otologic use. The authors use this laser and the argon laser most frequently in otologic cases.

During otologic laser surgery, constant suction is necessary for removal of smoke and vaporized tissue fragments. During procedures involving the middle ear, a speculum holder is helpful, especially if the hand-held laser probe is being used in one hand and the suction in the other hand. As with all laser surgery, appropriate eye protection of the patient, the surgeon, and other operating room personnel is important. Whenever the laser is not in actual use, it should be off or in the standby mode to minimize the risk of inadvertent actuation and subsequent damage.

If the laser energy is delivered through the microscope lens system, it is important that the focusing of the laser be calibrated prior to the surgery. It is also necessary for the safety of the surgeon's eyes that the protective shutter mechanism in the microscope is functional. The surgeon should remember that the laser is a heat-generating device that contributes to the deeper tissue damage ("footprint") created by the laser. The footprint is greater at higher power densities and longer pulse durations and is greater with Nd:YAG and argon lasers than with CO_2 lasers.

Myringotomy, cholesteatoma excision, ossicular reconstruction, tympanoplasty, adhesion lysis, granuloma excision, bleeding control, and vascular tumor removal are examples of laser application in tympanomastoid surgery.

It is important to reemphasize that laser use does not eliminate the need for proper exposure of the pathologic process. The sterile preparation of the ear is the same for laser and nonlaser techniques. Local anesthesia, if appropriate, is also used for laser otologic surgery.

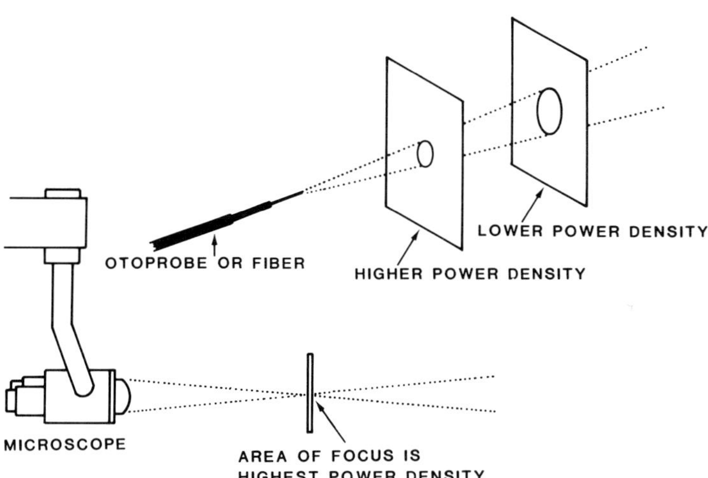

FIGURE 13–1. Power density with a fiber delivery system diminishes as the distance from the fiber tip to the tissue increases. The power density through a microscope system is greatest at the distance of finest focus.

The small fenestra stapedotomy has been shown to have comparable or even better hearing results than total stapedectomy.[1] Manipulation of the ossicular chain increases the risk of cochlear damage and sensorineural hearing loss in stapes surgery. Use of the laser to create the stapedotomy decreases ossicular manipulation. McGee described the successful application of the laser in stapedotomy surgery.[2]

In 1978, Perkins performed a laser stapedotomy, and subsequent cases confirmed the validity of laser stapedotomy as an acceptable technique capable of decreasing ossicular manipulation.[3]

Results of revision stapedectomy are much less satisfactory than results of primary stapedectomy. Adverse effects are reported to occur more commonly when the footplate region requires drillout or reopening.[4,5] The laser allows both of these procedures to be accomplished with less trauma. Significant comparative results are not yet reported.

Preservation of the facial nerve in acoustic neuroma surgery requires atraumatic tumor removal in a well-visualized, blood-free operative field. Lasers have been used in an attempt to accomplish better bleeding control and less traumatic tumor removal.

EXTERNAL AUDITORY CANAL

Membranous stenosis of the external auditory canal can be bloodlessly removed with the argon and KTP-532 lasers. With the argon laser, a 2 watt power setting at a 0.2 second duration in the single pulse mode is used. The thin bony plates can be removed in a similar way; however, complete bony atresia requires standard otologic drilling and curettage.

Secondary granulomas and fibrous stenosis of the reconstructed canal are nicely managed with the laser technique indicated above. Excess heat production can result in restenosis, so it is important to use the pulse mode rather than the continuous mode in performing these procedures.

TYMPANIC MEMBRANE

A laser can certainly be used to create a myringotomy; however, it has the disadvantages of increased cost and increased equipment. It can be useful in a highly vascular tympanic membrane, as a myringotomy can be created and the blood vessels coagulated so the tympanostomy tube is not filled with coagulum immediately after the procedure. In the atelectatic membrane there is also some observed tightening of the membrane with laser treatment.

Vascular tumors of the tympanic membrane, such as hemangiomas, can be effectively photocoagulated with an argon laser at a 1 to 2 watt power setting in a continuous mode or as a 1 watt setting and 0.1 second duration in the single pulse mode. Granulomas of the tympanic membrane can be removed with excellent hemostasis in a similar way.

The laser efficiently removes the circumferential margins of the tympanic membrane perforation. A moistened cotton pledget or absorbable gelatin sponge (Gelfoam) in the middle ear reduces inadvertent damage during the procedure. Tympanosclerotic plaques can also be removed from the tympanic membrane; however, this results in increased size of the perforation or the creation of a new perforation. A low power density can create a ''spot weld'' between the margins of the tympanic perforation and the underlying fascia graft. Care and low power density are important to avoid perforating the graft.

OSSICLES

Laser use in stapedectomy and stapedotomy surgery has the advantages of improved hemostasis with better visualization and decreased ossicular manipulation with lessened risk of cochlear damage. The most impressive advantage of the laser is seen in revision stapes surgery in which adhesions can be lysed, granulations removed, bleeding controlled, prosthesis removal facilitated, and a new stapedotomy created.

In performing laser stapedotomy, a standard tympanomeatal flap is elevated in the conventional way. Sufficient posterior bony canal wall removal is accomplished to visualize the pyramidal eminence with the stapedius tendon, the horizontal facial nerve canal, and the stapes (Fig. 13–2). The chorda tympani is preserved and may be retracted superiorly or inferiorly by freeing its attachments to the incus and malleus. Stapes fixation is confirmed by palpation.

If the argon laser is used, the power is set at 1 to 2 watts with the pulse duration set at 0.1 to 0.2 second. The higher settings are utilized for tissue vaporization of adhesions, tendons, and bones. The lower power settings are more effective for photocoagulating small blood vessels to decrease bleeding. An aberrant stapedial artery can be controlled with laser photocoagulation.

In primary stapedotomy, the stapedius tendon is then vaporized (Fig. 13–3). The posterior crus of the stapes is vaporized below the stapes suprastructure (Fig. 13–4). The char is removed with a fine pick and suction. If the anterior crus can be directly visualized, it is also vaporized with the laser (Fig. 13–5). If the anterior crus cannot be directly visualized, a special metallic mirror can be used to reflect the laser beam onto the anterior crus and accomplish this vaporization. The suprastructure of the stapes can then be removed from the lenticular process of the incus with a joint knife or with the laser.

The center of the stapes footplate is visualized. Blood vessels around the periphery of the footplate can be photocoagulated at this time to decrease bleeding when the stapedotomy is accomplished. The stapedotomy is then created by forming a charred rosette on the footplate (Fig. 13–6). The power setting for this part of the procedure is 2 watts at 0.1 second duration in the single pulse mode. The size of the stapedotomy to be created is determined by the diameter of the piston on the stapes prosthesis. Perilymph can be seen oozing through the stapedotomy char at this time. This char can be carefully removed with a small right-angled pick. Some surgeons do not disturb the char, but place the prosthesis directly through the charred region. The length of the prosthesis should be sufficient to allow the piston to penetrate the footplate, approximately 0.25 mm (Fig. 13–7).

The stapedotomy opening around the piston can be sealed with several drops of endogenous blood, mucosa from the promontory, vein or fascia, or gelatin sponge (Gelfoam). Some surgeons use no seal around the stapedotomy piston.

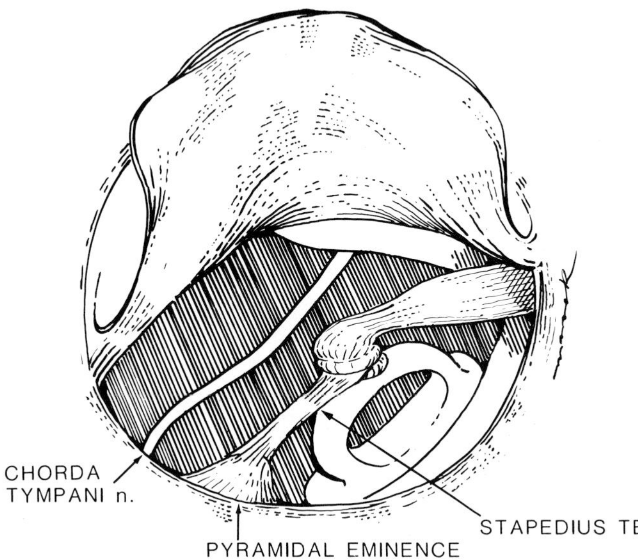

FIGURE 13–2. Tympanomeatal flap for stapedotomy exposure.

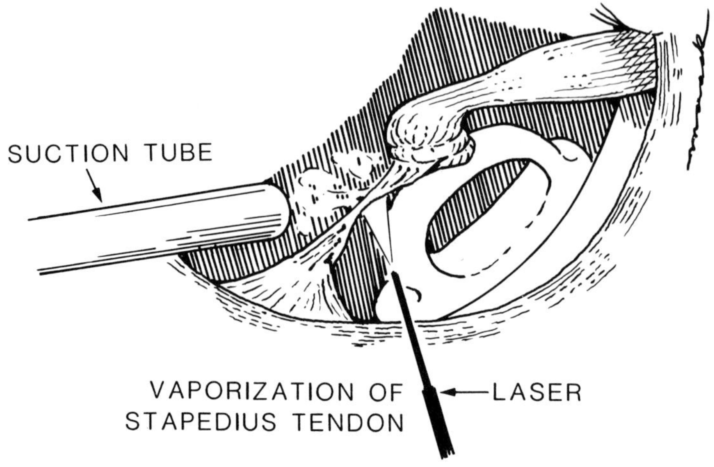

FIGURE 13–3. Hand-held argon laser probe vaporizing the stapedius tendon.

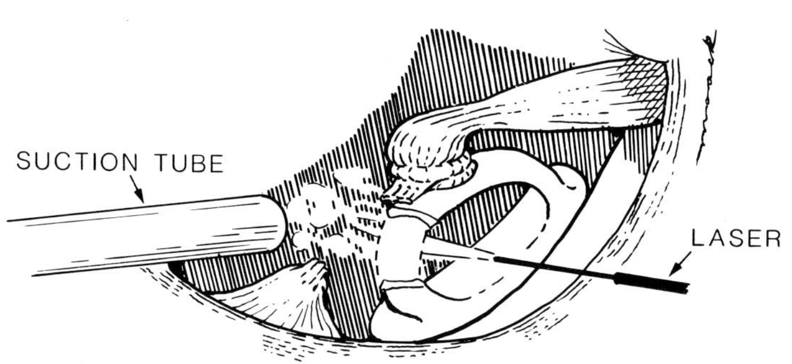

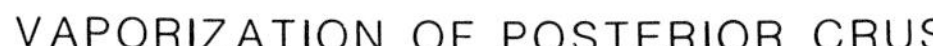

FIGURE 13–4. Argon laser vaporization of the posterior crus of the stapes.

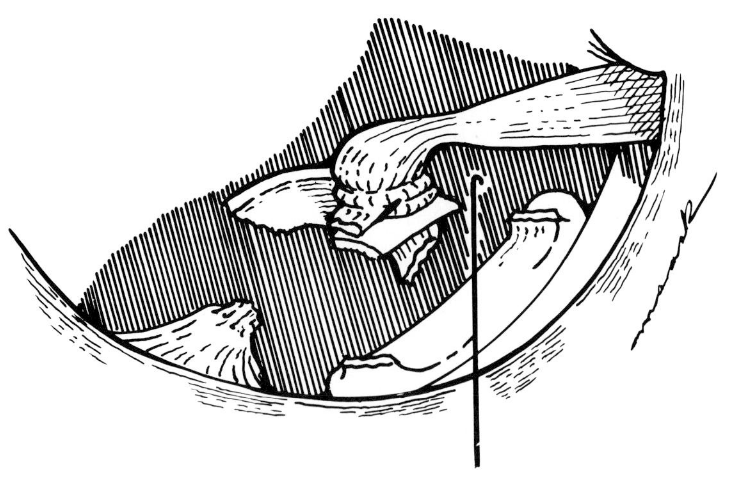

FIGURE 13–5. The anterior stapes crus can be vaporized and/or down fractured.

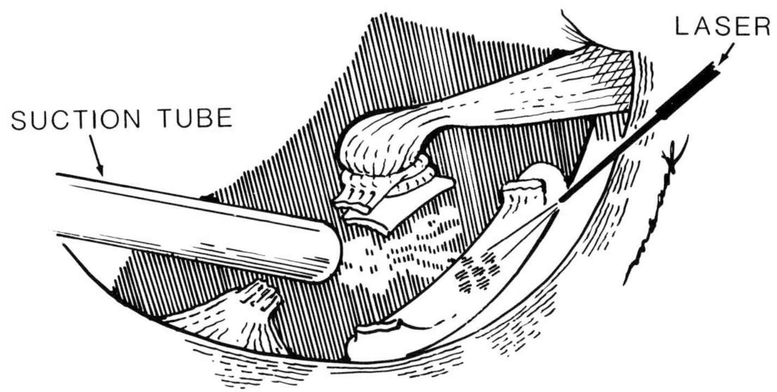

FIGURE 13–6. The stapedotomy is created in a rosette pattern.

If revision stapedotomy is being performed, the advantages of laser use are readily apparent. Adhesions can be lysed to allow more complete visualization of the ossicular chain. Granulomas can be removed from the footplate region. Tissue that has built up around the oval window and the stapes prosthesis can be vaporized with safer removal of the old prosthesis. A new stapedotomy can then be created for insertion of the new prosthesis.

Laser use in revision stapes surgery dramatically reduces the need for mechanical manipulation of the ossicular chain. It also significantly improves hemostasis for better overall visualization. It is important to remember that the saccule and the utricle are more likely to be adherent to the footplate region, thus placing them at greater risk.

Lesinki has recently reported on the potential damage to the structures of the vestibule when using the visible lasers in stapes footplate surgery and specifically in revision stapes surgery in which the footplate area may be covered by a neomembrane.[6] The visible laser energy can potentially penetrate the neomembrane and cause damage to the deeper-lying structures in the vestibule and also heat the temperature of the vestibular fluids to dangerous levels. It has been recommended that the CO_2 laser be utilized for an added safety margin in stapedectomy/stapedotomy revision procedures.

Malleus and/or incus fixation requires surgical visualization of the area of fixation for the laser to be effective. If the malleus head and the body of the incus are fixed in the attic, sufficient atticotomy must be performed to allow visualization of this area of fixation. The laser can then vaporize the fibrous adhesions and bony fixation points to allow mobilization of the ossicular

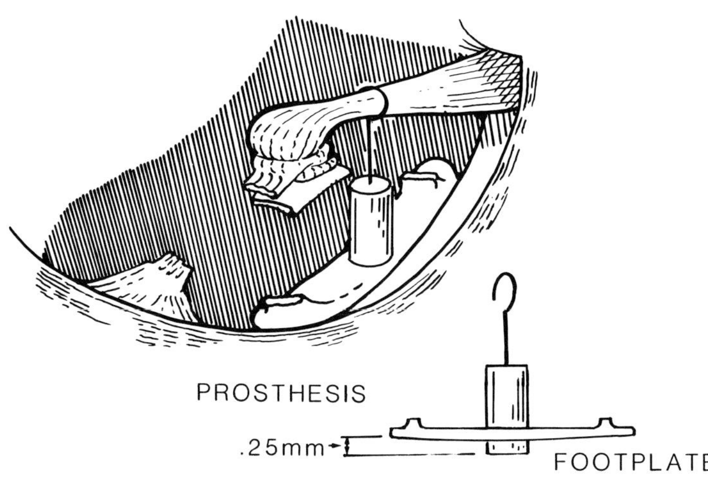

FIGURE 13–7. A wire piston prosthesis is used to reestablish ossicular continuity. The piston extends 0.25 mm into the vestibule.

chain. Gelatin film or silicone rubber sheeting is then placed between the ossicles and the attic wall to reduce the risk of recurrent fixation.

If mobilization of the ossicles in the attic cannot be accomplished, the laser can be used to vaporize the neck of the malleus and the long process of the incus to allow placement of a partial ossicular replacement prosthesis between the long process of the malleus and/or the tympanic membrane and the suprastructure of the stapes.

Fibrous union between the long process of the incus and the suprastructure of the stapes can be vaporized with the laser to allow placement of an appropriate graft between the long process of the incus and the stapes if lateral ossicular mobility is present. When the long process of the incus is too short to allow placement of such a graft, the laser can vaporize the long process of the incus to provide sufficient room for other ossicular replacement prostheses, homograft or autograft.

MIDDLE EAR

As indicated above in the discussion of ossicular surgery, the laser is effective in the atraumatic vaporization of middle ear adhesions around the ossicles and between the tympanic membrane and the medial wall of the middle ear cleft. Adhesions covering the niche of the round window can be carefully removed with the laser.

Cholesteatomas and other benign neoplasms of the middle ear cleft require complete surgical exposure and removal as in nonlaser surgery. Major advantages of the laser in this type surgery seem to be hemostasis in surrounding hypervascular inflammatory tissue and the vaporization of small pathologic remnants in delicate areas, such as around the stapes, over the facial nerve, and in the mouth of the eustachian tube. Laser use does not justify incomplete surgical exposure or incomplete excision of these lesions.

In the treatment of glomus tumors of the middle ear cleft and the mastoid, the laser can have some usefulness. The laser is successful in photocoagulating small peripheral feeding blood vessels and in vaporizing small remnants of tumor in delicate or precarious areas after the bulk of the tumor has been otherwise removed. The blood supply in most glomus tumors is so rich that primary excision of the glomus with the laser is not possible, as the laser cannot control the bleeding.

MASTOID

Chronic hypervascular inflammatory tissue around cholesteatomas and in the chronically inflamed mastoid is effectively treated with the laser (Fig. 13–8). As indicated in the discussion of glomus tumors above, the laser has limited usefulness in this tumor. Other vascular tumors such as eosinophilic granulomas can be successfully removed, utilizing the laser with good hemostasis.

The laser appears to have little benefit in standard cholesteatoma removal except for the photocoagulation and reduced bleeding or cholesteatoma removal in anatomically tight locations. It also has little obvious advantage in the performance of standard mastoidectomy procedures for endolymphatic sac surgery or cochlear implantation.

INTERNAL AUDITORY CANAL

After appropriate exposure of acoustic neuromas and other tumors of the internal auditory canal–cerebellopontine angle via a translabyrinthine or suboccipital approach, lasers can be used to photocoagulate the capsular blood vessels, incise the capsule, and vaporize the tumor. When the laser is utilized, it is important to identify carefully the facial nerve and to protect it from laser

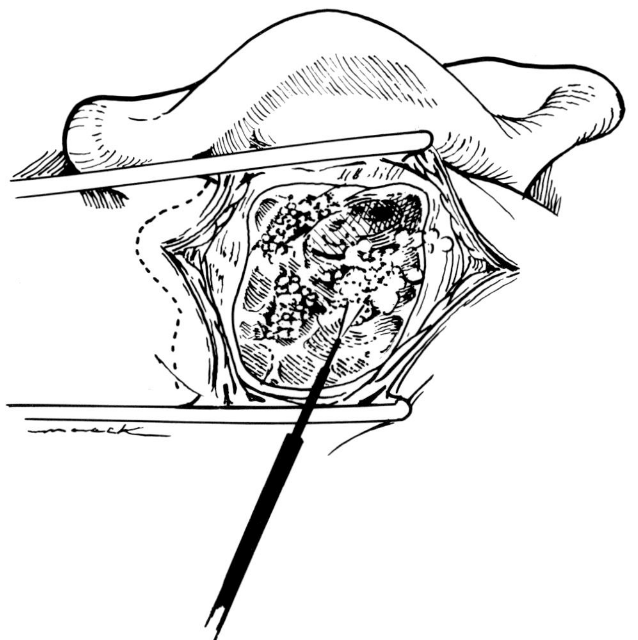

FIGURE 13–8. Mastoid granulations removed with an argon laser.

injury with a cottonoid or other protective device. Complete evacuation with constant suction of the products of vaporization is also important to reduce the potential risk of scattering viable cells.

Vestibular nerve section can certainly be accomplished with the laser, however, it appears to offer little significant advantage over other neurectomy techniques.

References

1. McGee TM: Comparison of small fenestra and total stapedectomy. Am J Otol Rhinol Laryngol 90:633, 1981.
2. McGee TM: The argon laser in surgery for chronic ear disease and otosclerosis. Laryngoscope 93:1177, 1983.
3. Perkins RC: Laser stapedotomy for otosclerosis. Laryngoscope 90:228, 1980.
4. Sheehy J, Nelson RA, House HP: Revision stapedectomy: A review of 258 cases. Laryngoscope 91:43, 1981.
5. Derlacki EL: Revision stapes surgery: Problems with some solutions. Laryngoscope 95:1047, 1985.
6. Lesinski GS, Stein JA: Stapedectomy revision with the CO_2 laser. Laryngoscope 99 (Supplement 46):13–19, 1989.

LASER THERAPY: FUTURE DIRECTIONS

R. Kim Davis

The purpose of this chapter is to summarize selected future directions presented in the preceding chapters and to make several observations about the future of laser surgery in otolaryngology–head and neck surgery. When the value of laser surgery is critically evaluated, several factors must be carefully considered. For laser therapy to have a legitimate place in the surgical armamentarium of this specialty, it must be able to confer a distinct advantage over other nonlaser forms of therapy that can accomplish the same surgical goal, or laser therapy must be able to achieve results not obtainable in other ways. Objective evaluation of these two factors may be more difficult than the face value of the statements indicates. In today's world of highly aggressive marketing, often based on anecdotal case reports or impressions, critical analysis of efficacy can be obscured.

Another area of needed careful analysis involves the evaluation of cost factors in addition to purely medical factors. Some nonlaser procedures that can be accomplished with good success rates and minimal morbidity may be done with equal success and slightly less morbidity using a laser technique. Whether the small change in morbidity justifies the additional expense of laser technique becomes an important question.

Future use of laser technology will likely involve three major areas: The first is the continuation of current laser techniques that are efficacious and safe with the hope of improving these procedures. Additionally, current laser technology will probably be extended to include procedures, which have not as yet been attempted by laser therapy. Finally, new laser technologies may well be developed that truly revolutionize the approach to certain disease entities. Although this is a speculative statement, the history of progress in medicine certainly justifies the anticipation of truly revolutionary methods to deal with old problems.

PERSPECTIVES ON CURRENT PROBLEM AREAS

The treatment of cancer has been and will continue to be one of the areas of greatest challenge. With nonlaser technologies, a predominating motivation has been to develop better or larger surgical techniques to eradicate the cancer. There are many examples of current clinical practice, however, in which the best solution has not been to conceive of a more elaborate or refined surgery, but rather to judiciously use multidisciplinary treatment, including radiation therapy, chemotherapy, and immunotherapy. A good example is the treatment of childhood sarcomas in which surgery clearly plays a lesser role in this decade than previously. At the same time, cure rates have increased. There are numerous pathologic conditions for which conservative surgical procedures coupled with other treatment modalities have clearly decreased patient morbidity. In the future laser therapy may play an important role in facilitating more precise surgery with less loss of normal tissue and less change in blood supply. Such precise laser surgery could then be coupled effectively with a systemic therapy such as chemotherapy or immunotherapy, which depends on an intact blood supply to the area of tumor.

Laser therapy is also continuing to have positive impact on the management of early laryngeal cancer. For many years, the standard therapy for early laryngeal cancer was irradiation therapy. This clearly is efficacious, and certainly in many, if not most cases, remains the standard treatment. There are, however, situations in which radiation therapy is overtreatment for some early laryngeal cancers. The use of the carbon dioxide (CO_2) laser has allowed highly precise endoscopic therapy to be delivered with minimal morbidity, decreased cost, and long-term cure rates at least equal to those with irradiation therapy. (The technique and rationale are discussed in Chapter 6.) As more surgeons become trained in appropriate laser surgery, more patients worldwide will be able to be treated in this manner. Future advances in laser endoscopy will then largely depend on more surgeons utilizing current laser techniques instead of revolutionary breakthroughs in laser technique or technology.

The CO_2 laser may also have future application in the treatment of supraglottic cancer. Initial studies are confirming the efficacy of using the CO_2 laser as a cytoreductive therapy prior to definitive radiation therapy. This allows precise tumor excision as well as airway stabilization before irradiation. Although may patients with stage I and stage II cancer may have excellent rates of response to irradiation alone, the resulting supraglottic edema makes follow-up difficult. Judicious use of the CO_2 laser preoperatively in cytoreduction of these lesions clearly opens the airway and allows subsequent follow-up to be more precise. It also decreases the magnitude of the postirradiation edema. This type of approach in the future will depend on more precise laser surgery techniques coupled with the nonsurgical modality of irradiation therapy.

Palliation of tracheobronchial and esophageal cancer was addressed in this book. It reflects true advances in which selected patients are highly benefited by laser technology. Many patients have received significant palliation, particularly in the tracheobronchial system, with techniques developed in the last 10 years. It certainly seems probable that refinements in these techniques will benefit future patients.

Future advances will be seen in the thermal application of lasers attributable to refinements of laser technology. An excellent example is the use of the microspot laser technique described in Chapter 3. Precision surgery with the CO_2 laser allowed by use of a microspot coupled with superpulse techniques allows extremely high power densities to be carefully delivered. This presents new possibilities for precise tissue excision, endoscopic flap development, and laser welding techniques, which are just starting to be used. This potentially reopens the door to numerous laryngeal laser applications. Conventional CO_2 laser therapy initially seemed to confer advantage, but ultimately was shown to have minimal advantage over other techniques because of thermal damage to adjacent normal tissue. The microspot technique largely circumvents this problem. With refinement, this technique may have actual advantage in the future. Additionally, as new delivery systems are developed to include fiberoptic delivery of the CO_2 laser, a wide range of thermal applications in endoscopic surgery can be anticipated.

One area of current enthusiastic application of laser technique involves the use of argon, neodymium:yttrium-aluminum-garnet (Nd:YAG), and potassium-titanyl-phosphate (KTP) lasers in tissue incision. The KTP laser is being proposed as an instrument with wide application in soft tissue excision with which hemostasis is gained simultaneously with tissue excision. Use of the argon beam photocoagulator is being proposed as a better method of tissue incision with hemostasis than other current techniques. Additionally, use of the Nd:YAG laser with contact probes and sapphire tips to allow tissue excision with similar hemostatic advantage is also being advocated. Controlled studies clearly are yet needed to define whether these techniques have major advantage over electrocautery or other thermal techniques, such as the Shaw scalpel. Each surgeon will need to exercise great judgment and intellectual honesty to determine if enough benefit is gained by laser incision to justify the greater expense involved in these applications. This may be case in which clinical enthusiasm has preceded careful, controlled studies, and caution must be enjoined.

Future advances could be made in nasal and paranasal sinus applications of lasers. To date, laser technology can be used in selected instances as detailed in Chapter 11. However, laser therapy has not made a major impact. On the other hand, with improvements in general sinus treatment techniques, such as endoscopic surgery, laser therapy may be demonstrated to confer advantage owing to the fiberoptic delivery potential and the hemostatic properties of several lasers.

Use of laser technology in otology represents a clinical situation in which a different advantage may be seen. Laser stapedotomy, as detailed in Chapter 13, is gaining greater acceptance. The advantage of this technique involves the benefits of carefully controlled tissue excision with minimal trauma to adjacent structures. Although stapedectomy has been done with great precision and excellent results by many trained individuals over time, the number of patients needing this particular therapy has decreased. Related to that, the opportunities for newer surgeons to learn this technique are more limited. As this is indeed highly precise surgery, which must be carefully done by traditional techniques, the number of surgeons who are well trained in these techniques is clearly decreasing. The application of laser technology may allow training in careful, precise techniques to be more readily acquired in the context of a more limited operative experience. Such laser therapy must be as precise as conventional techniques, but may be more readily acquired as a skill when learning laser technique. This principle of newer laser technologies' allowing safe surgery to be learned by more physicians could pertain to other areas of practice.

Another exciting aspect of laser therapy involves the plastic surgical applications. This is well detailed in Chapter 12. This area of current laser therapy may well be in the stage of current wide application of lasers, which will be more highly refined in the future. Use of the argon laser and the Nd:YAG laser in treating vascular malformations has gained some application. At the same time, the advances in the biophysics of lasers have offered the argon ion pumped dye laser, the copper vapor laser, and the flashlamp pumped dye lasers. These lasers may confer advantages beyond those initially derived from the argon or the Nd:YAG laser. Clearly, the wide clinical application of these lasers is only beginning. The potential and future benefit of these lasers is detailed throughout this text.

FUTURE DEVELOPMENT

Most of the comments in this chapter concern the application of currently available lasers to clinical entities already being treated. Certainly the future of laser surgery will extend well beyond this current scope of medical therapy. When high energy pulsed lasers are applied to tissue for extremely short periods, a new realm of laser therapy can be envisioned. Such therapy results in true molecular surgery in which chemical bonds may be broken or electrons stripped from atoms, producing nonthermal effects. Molecular or genetic surgery could have application in the practice of otolaryngology–head and neck surgery.

Another future development in laser technology will likely employ photodynamic therapy. Although the initial clinical trials with the hematoporphyrin photosensitizers have shown few areas of actual advantage in cancer therapy, current research projects in the application of porphyrin phototherapy to limited mucosal disease and as an adjuvant intraoperative therapy hold interest if not promise. Application of porphyrin photodynamic therapy to noncancer problems, such as multiple respiratory papillomatosis, also holds future potential. As newer photosensitizers, such as rhodamine dye, are developed they will surely have application. Extension of photodynamic therapy to noncancer modalities also holds potential interest. Viral and bacterial inactivation is one such method in which current research indicates future potential.

In summary, the future of lasers in otolaryngology–head and neck surgery is indeed bright. Progress will depend on critical and thoughtful research coupled with highly judicious clinical application. As long as lasers are used in appropriate situations, laser applications will increase, and patient benefit will be seen.

INDEX

Note: Page numbers in *italics* refer to illustrations;
page numbers followed by t refer to tables.